Study Guide to Accompany Craven and Hirnle's

Fundamentals of Nursing

HUMAN HEALTH AND FUNCTION

FIFTH EDITION

Study Guide to Accompany Craven and Hirnle's

Fundamentals of Nursing

HUMAN HEALTH AND FUNCTION

FIFTH EDITION

Joyce Young Johnson, PhD, RN, CCRN
Dean and Professor, College of Health Professions Department of Nursing
Albany State University
Albany, Georgia

Bennita W. Vaughans, RN, MSN
Performance Improvement Coordinator
Central Alabama Health Care System

Phyllis Prather-Hicks, RN, BSN
Nursing Instructor
Harrisburg Community College
Harrisburg, Pennsylvania

Lippincott Williams & Wilkins
a Wolters Kluwer business
Philadelphia • Baltimore • New York • London
Buenos Aires • Hong Kong • Sydney • Tokyo

Senior Acquisitions Editor: Quincy MacDonald
Managing Editor: Doris S. Wray
Senior Production Editor: Marian A. Bellus
Director of Nursing Production: Helen Ewan
Managing Editor / Production: Erika Kors
Art Director: Doug Smock
Design Coordinator: Brett MacNaughton
Manufacturing Manager: William Alberti
Compositor: TechBooks
Printer: Victor Graphics

5th Edition

9 8 7 6 5 4 3 2 1

ISBN 0-7817-7476-4

Care has been taken to confirm the accuracy of the information presented and to describe generally accepted practices. However, the author, editors, and publisher are not responsible for errors or omissions or for any consequences from application of the information in this book and make no warranty, express or implied, with respect to the content of the publication.

The author, editors, and publisher have exerted every effort to ensure that drug selection and dosage set forth in this text are in accordance with the current recommendations and practice at the time of publication. However, in view of ongoing research, changes in government regulations, and the constant flow of information relating to drug therapy and drug reactions, the reader is urged to check the package insert for each drug for any change in indications and dosage and for added warnings and precautions. This is particularly important when the recommended agent is a new or infrequently employed drug.

Some drugs and medical devices presented in this publication have Food and Drug Administration (FDA) clearance for limited use in restricted research settings. It is the responsibility of the health care provider to ascertain the FDA status of each drug or device planned for use in his or her clinical practice.

LWW.com

Preface

As today's healthcare environment becomes more challenging and dynamic, nursing education becomes more complex and demanding. *This Study Guide to Accompany Fundamentals of Nursing: Human Health and Function, Fifth edition*, provides exercises to assist you with learning and applying the concepts and principles presented in the text. The major focus of *Fundamentals of Nursing* and, thus, this *Study Guide* is providing a solid foundation for using the nursing process to provide safe, effective nursing care.

The study guide is divided into chapters that correspond to the text. The answer key in the back of this book provides answers to the questions in the chapters to give you immediate feedback.

For the most part, each chapter in the study guide contains the following elements.
Chapter Overview: A summary of the content in the textbook chapter.
Learning Objectives: A list of learning goals that you will be able to meet after you read the textbook and work through the exercises in this study guide.
Mastering the Information: exercises to assist you in learning content. A brief description of these item types follows:

- *Matching:* Questions that most often address the definitions of key terms or the meaning of key concepts.
- *True or False:* Questions that are answered by knowing whether the statement is true or false. In the answer key, the false statements are corrected so you will know what part of the statement was in error and what information is accurate.
- *Fill in the Blank*: Questions that require you to supply the missing information. The answers may be as short as one or a few words or as long as a short paragraph. Where a more lengthy answer is required, several lines are provided. Where answers of one or a few words are required, a single line is provided.

Applying Your Knowledge: Includes a case study and exercises to help you apply the information through critical inquiry and critical exploration while answering questions designed specifically to allow you to analyze client situations while applying essential concepts. These learning exercises provide individual and clinical activities that will broaden your knowledge and understanding of the content covered in the chapter.
Practicing for NCLEX: Practice NCLEX-style questions, including alternative format quesitons (new to this edition!).

The various types of questions and exercises in the *Study Guide* are designed to help you better understand the material presented in *Fundamentals of Nursing: Human Health and Function.* It is hoped that some of the exercises will prompt discussion with other students and instructors. Together, the text and *Study Guide* provide you with the opportunity to fully explore and learn about the fundamentals of nursing care.

Joyce Young Johnson, PhD, RN, CCRN
Bennita W. Vaughans, RN, MSN
Phyllis Prather Hicks, RN, BSN

Dedication

To God be the glory for this and all works in my life. To my husband, Larry and my children, Virginia and Larry Jr. for the love and support that gives me strength and inspiration I need. To my mother, Dorothy Young, and in memory of my father, Riley H. Young Sr., who instilled a strong sense of purpose in me. To my family and friends who believe in me and keep me lifted up in prayer, thank you! — Joyce

First and foremost, to my dear Lord and personal savior, through whom all things are possible, thanks for empowering me. To my husband, Charles thanks for your love and unending support. To my son Kedrick, whom I am so proud of, thank you for your love and cooperative spirit. To my daughter, Kendra, my number one cheerleader, thanks for the joy and happiness you bring to my life. To Charles and Gertie Vaughans, my in-laws, who are as close to parents as is possible and in loving memory of my parents Benjamin and Juanita whom I dearly miss. — Bennita

Count it all joy! Thanks be to the Most High God for my husband, Rick and our children; Felicia, Stephanie, Georgi, and Gabriel. I am grateful for my friend and fellow nursing professional, Joyce Young Johnson.

A special acknowledgment to the nursing professionals at Harrisburg Area Community College and my team members in the CVOR at The Ortenzio Heart Center in Camp Hill, Pa. For your enthusiasm, encouragement, and commitment to the very best in healthcare ideals, thank you! — Phyllis

To our students, the next generation of nurses and nurse educators
– Joyce, Bennita, and Phyllis

Acknowledgements

We would like to thank everyone at LWW who helped throughout the production of this edition of the *Study Guide*. We owe special thanks to Doris Wray, Claudia Vaughn, and our editor Quincy McDonald who helped to make this project a success.

Contents

SECTION I

Conceptual Foundations of Nursing

UNIT I

The Delivery of Nursing

CHAPTER 1

The Changing Face of Healthcare

CHAPTER OVERVIEW

Chapter 1 introduces the reader to the "changing face" of healthcare by presenting a brief overview of key aspects of nursing and healthcare delivery. Stories of several nurses practicing in a variety of settings are presented to provide real-life examples of the topics introduced.

LEARNING OBJECTIVES

After mastering the content in this chapter, you should be able to do the following:

1. Describe how nursing practice has shifted from an institution-based to a community-based paradigm.
2. Discuss how nurses have developed more independent practice during the last 50 years.
3. Explain how nurses must collaborate with other disciplines to care for clients.
4. Articulate how socioeconomic trends influence care delivery.
5. Describe how personal views and experiences influence nursing practice.
6. Identify how critical thinking is integral to nursing education and practice.

■ Mastering the Information

MATCHING

Match the terms in Column II with a definition, example, or related statement from Column I. Place the letter corresponding to the answer in the space provided. (Use each letter only once; some letters may not be used.)

COLUMN I

1. ______ Prioritize specific calls in order of importance
2. ______ The public's expectation that it will have a voice in determining the type, quality, and cost of healthcare it receives
3. ______ Has broadened the possibilities in healthcare and significantly altered the profile of the hospitalized patient.
4. ______ Refers to a person's ability to find and receive care from a healthcare provider.
5. ______ Reflect a much more diverse population; many have pursued other paths before choosing nursing as a career
6. ______ A hallmark of good ambulatory care

COLUMN II

a. Access to healthcare services
b. Client and family education
c. Triage
d. Technologic advances
e. Consumerism
f. Today's students

TRUE–FALSE

Indicate if the following statements are true or false.

______ 1. Virginia's story reveals that nurses should focus on one aspect of care delivery and one client population.

______ 2. Liz's story illustrates how public policy and procedure evolve with economic concerns and the public's need.

______ 3. Jenny's story relates that staff conferences can be effective in resolving tension between clients and staff.

______ 4. Bill's story reveals the difficulties in working in a nursing home and the need for practice in a hospital first.

______ 5. Denise's story relates the fact that nurses work with the most vulnerable people in society and often meet them at their most intimate and painful moments.

______ 6. Linda's story reveals how nursing can be a stepping stone to an executive position requiring no nursing skills.

______ 7. Sharon's story indicates that nurses can serve as advocates with lawmakers, focusing on important healthcare issues.

FILL IN THE BLANK

Supply the missing term or the information requested.

1. The stories of the nurses reveal that nursing practice is often influenced by political, ________________, and ________________ realities.
2. During the past 50 years, nursing has undergone dynamic changes in its ________________ of practice.
3. Nurses are the healthcare professionals who physically ________________ clients, ________________ with various team members, ________________ plans of care, and ________________ plans with clients.
4. Healthcare services focus on varied areas, with some concentrating on health ________________ and disease ________________, and others focusing on diagnosis and treatment, rehabilitation or ________________ ________________.
5. Today, many citizens view equal access to healthcare as everyone's ________________.

■ Applying Your Knowledge

CASE STUDY

Janelle S. is a 47-year-old widow who lives alone in Summitsville, population 7937. Every day she drives 12 miles to work in the nearest manufacturing plant. Two weeks ago, Janelle traumatically amputated her index and ring fingers on her dominant hand.

As the nurse caring for Janelle, discuss three potential nursing care issues that you plan to address.

CRITICAL INQUIRY EXERCISE

Your school program has several required courses and some elective courses. You notice that some courses have a large number of credit hours, whereas others have only a small number. Your faculty advisor has asked you about the order in which you would like to take your clinical courses, which include medical–surgical nursing, maternal-child health nursing, and psychiatric–mental health nursing. You may also choose when to take your course concentrating on the area of nursing in which you wish to practice.

1. Discuss why some courses might have more credit hours assigned to them than others.
2. What elective courses might be most beneficial in your journey to become a nurse, and in what way might they help you?
3. Considering you know the area of nursing in which you wish to practice, how might you prioritize your clinical courses and why?
4. What questions might you ask about the program of study before deciding the order in which you will take courses?

CRITICAL EXPLORATION EXERCISE

1. Perform an assessment of your curriculum to determine what information you will receive about the changing face of healthcare during your nursing program.
2. Interview two faculty members (one new and one who has been with the program more than 5 years); ask them to tell you their stories about starting nursing practice through becoming faculty. Compare and contrast the stories.
3. Begin a log or journal of your experiences in the nursing program and related experiences (work, family encounters) to begin your story of your life in nursing and healthcare delivery.
4. Search the Internet and note the number of sites that relate to "nursing education." Visit one site and note the major topics mentioned on the site's home page.
5. Perform a review on the most recent National Sample Survey of Registered Nurses conducted by the U.S. Department of Health and Human Services. Note the number of nurses holding an RN license in the United States, the average age of nurses, their employment status, and average salary.

■ Practicing for NCLEX

MULTIPLE CHOICE QUESTIONS

Circle the letter that corresponds to the best answer for each question.

1. The stories in this chapter reveal that:
   a. nursing education is not an important aspect of nursing care.
   b. in reality, clients have very little input into their care.
   c. intricate relationships link the needs of clients and the healthcare system.
   d. technologic changes will soon make nursing unnecessary in healthcare delivery.
2. The two factors that combine to give nurses a unique place within the healthcare delivery system are which of the following?
   a. Time and money
   b. Doctors and clients
   c. Hospitals and doctors
   d. Needs and resources
3. If a population, such as the elderly, is being given less and less access to healthcare, which of the following nursing functions may have the greatest impact?
   a. Begin to provide transportation to local elderly clients to increase access
   b. Advocate for the elderly by lobbying the legislature
   c. Teach elderly clients to seek healthcare in surrounding areas
   d. Report the need for access to the physicians in the area
4. Peter, age 45 years, is being discharged from the hospital. He will have tubes and drains he must care for, and his wife works 12 hours a day to pay bills and maintain the house. Peter has a chronic condition that will require additional surgery in the future. Peter might benefit most from which of the following?
   a. A longer hospital stay
   b. Case management
   c. Placement in a nursing home
   d. Consumerism

FILL IN THE BLANK

Complete the following fill-in-the-blank exercises.

1. Healthcare providers are being asked to ________________ on their services and to relate these costs to ________________.
2. Changes in the healthcare industry have led to the ________________________________ of nursing practice.
3. Clients, their families, and other members of the healthcare team rely on nurses for ________________, critically ____________________________________.
4. Nursing operates within a ________________________ of client needs and resources.
5. ________________________________ and awareness are necessary for advancing nurse practice and creating a healthy community.

MULTIPLE-ANSWER MULTIPLE CHOICE

Circle the letter(s) corresponding to the appropriate answer(s). Select all that apply.

1. Considered a key skill in nursing, this tool enables development of one's own concept of nursing:
   a. Triage
   b. Consumerism
   c. Nursing education
   d. Critical thinking
   e. Cultural diversity

2. The advent of managed care organizations (MCOs), which promote prevention and treatment of illness, fostered which of the following?
   a. Workplace benefits
   b. Consumer movement
   c. Ambulatory care facilities
   d. Cultural diversity
   e. Nursing expertise

3. Clients may have a reasonable expectation of staying overnight in healthcare facilities designated as:
   a. hospitals
   b. ambulatory care centers
   c. skilled nursing facilities
   d. medical centers
   e. outpatient clinics

4. Nursing education that required mandatory time spent working at the hospital with which the school was affiliated was most likely to occur within which of the following time frames?
   a. a decade ago
   b. 50 years ago
   c. during the 1980s
   d. during the era of Clara Barton
   e. about the time of World War II

5. Effective nursing is characterized by which of the following traits?
   a. the ability to think critically
   b. adaptation to new circumstances as necessary
   c. the ability to perform complex, technologically advanced nursing tasks
   d. the administration of quality care
   e. cultural diversity and awareness

CHAPTER 2

Community-Based Nursing and Continuity of Care

CHAPTER OVERVIEW

Chapter 2 discusses the different components of the American healthcare system and the rapid changes that are occurring, with emphasis on community-based nursing. The effects of these changes on both the consumer and healthcare providers are discussed.

LEARNING OBJECTIVES

After mastering the content in this chapter, you should be able to do the following:

1. Discuss what is meant by community-based healthcare.
2. Identify three levels of healthcare and the services under each.
3. List various healthcare providers and the services given by each.
4. Identify the role of various settings for community-based healthcare.
5. Explain how financial considerations have influenced the growth of community-based healthcare.
6. Determine the focus of nursing care in all settings and situations.
7. Discuss forms of community-based nursing practice, both traditional and more recent.
8. Identify the importance of continuity of care.
9. Explain the nurse's role in the processes of admission and discharge planning.

■ Mastering the Information

MATCHING

Match the terms in Column II with a definition, example, or related statement from Column I. Place the letter corresponding to the answer in the space provided.

COLUMN I

1. ______ Includes acupuncture, acupressure, hypnosis, and herbal treatments
2. ______ People at risk who require complex care are most likely to be in need of this
3. ______ Assembling and directing activities to provide services harmoniously
4. ______ Often a critical link between underserved or high-risk populations and the formal healthcare system
5. ______ System that provides for delivery of health services without disruption, regardless of movement between settings

COLUMN II

a. Complementary and alternative healthcare
b. Coordination
c. Continuity of care
d. Case management
e. Lay health workers

COLUMN I

1. ______ Emergency room
2. ______ Health fair
3. ______ Rehabilitation facility
4. ______ Intensive care unit
5. ______ Blood pressure screening
6. ______ Extended care facility
7. ______ X-ray department
8. ______ Hospice

COLUMN II

a. Primary
b. Secondary
c. Tertiary

TRUE–FALSE

Indicate if the following statements are true or false.

_______ 1. According to the Healthcare Forum (1994), the desire for affordable healthcare is greater than the desire for quality or easy access to healthcare.

_______ 2. The NLN in 1992 predicted that the center of healthcare in the future will not be the hospital but the home.

_______ 3. The majority of current resources exist within the category of secondary care.

_______ 4. Certification combines features of licensing and accreditation.

_______ 5. As site and type of intervention in nursing care vary, the focus of the nurse varies as well.

_______ 6. One form of community-based nursing practice, known as community nursing centers, recognizes the chief management role of nursing staff.

FILL IN THE BLANK

Supply the missing term or the information requested.

1. American consumers are moving toward an approach to health that emphasizes _______________ "creating" health.
2. Community-based healthcare is directed toward a _______________ group within the community.
3. For most in-hospital clients, the primary goal of the nurse is _______________ _______________ and _______________ stabilization.
4. Home healthcare nurses focus on complex _______________ health situations or _______________ care assistance.
5. Effective wellness programs must be _______________ and oriented to the whole _______________.

■ Applying Your Knowledge

CASE STUDY

Rita Valdez, age 30 years, has three children, ages 3, 5, and 10 years. Her 10-year-old child has asthma. She and her husband both work but have no health insurance. Mrs. Valdez wishes to know what resources are available in her community that she might use for healthcare for her family. She knows the children will need immunizations and physicals, and her 10-year-old child needs monitoring for asthma.

1. Outline the additional assessments needed for Mrs. Valdez and her family to determine their healthcare needs.
2. Discuss the community-based facilities available to help Mrs. Valdez and her family to maintain health.
3. Design a plan that indicates sources that would support the Valdez family through an acute illness episode and with monitoring of a chronic illness.

CRITICAL INQUIRY EXERCISE

1. Determine the variety of levels of healthcare—primary, secondary, tertiary—available in the community in which you reside. How does the availability, or lack thereof, affect the healthcare of your immediate family?
2. List courses in your curriculum that directly relate to primary and tertiary healthcare delivery systems.
3. Interview a community health nurse with at least 10 years' practice. Compare changes in terminology, the role of nurses, expectations of clients, and support services available then and now.

CRITICAL EXPLORATION EXERCISE

Determine the community health organizations available in your community.

Ascertain whether they are national, regional, state specific, or local.

Attempt to determine one organization that serves a population unique to your area.

■ Practicing for NCLEX

MULTIPLE-CHOICE QUESTIONS

Circle the letter that corresponds to the best answer for each question.

1. Akita Jackson, RN, is the chief manager in a center where nurses are the primary providers clients see when visiting the center. Nursing staff are also accountable and responsible for client care and professional practice. Ms. Jackson most likely practices in a:
   a. hospital-sponsored satellite.
   b. community nursing center.
   c. secondary healthcare system.
   d. wellness program.

2. Ms. Jackson is an advanced practice nurse working independently in a group practice. Which of the following categories best describes Ms. Jackson?
   a. nurse educator
   b. nurse midwife
   c. nurse practitioner
   d. nurse provider

3. Which of the following best describes discharge planning?
   a. Discharge plans are based on institutional goals or needs.
   b. Basic discharge plans involve referral to community resources.
   c. Simple referral involves use of a discharge planner.
   d. Complex referral involves interdisciplinary collaboration.

FILL IN THE BLANK

Supply the missing term or the information requested.

1. Nurses have delivered nursing care in the home setting since ________________.
2. A ________________ helps to determine the most comprehensive service delivery.
3. A referral to the ________________ is appropriate for coordinating placement of the client in a ________________.
4. Changes in the healthcare system result in changes in the delivery of ________________.
5. Community nursing centers deliver healthcare to a ________________.

MULTIPLE-ANSWER MULTIPLE CHOICE

Circle the letter(s) corresponding to the appropriate answer(s). Select all that apply.

1. When clients are admitted to any healthcare setting, the client and family need to know which of the following:
   a. How to obtain assistance
   b. Physical environment and healthcare arrangements
   c. Basic care equipment
   d. Location of emergency equipment and policy manuals
   e. Frequency of contact with care provider

2. Most current sources and services fall in the arena of which of the following types of healthcare?
   a. Primary
   b. Secondary
   c. Tertiary
   d. Quarterly

3. A referral to the local health department of a high-risk mother is an example of which of the following discharge plans?
   a. First or basic
   b. Second or simple
   c. Third or complex
   d. Fourth or challenging

4. One popular, voluntary approach to quality measurement involves:
   a. Licensing
   b. Certification
   c. Accreditation
   d. Data analysis

UNIT II

Concepts Essential for Professional Nursing

CHAPTER 3

The Profession of Nursing

CHAPTER OVERVIEW

Chapter 3 defines and discusses professional nursing practice and the evolution of nursing. Nursing education preparation and career opportunities, nursing organizations, and current and future trends in nursing practice are discussed.

LEARNING OBJECTIVES

After mastering the content in this chapter, you should be able to do the following:

1. Describe the evolution of professional nursing.
2. Identify distinct pathways for entrance into professional nursing practice.
3. Discuss the influence of nursing's historic development on contemporary views of professional nursing.
4. Explain types of graduate educational programs in nursing.
5. Identify roles and responsibilities of professional nursing within the healthcare delivery system.
6. Describe career development opportunities and expanded nursing roles.
7. Describe the purpose and function of professional nursing organizations.
8. Discuss the impact of current and future social trends on professional nursing practice.

■ Mastering the Information

MATCHING

Match the terms in Column II with a definition, example, or related statement from Column I. Place the letter corresponding to the answer in the space provided. (Use each letter only once; some letters may not be used.)

COLUMN I

1. ______ The American Red Cross and Nurse Corps of the U. S. Army established
2. ______ Hippocrates, the father of medicine, credited with recognizing a need for nurses
3. ______ Florence Nightingale improved health laws, reformed hospitals, and re-established nursing as a profession
4. ______ Revolutions and epidemics resulted in expansion of nursing roles
5. ______ Revival of learning contributed to recognition of the need for sound educational preparation in nursing
6. ______ University-based educational preparation in nursing supported with publication of the Goldmark Report
7. ______ Crusades resulted in the establishment of military nursing orders and the recruiting of men into nursing

COLUMN II

a. Pre-Christian era
b. Early Christian era
c. Greeks' contribution
d. The Middle Ages
e. The Renaissance
f. The American Civil War period
g. Nursing in the 18th century
h. Nursing in the 19th century
i. Nursing in the 20th century

COLUMN I

1. ______ A certified nurse who provides independent care for women during normal pregnancy, labor, and delivery
2. ______ Usually a doctoral-prepared nurse who refines nursing knowledge and practice through investigation of nursing problems
3. ______ A master's-prepared nurse with advanced experience and expertise in a specialized area whose roles include clinician, educator, manager, consultant, and researcher
4. ______ A nurse with advanced education (at least a master's degree) who functions with more independence and is highly skilled in nursing assessments, performing physical examinations, counseling, teaching, and treating minor health problems

COLUMN II

a. Clinical nurse specialist
b. Nurse midwife
c. Nurse practitioner
d. Nurse researcher

FILL IN THE BLANK

Supply the missing term or the information requested.

1. List the three major educational routes leading to registered nursing licensure.
   a. ______________________________
   b. ______________________________
   c. ______________________________
2. List three current issues affecting the nursing profession.
   a. ______________________________
   b. ______________________________
   c. ______________________________
3. List and briefly discuss four responsibilities of the professional nurse.
   a. ______________________________
   b. ______________________________
   c. ______________________________
   d. ______________________________
4. A nurse who communicates the client's needs and concerns and ensures that the client understands the treatment is functioning as a ______________.
5. Nursing functions include activities that the nurse performs ______________, in response to a physician-prescribed intervention, or ______________, which are initiated as nurse-prescribed interventions.

TRUE–FALSE

Indicate if the following statements are true or false.

______ 1. The practice of nursing within a state is regulated by the American Nurses Association.

______ 2. The main purpose of the National League for Nursing is to ensure that the public need for nursing will be met.

______ 3. The associate degree nursing programs were the first educational preparation available for registered nurses.

______ 4. The question of whether nursing is a profession has been an ongoing debate.

■ Applying Your Knowledge

CASE STUDY

Susan B is in her first year of a 4-year university and has been considering changing her major to nursing.

She asks you, a nurse for 2 years working on a busy surgical floor in an urban hospital, about the training required, as well as the role and responsibilities of a nurse.

1. How would you describe the role of a staff nurse in such a setting?
2. What words would you use to describe the responsibilities of a nurse?
3. What are some advanced level options for a nurse with a bachelor's degree?

CRITICAL INQUIRY EXERCISE

Malcolm completed a diploma program in nursing 5 years ago. He wishes to become a professional nurse and in the future plans to become a nurse practitioner.

1. Considering the various nursing education programs, outline the alternative ways Malcolm could meet his goals.
2. Contrast the type(s) of state or national certification or licensure examination(s) Malcolm must take as he proceeds to become a professional nurse and then a nurse practitioner with the examinations a generic nursing student (with no prior nursing education) with the same career path must take.
3. Compare and contrast the care Malcolm will provide as a professional nurse with the care he will provide as a nurse practitioner.

CRITICAL EXPLORATION EXERCISE

1. Interview nurses in various practice settings. Collect information regarding job descriptions, nursing responsibilities, and educational preparation.
2. Write a brief paper stating your ideas or beliefs about nursing in the future, entry-level nursing, nursing as a profession, and the definition of nursing.
3. Search the web home page or newsletter of a nursing organization. Submit a brief summary of one current nursing event report on a trend or issue affecting the nursing profession.

■ Practicing for NCLEX

MULTIPLE CHOICE QUESTIONS

Circle the letter that corresponds to the best answer for each question.

1. The American Red Cross was founded by which of the following?
   a. Clara Barton
   b. Dorothea Dix
   c. Linda Richards
   d. Jean Watson

2. Which of the following is a professional organization in which membership is open only to registered professional nurses?
   a. National League for Nursing
   b. International Council of Nurses
   c. American Holistic Nurses Association
   d. American Nurses Association

3. According to the American Nurses Association policy statement in 1985, the two levels of educational preparation are:
   a. practical nurse and associate degree programs.
   b. associate degree and diploma programs.
   c. associate degree and baccalaureate degree programs.
   d. baccalaureate degree and diploma programs.

4. A national accrediting body for nursing programs would correctly be identified as the:
   a. Commission on Collegiate Nursing Education.
   b. Canadian Nurses Association.
   c. International Council of Nurses.
   d. Nurse Consultant Association.

5. The American Nurses Association identifies which of the following as standards of nursing care?
   a. Performance appraisal
   b. Collegiality
   c. Research
   d. Outcome identification

FILL IN THE BLANK

Complete the following fill-in-the-blank exercises. Identify the following nursing skills or activities as **collaborative** *or* **independent** *functioning.*

1. Assisting a client to turn ________________
2. Providing a safe environment ________________
3. Administering a pain medication ________________
4. Providing client teaching/counseling ________________
5. Applying cream to a surgery incision ________________

MULTIPLE-ANSWER MULTIPLE CHOICE

Circle the letter(s) corresponding to the appropriate answer(s). Circle all that apply.

1. Which of the following roles is important to the provision of responsible nursing care?
   a. Caregiving
   b. Client advocacy
   c. Communication
   d. Education
2. Of the following choices, which is the name for the oldest international organization of professional nurses?
   a. Sigma Theta Tau International
   b. International Council of Nurses
   c. National League for Nursing
   d. Canadian Nurses Association
3. Which of the following statements about the Volunteer Nurse Corps is true?
   a. Developed during World War I
   b. Established in the 19th century
   c. Evolved into the Army Nurse Corps
   d. Developed during the Spanish/American War
4. Which of the following best describes one of the aspects of the NSNA?
   a. International
   b. Philanthropic
   c. Autonomous
   d. Membership by invitation only
5. Which of the following statements regarding associate degree nursing programs is correct?
   a. Initially developed in response to the nursing shortage
   b. Graduates receive college credit for 2 years
   c. Graduates may sit for state board licensure for RNs
   d. Schools are located all over North America

CHAPTER 4

Nursing Theory and Conceptual Frameworks

CHAPTER OVERVIEW

Chapter 4 discusses nursing theory and conceptual frameworks. An overview of nursing theory and a synopsis of major non-nursing theories used in nursing are provided. The use of functional health patterns as a framework for nursing is discussed.

LEARNING OBJECTIVES

After mastering the content in this chapter, you should be able to do the following:

1. Define nursing theory and conceptual framework.
2. Recognize major nursing theories and their relevance to nursing practice.
3. Identify the four major concepts of nursing theories.
4. Discuss the relationship between nursing theories and non-nursing theories.
5. Summarize non-nursing theories and their use in nursing.
6. Discuss the relationship of functional health pattern typology to nursing.

■ Mastering the Information

MATCHING

Match the terms in Column II with a definition, example, or related statement from Column I. Place the letter corresponding to the answer in the space provided.

COLUMN I

1. ______ A feeling of belonging
2. ______ A sense of predictability and routine
3. ______ A need to develop one's maximal potential
4. ______ A need to maintain thermoregulation

COLUMN II

a. Safety needs
b. Physiologic needs
c. Love needs
d. Esteem needs

COLUMN I

1. ______ The shift of behavior toward a new and more healthful pattern
2. ______ The recognition of the need for change and the dissolution of previously held patterns of behavior
3. ______ The long-term solidification of the new pattern of behavior

COLUMN II

a. Unfreezing
b. Refreezing
c. Movement

TRUE–FALSE

Indicate if the following statements are true or false.

______ 1. A conceptual framework contains highly specific and distinct concepts and propositions.

______ 2. Maslow's theory relates to a hierarchy of needs.

______ 3. Nursing research should be unrelated to theory.

______ 4. Gordon's functional health patterns are unique but interrelated to each other.

______ 5. General systems theory describes human systems as open and dynamic.

FILL IN THE BLANK

Supply the missing term or the information requested.

1. Discuss the relationship of nursing theories to nursing knowledge, practice, and research.
2. A client's ______ and ___________ should be considered by the nurse in holistic practice.
3. Discuss the focus of Gordon's (1994) health perception-health management pattern.
4. A _________ is defined as a set of concepts and the propositions that integrate them into a meaningful configuration.
5. The four major concepts that nursing theories define are:
   a.
   b.
   c.
   d.

■ Applying Your Knowledge

CASE STUDY

Mr. L. E. was just received from the emergency room (ER) by stretcher with a diagnosis of congestive heart failure (fluid in the lungs because of heart failure) and hypertension (high blood pressure). He is alert, very anxious, and short of breath with "noisy" breath sounds. He has a urinary catheter, and low urine output is noted. His heart rate is 140 beats per minute, and his blood pressure is 198/102 mm Hg. His wife states, "He doesn't take his medicine. I think he just wants to die. I don't know if I can help him any more."

1. Explain what Mr. L. E.'s most important needs would be as you receive him from the ER.
2. Identify additional data you would collect to address Mr. L. E.'s needs in a holistic way using a functional health approach.
3. Discuss other concerns the nurse could help Mr. L. E. and his wife address when Mr. L. E.'s heart failure and high blood pressure are under control.

CRITICAL INQUIRY EXERCISE

1. Identify and review your nursing program's conceptual model of nursing.
2. Explore if your nursing program or local hospital uses a nursing theory or collection of theories as a basis for practice.
3. Pick a nursing theorist and perform an Internet search; note the results.

■ Practicing for NCLEX

MULTIPLE CHOICE QUESTIONS

Circle the letter that corresponds to the best answer for each question.

1. Roy's adaptation model, Neuman's healthcare model, Johnson's behavioral model, and Parse's theory for nursing have in common their use of which of the following non-nursing theories?
   a. General systems theory
   b. Maslow's human needs theory
   c. Change theory
   d. Henderson's spiritual needs theory

2. Your client has several concerns, including decreased self-esteem, isolation from family, malnutrition, and anxiety regarding hospitalization. Although you know the client may have different priorities, according to Maslow's hierarchy of needs, which of the following concerns would you list as most important?
   a. Anxiety
   b. Decreased self-esteem
   c. Isolation from family
   d. Malnutrition

3. Dale Smith, 21 years old, is admitted to the hospital with a broken leg. Although all areas would be assessed, which functional health pattern would be most directly affected?
   a. Activity and exercise
   b. Cognitive–perceptual
   c. Nutrition/metabolic
   d. Values and beliefs

4. Mrs. Pallet has received a diagnosis of asthma (lung spasms) and must stop smoking. She and her husband are both smokers. Considering change theory, which of the following is true?
   a. Mr. and Mrs. Pallet should be told to stop smoking immediately, with no exploration of why they smoke.
   b. Mrs. Pallet will undergo a process of refreezing as she resumes her usual smoking habits.
   c. Mrs. Pallet's success in not smoking will be influenced by her husband's opinion regarding not smoking.
   d. Mr. and Mrs. Pallet's shift of behavior toward smoking less is the process of unfreezing.

5. Dorothea Orem's theory would support which of the following nursing strategies?
   a. include performing all daily activities for the client
   b. avoid upsetting the client by teaching about medications
   c. involve making decisions for the client to lower anxiety
   d. promote the client's assuming responsibility for self-care

FILL IN THE BLANK

Supply the missing term.

1. According to Lewin, _______________ is the recognition of the need for change and the dissolution of previously held patterns of behavior.
2. The body monitors and maintains its temperature through sensors in the skin, the _______________, and the effector system.
3. The general state of a person's well-being is addressed by the term _______________.
4. _______________ _______________ provides the foundation for nursing knowledge.
5. _______________ is the shift of behavior toward a new and more healthful pattern.

MULTIPLE-ANSWER MULTIPLE CHOICE

Circle the letter(s) corresponding to the appropriate answer(s). Select all that apply.

1. Which of the following theories asserts that "human systems are open and dynamic"?
   a. Von Bertalanffy's theory
   b. Change theory
   c. Nightingale's *Notes on Nursing*
   d. General systems theory
   e. Maslow's hierarchy

2. The development and future direction of nursing research should be guided by which of the following?
   a. Nursing theory
   b. Maslow's hierarchy
   c. Self-actualization
   d. General systems theory
   e. Change theory

3. The theory of the stages of change involving freezing, movement, and unfreezing was developed by this theorist:
   a. Maslow
   b. Hall
   c. Gordon
   d. Lewin
   e. Barnum

CHAPTER 5

Values

CHAPTER OVERVIEW

Chapter 5 examines and summarizes the basic concept of values. Concepts closely related to the evolution of values are also discussed. Emphasis is placed on the role that values play during nurse–client interactions.

LEARNING OBJECTIVES

After mastering the content in this chapter, you should be able to do the following:

1. Define values and related concepts.
2. Identify sources of professional nursing values.
3. Relate values with functional health patterns.
4. Examine values conflict and resolution in nursing care situations.
5. Integrate values assessment into nursing care.
6. Appreciate the impact of values in such situations as the initial assessment and discharge planning.

■ Mastering the Information

MATCHING

Match the terms in Column II with a definition, example, or related statement from Column I. Place the letter corresponding to the answer in the space provided.

COLUMN I

1. ______ Characterized by identification of behaviors that elicit reward or punishment
2. ______ Characterized by conformity to expectations and behaviors of others
3. ______ Values involving correct behavior, such as having a sense of right or wrong
4. ______ Value indicated by a behavior only performed when the person sets it as a goal
5. ______ Value that will not become "real" until the person acts
6. ______ Value indicated by a behavior that is performed out of habit

COLUMN II

a. Foundation value
b. Focus value
c. Moral
d. Preconventional
e. Conventional
f. Future value

COLUMN I

1. ______ Adaptability/flexibility
2. ______ Vital signs
3. ______ Problem solving
4. ______ Awareness of total picture
5. ______ Counseling
6. ______ Creativity
7. ______ Hygiene assistance
8. ______ Human dignity
9. ______ Research/originality/knowledge
10. ______ Wonder/curiosity

COLUMN II

a. Instrumental skill
b. Interpersonal skill
c. Imaginal skill
d. System skill

FILL IN THE BLANK

Supply the missing term or the information requested.

1. ______________, ______________, and ______________ are value indicators.

2. According to the American Nurses Association *Code for Nurses*, the central value underlying standards of practice in nursing is _______________.
3. Identify three of five ways in which children learn values.
   a.
   b.
   c.
4. Values in nursing are developed through _______________, _______________, and _______________.
5. Differentiate between value clarification and value inquiry. _______________
6. Identify and briefly discuss the three levels of information of which the nurse needs to be aware when assessing values related to functional health.
   a.
   b.
   c.

TRUE–FALSE

Indicate if the following statements are true or false.

______ 1. All human interactions are value based.

______ 2. The only indicator of a person's values is the person's belief system.

______ 3. When involved in a situation of value conflict, the nurse should first examine his or her own values.

______ 4. A client's cultural background would have no relevance when conducting a nutritional assessment.

______ 5. Time, nature, relationships, and activity modes are four value orientations that are useful in understanding the meaning of behaviors across cultures.

▪ Applying Your Knowledge

CASE STUDY

Joshua M. is a 13-year-old client on the pediatric unit of your hospital. You are the nurse taking care of him as he recovers from orthopedic surgery; you are concerned that the dietitian/nutritionist continues to include foods in his plan that are a combination of beef and cheese or chicken salad with hard-boiled eggs. You know that Joshua and his family keep a kosher diet.

1. What are some of the value issues that may be affecting the nutritionist's choices?
2. What attitudes and beliefs may be involved in her interactions with Joshua and his family?

CRITICAL INQUIRY EXERCISE

You are the nurse in a health clinic located near a reservation. Most of the client population is Native American. There are several educational seminars being presented to promote health. Mr. Appachutu is not attending the health seminars but sits silent in the lobby. You approach Mr. Appachutu to determine his needs. He tells you, "The doctor in the city said my leg has to be cut off." After listening to Mr. Appachutu, you review his file. The history assessment included the following subjective data: "The body should be treated with respect, and harmony between the body halves should exist. If not, illness occurs." Mr. Appachutu has a history of diabetes mellitus and vascular disease.

1. This chapter discusses value conflicts that are likely to occur with human interaction. Discuss how the four definitions of resolution may be applied to Mr. Appachutu's situation to resolve the conflicts among cultural beliefs, values, and health needs.
2. You reviewed Mr. Appachutu's history form but determined that interaction with the client also will provide value indicators. Discuss additional value assessment data you could obtain to assist Mr. Appachutu.
3. You researched Native American culture and uncovered data that reflect the following:
   - Belief of harmony
   - Present time orientation
   - Family-oriented beliefs imposed on children

Using this information, discuss the cultural value orientation theory and its application to Mr. Appachutu.

CRITICAL EXPLORATION EXERCISE

1. Identify four values that you have as a person. Tell how each has contributed to your decision to pursue nursing as a career.
2. You were taking care of 6-year-old Tommy Lewis yesterday. The doctor ordered Tommy to be begin taking ampicillin 250 mg every 6 hours. You were waiting for the medication to come from the pharmacy so that you could give the first dose. The medication did not arrive before you left, so you did not give the medication. Today the charge nurse approaches you and tells you that you forgot to sign the medication administration sheet for the dose of medicine you gave Tommy yesterday. Tommy has not experienced any adverse reactions as a result of having missed this dose of medication.
   - What would you do in this situation?
   - What personal and professional values affect your decision?
   - How do these values affect your decision?
3. Perform an online computer search for information on value conflicts related to nursing care situations.

■ Practicing for NCLEX

MULTIPLE CHOICE QUESTIONS

Circle the letter that corresponds to the best answer for each question.

1. A belief is
   a. an idea that is accepted as true.
   b. a person's disposition toward an object or situation.
   c. a reflection of a person's mindset.
   d. synonymous with a value.

2. The person who would have the most difficult time adjusting to a health problem that results in mandatory job retirement is
   a. one who believes in "harmony with others."
   b. one who has a "present orientation."
   c. one who thrives on collateral relationships.
   d. one whose activity orientation is "doing."

3. Children begin to demonstrate an understanding of right and wrong during
   a. toddlerhood.
   b. the preschool years.
   c. the school-age years.
   d. adolescence.

4. Internalization of personal values is more likely to occur when
   a. the individual recognizes the importance of others' viewpoints and becomes less egocentric.
   b. the individual is confident in relying on his or her feelings, beliefs, and behaviors as guides for decision making.
   c. the individual recognizes the relationship between personal behavior and rewards or punishment.
   d. the individual expands his or her horizon of experiences beyond the family.

5. An attitude is
   a. an idea that is accepted as true.
   b. an observable behavior.
   c. a standard that endures over a period of time.
   d. one's disposition toward an object or situation.

FILL IN THE BLANK

Supply the missing term.

1. Children may learn values by ________________ the behavior of significant others.
2. The most important indicator of a value is a person's ________________.
3. Conventional behaviors are characterized by ________________ to expectations and behaviors of others.
4. As adults invest in careers and families they focus on ________________ and ________________.
5. Cognition and ________________ involve all five senses, as well as memory, ________________, and decision making.

MULTIPLE-ANSWER MULTIPLE CHOICE

Circle the letter(s) corresponding to the appropriate answer(s). Select all that apply.

1. Value indicators include which of the following:
   a. Behaviors
   b. Physiologic principles
   c. Attitudes
   d. Measurable outcomes
   e. Beliefs

2. Certain functional health patterns are common to which of the following?
   a. Diabetics
   b. Healthy adults
   c. Children
   d. Bilateral amputees
   e. Elderly populations

3. Examples of interpersonal skills include which of the following?
   a. Creativity
   b. Respect
   c. Counseling
   d. Bathing clients
   e. Problem solving

4. Examples of focus values would include which of the following?
   a. Sheila cleans her room to avoid having her "online" privileges revoked.
   b. John takes out the trash every Thursday morning.
   c. Kramer plans to stop smoking before his vacation.
   d. Cheryl goes to the gym twice a week in order to lose 15 pounds by Thanksgiving.
   e. Ellen is studying for the online NCLEX examination, so she does not attend the office party.

5. The age of peer influence and identification reaches its greatest persuasiveness at which of the following developmental stages?
   a. Toddlerhood
   b. Adolescence
   c. Newborn
   d. Young adulthood
   e. Infancy
   f. Older adulthood

CHAPTER 6

Ethical and Legal Concerns

CHAPTER OVERVIEW

Chapter 6 examines and summarizes basic legal and ethical principles as they relate to the nursing profession. Emphasis is placed on strategies for addressing ethical dilemmas and ensuring legal protection.

LEARNING OBJECTIVES

After mastering the content in this chapter, you should be able to do the following:

1. Define key terms in the chapter.
2. Differentiate morals from values.
3. Explain ethical philosophy.
4. Discuss the principles and rules of healthcare ethics.
5. Describe a systematic approach for resolving ethical dilemmas.
6. Analyze an ethical dilemma, citing ethical principles.
7. Explain licensure.
8. Describe standard of care.
9. Explain and give examples of crimes and torts.
10. Compare and contrast crimes and torts, citing appropriate examples.
11. Define four elements of negligence.
12. Describe legal protections for nurses; cite measures to be taken.

■ Mastering the Information

MATCHING

Match the terms in Column II with a definition, example, or related statement from Column I. Place the letter corresponding to the answer in the space provided. (Use each letter only once; some letters may not be used.)

COLUMN I

1. ______ Intentional or unintentional acts that are subject to action in a civil court
2. ______ Documents by which clients communicate their wishes to healthcare providers
3. ______ Doing or promoting good
4. ______ The branch of philosophy dealing with standards of conduct and moral judgment
5. ______ Means "telling the truth"
6. ______ The threat of touching another person without his or her consent
7. ______ Any wrong punishable by the state that involves evil intent or a criminal act
8. ______ Negligence on the part of a professional

COLUMN II

a. Advance directives
b. Assault
c. Beneficence
d. Crime
e. Ethics
f. Malpractice
g. Torts
h. Veracity

COLUMN I

1. ______ Focuses on a person's physical and neurologic functioning
2. ______ Consent or refusal of treatment alternatives
3. ______ Considers the client's diagnosis and condition
4. ______ Includes matters of costs, policies, and family situations

COLUMN II

a. Quality of life
b. Indications for medical intervention
c. Contextual features
d. Patient preference

TRUE–FALSE

Indicate if the following statements are true or false.

_____ 1. Torts must be accidental acts to qualify for damages.

_____ 2. A just decision is based on equal treatment according to client need and a fair distribution of resources.

_____ 3. The concept of double effect means that an action can produce helpful and harmful outcomes.

_____ 4. The American Nurses Association National Action Agenda delineates the primary conduct and responsibilities nurses are expected to maintain in their practice.

_____ 5. Frameworks in ethics provide a systematic way of organizing reasons that serve as a basis for deciding the best and right action to take.

_____ 6. The major type of law that governs nursing is civil law.

_____ 7. Local criminal laws are the primary guidelines for the standard that nursing care should meet.

_____ 8. One way to avoid malpractice litigation is to follow the current standard of nursing care demonstrated at a specific agency or facility.

_____ 9. Liability denotes legal responsibility to pay damages.

_____ 10. A healthcare agency may be held responsible for a nurse's negligence under the doctrine of respondent superior.

FILL IN THE BLANK

Supply the missing term or the information requested.

1. Emotions affect how people _____________ and ___________ in any situation.
2. The major principles of healthcare ethics are _______________, _______________, _______________, and _______________.
3. In addition to the major principles of healthcare ethics, four principles that guide the behavior of healthcare professionals are __________, __________, __________, and ______________.
4. Identify the four conditions that must be present to prove negligence.

   a.

   b.

   c.

   d.
5. _______________ are standards of right and wrong that help individuals judge what is correct action, whereas _______________ are ideas or beliefs an individual considers important and about which he or she feels strongly.
6. Identify the elements to be covered in order for a consent to be "informed."

   a.

   b.

   c.

   d.

   e.

■ Applying Your Knowledge

CASE STUDY

You are the in-service educator for a burn unit. A client admitted with second-degree burns reports painful urination. Two urine specimens have been sent to a laboratory. On the third day, the client continues to complain and passes bloody urine and mucus. The physician was notified on the first day of the complaint but does not examine the client or prescribe treatment. You again report the situation to the physician. The physician examines the client, who reports the same symptoms. The physician tells you that no treatment can be prescribed without the urine culture reports.

1. Explain what a nurse should do when a collaborative problem is not being addressed or when he or she disagrees with a physician's actions.
2. Describe the options a nurse has if he or she thinks a physician is following an unsafe practice.
3. Describe the process for monitoring individual and team competence and include information regarding the reporting of errors made during the delivery of nursing care.

CRITICAL INQUIRY EXERCISE

During a clinical experience, review the nurses' notes for an assigned client. Evaluate documentation for legal soundness. Include the following points:

- Thoroughness and data gaps
- Legibility
- Method of error correction
- Presence or absence of judgment statements

CRITICAL EXPLORATION EXERCISE

Before attending a clinical experience, review the American Nurses Association *Code for Nurses.* During the clinical experience, complete the following activities:

- Observe the behavior of the nurses working in the area for consistency and inconsistency with the *Code for Nurses.*
- Evaluate your behavior for consistency or inconsistency with the *Code for Nurses.*

■ Practicing for NCLEX

MULTIPLE CHOICE QUESTIONS

Circle the letter that corresponds to the best answer for each question.

1. You have just entered Mr. Bradford's room and observed him lying on the floor next to the bed. The side rails on the bed are down. When you ask Mr. Bradford what happened, he replies, "I was asleep and the next thing I knew I was on the floor." Which of the following samples of documentation is most appropriate for this situation?
   a. Mr. Bradford fell out of bed while asleep. Both side rails were left down.
   b. Mr. Bradford was found lying on the floor next to his bed. When asked what happened, he stated, "I was asleep and the next thing I knew I was on the floor."
   c. Lying on the floor, side rails down. Rolled out of bed while asleep.
   d. Lying on floor next to bed. No complaints verbalized. Side rails down. Appears to have fallen out of bed while asleep.

2. The correct way of indicating charting errors is to:
   a. White out the error and replace it with the correct information.
   b. Make one straight line through the word and initial the correction.
   c. Complete an incident report, and document the error on the report, not in the chart.
   d. Make a late entry in the chart, put the current time, and state the correction that should be made.

3. Mr. Tyna suffered a massive heart attack and was placed on life support. Before this incident, Mr. Tyna had completed a living will or durable power of attorney for healthcare while in a mentally alert and healthy state requesting that he not be kept alive with life support equipment. Which of the following statements is correct about his situation?
   a. Mr. Tyna can be removed from life support because he was mentally alert when he completed the living will, and he is now unable to talk while he is on a respirator and recovering from the heart attack.
   b. Mr. Tyna's "surrogate decision maker" would make decisions with the healthcare team regarding whether Mr. Tyna's condition is terminal, and his wishes regarding life support would be honored at this time.
   c. Mr. Tyna can be removed from life support because a massive heart attack always results in death.
   d. Mr. Tyna should remain on life support because a massive heart attack is very seldom life threatening, and the recovery rate is high.

4. The Patient Self-Determination Act of 1990 requires that agencies admitting clients:
   a. educate nurses about their role in witnessing a living will.
   b. inform nurses of the client preferences regarding traumatic treatments.
   c. abolish "no code" status for all clients.
   d. inform clients about their rights regarding end-of-life decisions.

5. The student initiating strategies to address an ethical dilemma would be in error and demonstrate a need for additional study if one strategy used was:
   a. clarifying any misunderstandings in the situation.
   b. analyzing the case by organizing the facts.
   c. identifying outcomes by which to plan care.
   d. using personal values to determine interventions.

FILL IN THE BLANK

Supply the missing term or the information requested.

1. Quality of life issues focus on a person's physical and ________________ functioning.
2. The principle of ________________ ________________ protects the client's right of self-determination.
3. Malpractice cases are a type of ____________ law that tends to involve nurses.
4. The legal responsibility to pay damages is known as ________________.
5. Professionals may be protected from liability under specific circumstances. This legislation is referred to as the ______________ ________________________ ______________.

MULTIPLE-ANSWER MULTIPLE CHOICE

Circle the letter(s) corresponding to the appropriate answer(s). Circle all that apply.

1. Nurses may minimize the risk of legal problems, such as malpractice, in several ways. Which of the following may be applicable?
   a. Utilize continuing education opportunities
   b. Inform clients and families of your malpractice coverage
   c. Stay abreast of new trends
   d. Be familiar with regulations governing nursing and other ancillary staff
   e. Document any acts of malpractice in the nurses' notes

2. The Uniform Anatomical Gift Act is in effect in which of the following states?
   a. California
   b. Georgia
   c. Alaska
   d. New York
   e. Kansas
   f. Tennessee
   g. Pennsylvania

3. Advanced directives may be rescinded under which of the following set(s) of circumstances?
   a. Within 72 hours of signing the document
   b. At any time
   c. Whenever the client changes his/her mind
   d. 30 days after signing the document
   e. For any reason the client chooses

4. False communication that results in an injury to a person's reputation through printed media is considered which of the following?
   a. Defamation of character
   b. Libel
   c. Slander
   d. Verbal battery
   e. Verbal assault

5. Confidentiality requires that information about a client be kept private. Which of the following statement(s) is also true of confidentiality?
   a. It is a legal obligation.
   b. Client information may be discussed with family members outside the clinical setting.
   c. A nurse has a professional duty to maintain client confidentiality..
   d. Client information may be discussed with colleagues in no clinical care areas.
   e. Information can be released to specific parties when the client signs a consent for release of information.

CHAPTER 7

Nurse Leader and Manager

CHAPTER OVERVIEW

Chapter 7 discusses the management process and the leadership concept. The skills required for effective management are reviewed. The use of management skills by practitioners and administrators is explored.

LEARNING OBJECTIVES

After mastering the content in this chapter, you should be able to do the following:

1. Explain the differences between leadership and management.
2. Describe the three areas of resource management.
3. Identify three skills required for effective management.
4. List interventions that can control perceptions and reactions to change.
5. Describe common clinical practice, management, and education roles in nursing.
6. Characterize leadership and management functions used in common nursing roles.
7. Describe the three most popular models of nursing care delivery.
8. Explain why problem solving, management, and nursing processes are similar.

■ Mastering the Information

MATCHING

Match the terms in Column II with a definition, example, or related statement from Column I. Place the letter corresponding to the answer in the space provided. (Use each letter only once; some letters may not be used.)

COLUMN I

1. ______ Focuses on influencing others to strive for a vision or goal or to implement change
2. ______ Functions as a care provider, client advocate, decision maker, team member, communicator, and educator
3. ______ Has the disadvantage of care that is fragmented
4. ______ Involves the development of a 24-hour nursing plan
5. ______ Uses a predetermined critical pathway
6. ______ Master's prepared nurse usually practicing in hospitals, clinics, home health, or private practice
7. ______ Includes the team leader and charge nurse
8. ______ Supervisors who are responsible for interdepartmental problem solving

COLUMN II

a. Clinical nurse specialist
b. Leadership
c. Managed care
d. Management
e. Middle manager
f. Nurse practitioner
g. Primary nursing
h. Staff nurse
i. Team nursing
j. First-line managers

TRUE–FALSE

Indicate if the following statements are true or false.

______ 1. Change is usually welcomed by staff members.

______ 2. Clinical nurse specialists practice primarily in the community.

______ 3. The charge nurse makes management decisions for a particular work shift.

______ 4. Managed care requires the nurse to instruct physicians in patient care.

FILL IN THE BLANK

Supply the missing term or the information requested.

1. Managers must manage ____________, ____________, and ____________ resources.
2. Briefly discuss the major differences in the primary focus of leadership and management. ____ ____ ____________________________.
3. Discuss the most appropriate leadership style to be used in an emergency situation, and explain why this might be effective. ____ ____.
4. Discuss the differences between team nursing and primary nursing, and state one advantage and disadvantage of each. ____ ____ ____________.
5. Three skills needed for effective management are ______________, ______________, and ______________.
6. Describe the difference between the team leader and the charge nurse. ____ ______________.
7. In the ________________ delivery model, the primary nurse uses a predetermined critical pathway to establish and monitor the extent and timing of care.

■ Applying Your Knowledge

CASE STUDY

As nurse manager for the cardiac unit, you have just returned from a budget meeting with Stella D., the nurse executive for your medical center. You have been informed that your operating budget for the year has been cut by approximately $85,000. You are responsible for considering methods of compensating for this loss.

Approach this problem as a leader with a directive style and with a participative style.

CRITICAL INQUIRY EXERCISE

You are a new charge nurse on the 3-to-11 shift. You graduated a year ago, and your staff includes two new nursing graduates who finished orientation a month ago. An hour before the shift ends, one of the new nurse's clients has a cardiac and respiratory arrest. The nurse states, "I know I should control the code for my client. If you help me, I am sure I can do it."

1. Discuss your responsibilities as charge nurse in this situation.
2. Identify the type of leadership you would provide as charge nurse during this situation, and discuss how your leadership might differ if the clients on the unit had nonemergent problems.
3. List and explain the teaching activities that might occur with the graduate nurses in the above situation.

CRITICAL EXPLORATION EXERCISE

Recall a change that recently occurred in your personal or professional life. Describe the following:

1. How you reacted to the change initially.
2. How you reacted to the change 1 month later.
3. Ways in which you believe difficulties/challenges associated with the change could be improved.

■ Practicing for NCLEX

MULTIPLE CHOICE QUESTIONS

Circle the letter that corresponds to the best answer for each question.

1. When the nurse manager is deciding what to do, when, where, how, by whom, and with what resources, which of the following management processes is being performed?
   a. Controlling
   b. Directing
   c. Planning
   d. Organizing

2. Peggy, a registered nurse, worked with her staff in the development of objectives to establish priorities for procedures on her unit. Which of the following management processes does this exemplify?
   a. Directing
   b. Organizing
   c. Controlling
   d. Planning

3. The nurse executive who does not include staff members in the decision-making process is practicing which of the following leadership styles?
   a. Democratic
   b. Directive
   c. Participative
   d. Republican

4. Paula is very effective at inspiring and motivating her staff to give highly skilled, efficient nursing care. Which of the following leadership styles does she most likely exhibit?
   a. Controlling leadership
   b. Directive management
   c. Participative leadership
   d. Strong management

5. The staff nurse must gather data related to client needs and analyze the data to determine possible solutions. Which of the following styles most closely resembles this type of management skill?
   a. Controlling
   b. Decision making
   c. Directing
   d. Problem solving

6. Nurse managers recognize that to achieve effective communication, some techniques are more effective than others. Of the following, which choice would be most the effective listening style?
   a. Attempt to judge the meaning of the speaker's words as the words are being spoken
   b. Avoid questioning the speaker regarding the meaning of statements
   c. Formulate responses as the speaker talks to avoid an uncomfortable delay in the conversation.
   d. Give full attention to what the speaker is saying verbally and nonverbally.

7. Which of the following choices should nurse managers encourage to decrease resistance to the change process?
   a. Avoid changes that might be perceived as learning opportunities.
   b. Assess the implications of any change for themselves and their followers.
   c. Limit the information to staff regarding the change being made.
   d. Use a directive leadership style when initiating the change.

FILL IN THE BLANK

Supply the missing term or the information requested.

1. Considering the consequences of each possible solution before choosing a particular one is considered step number ____________ in the problem-solving process.
2. The second step in the problem-solving process is to ________________the possible solutions.
3. Finally, at step number ____________ of the problem-solving process the nurse will evaluate the results.
4. The first step in the problem-solving process is to both ________________ and ________________ the problem.
5. Implementing the solution is considered the ________________ step in the problem-solving process.

MULTIPLE-ANSWER MULTIPLE CHOICE

Circle the letter(s) corresponding to the appropriate answer(s). Select all that apply.

1. Once a task has been identified for delegation to assistive personnel, which of the following statements best describes the skill set *most* necessary?
   a. The assistant is knowledgeable.
   b. The assistant is competent.
   c. The assistant is dependable.
   d. The assistant is attentive.

2. As a member of a primary nursing team, the RN assumes responsibility for developing a client plan of care that encompasses a time span of
   a. 12 hours.
   b. 24 hours.
   c. 48 hours.
   d. 72 hours.

3. Leadership between the levels of nurse manager and nurse executive may include managers with titles that may include which of the following?
   a. Supervisor
   b. Director
   c. Vice president
   d. Assistant nurse manager
   e. Charge nurse

4. RNs who are involved in primary nursing assume responsibility for developing a plan of care that encompasses which of the following time periods?
   a. 8-hour shift
   b. 12-hour shift
   c. 24-hour shift
   d. Day/evening rotation
   e. Day/night rotation
   f. Day/evening/night rotation

5. As managers, nurses need to be skilled in which of the following?
   a. Problem solving
   b. Planning
   c. Communicating
   d. Delegating
   e. Managing change

CHAPTER 8

Nursing Research: Evidence-Based Care

CHAPTER OVERVIEW

In Chapter 8 the role of research in the improvement of nursing practice and its significance in the building of the nursing profession is discussed. The roles of different levels of nursing personnel in the research process are presented and explored.

LEARNING OBJECTIVES

After mastering the content in this chapter, you should be able to do the following:

1. Trace the historical appreciation of nursing research.
2. Explain the contributions of evidence-based research to nursing practice.
3. Review the research process for the beginning professional nursing student.
4. Summarize legal and ethical issues related to nursing research.

■ Mastering the Information

MATCHING

Match the terms in Column II with a definition, example, or related statement from Column I. Place the letter corresponding to the answer in the space provided.

COLUMN I

1. ______ A clear and unambiguous expression of a relationship between variable
2. ______ The plan for collection and analysis of data
3. ______ The process of selecting published material that substantiates the concepts to be studied
4. ______ The conceptual frame of reference for the study that gives clues on how to study the problem
5. ______ Protects the subject so that even the researcher cannot link the subject with the information provided
6. ______ A set of interrelated propositions that attempt to present or systematically explain some phenomenon
7. ______ Properties that differ from each other
8. ______ Ensures that the subject's identity will not be linked with the information they provide

COLUMN II

a. Anonymity
b. Confidentiality
c. Literature review
d. Problem statement
e. Research design
f. Theory
g. Method
h. Variables
i. Hypothesis
j. Qualitative research

TRUE–FALSE

Indicate if the following statements are true or false.

______ 1. Nursing research was not used in Florence Nightingale's era.

______ 2. The development of master's programs in nursing contributed to an increase in nursing research.

______ 3. Nursing research investigations have had little effect on the quality of nursing care.

______ 4. The National Center for Nursing Research established the National Institutes of Health to expand nursing research.

______ 5. The cost of the research process sometimes outweighs the value of the research.

FILL IN THE BLANK

Supply the missing term or the information requested.

1. Describe the focus of nursing research.

   ____

2. Nursing research is ________________ to that of any other discipline in which practitioners are interested in seeking the truth.
3. State three of the four pieces of information a researcher must provide to human subjects.
   a. ______________________________
   b. ______________________________
   c. ______________________________
4. Discuss three of the four holistic properties of nursing research.
   a. ______________________________
   b. ______________________________
   c. ______________________________

■ Applying Your Knowledge

CASE STUDY

As a perioperative nurse in a moderate-size farming community, you have noticed that many of your clients use herbal and "home" remedies that are important in their health maintenance routine. During your preoperative interview/assessment, you ask whether herbal supplements are a part of the daily regimen of your clients. Your curiosity has led you to research herbal supplements and clotting/platelet relationships after you began to notice a tendency to continue to bleed in some clients who regularly ingest certain supplements.

As a nurse interested in continuing a formalized study of your observations, what would be the next four steps in the research process?

CRITICAL INQUIRY EXERCISE

You are a nurse assigned to a rehabilitation service for children with head trauma. All of the children are school age. However, little is being done in the way of formal education for the children. Your colleague wants administration to hire a nurse to determine how much the children can learn.

1. Outline the steps needed to determine a valid answer to the question of how much the children can learn.
2. Explain the role of nurses at different levels of practice who might participate in the research.
3. Describe the involvement of the children and their parents.

CRITICAL EXPLORATION EXERCISE

1. Write a short essay exploring an identified research problem in terms of the following:
   - Potential benefits of research results to the nursing profession.
   - Possible problems encountered in the process of general information gathering.
2. Use your computer to conduct a search of the literature on a topic that you identify as a nursing research topic.
3. Identify an area of nursing research based on your observations of client needs. Determine whether your topic has previous research information that you may potentially validate.

■ Practicing for NCLEX

MULTIPLE CHOICE QUESTIONS

1. Which of the following statements is true about nursing research?
   a. Clinical research decreases the need for standards of nursing care.
   b. Research involves inquiry into problems in nursing practice.
   c. Research results should not be used in practice immediately after the study is completed.
   d. The research process will change the relationships among the variables being studied.

2. The statement that best defines the purpose of the National Center for Nursing Research is which of the following?
   a. Prevent the mitigation of the effects of chronic illness
   b. Remove nursing from the sphere of scientific investigation
   c. Replace the nursing process with research methodology
   d. Support research into client-care and disease prevention.

3. Which of the following statements about a dependent variable is most accurate?
   a. It has a presumed effect on another variable.
   b. It is manipulated by the researcher in an experimental study.
   c. It is the variable the researcher is attempting to explain
   d. It occurs naturally before or during the study.

4. A literature review should best be described as
   a. brief and limited.
   b. broad and theoretical.
   c. general and contextual.
   d. systematic and exhaustive.

5. Which of the following is the first step in the research process?
   a. Analyze and manage the data
   b. Define the specific clinical problem
   c. Make a nursing diagnosis
   d. Identify problem areas

6. Which of the following is the final step in the research process?
   a. Define the specific problem
   b. Disseminate the findings
   c. Make a nursing diagnosis
   d. Plan an intervention

7. Which of the following might prevent the conducting of a research study?
   a. Costs for conducting the study are low compared with the potential benefits form the research.
   b. In order to gather data for the research, excessive risk to the subject is required.
   c. The identified problem is covered in the literature.
   d. The research problem is based on untested nursing theories.

8. The nurse who is beginning to practice usually participates in research at which of the following stages?
   a. Statistical design
   b. Findings dissemination
   c. Treatment administration
   d. Hypothesis formation

9. The Nuremberg Tribunal did which of the following?
   a. Addressed the process for selecting research problems
   b. Allowed injury to subjects only when necessary to obtain accurate data
   c. Defined the steps for nursing research
   d. Developed a statement listing the rights of research subjects.

10. A primary reason that the conclusions or findings from nursing research studies should be disseminated is so that
    a. other disciplines will recognize nursing research efforts.
    b. findings can be validated through additional research.
    c. the researcher can be given credit for creating new knowledge.
    d. the research process used can become a matter of record.

FILL IN THE BLANK

Supply the missing term or the information requested.

1. A nurse with a ________________ degree may analyze and reformulate nursing practice problems.
2. Nurses with doctoral degrees may ________________ investigations to evaluate the contribution of nursing activities to client well-being.
3. Evidence-based practice is an outcome of ___________________ research.
4. ________________, or properties that vary from each other, are the focus of research studies.
5. The focus of nursing research must be on a _____________ that makes a difference in improving client care.

MULTIPLE-ANSWER MULTIPLE CHOICE

Circle the letter(s) corresponding to the appropriate answer(s). Select all that apply.

1. Nurses interested in research will *most* likely be involved
   a. in healthcare settings.
   b. inside laboratory settings.
   c. outside laboratory settings.
   d. in corporate settings.

2. The concept of evidence-based practice (EBP) has been evolving for about
   a. 10 years.
   b. 20 years.
   c. 30 years.
   d. 40 years.
   e. 50 years.

3. Nursing research is considered to be a step-by-step process that includes
   a. formulating a problem statement.
   b. protecting the findings as intellectual property.
   c. reviewing the literature.
   d. defining ideas.

4. Researchers determine how to study the problem, which is also referred to as which of the following?
   a. Variable
   b. Method
   c. Hypothesis
   d. Design
   e. Review

UNIT III

The Nursing Process: Framework for Clinical Nursing Therapeutics

CHAPTER 9

Nursing Process: Foundation for Practice

CHAPTER OVERVIEW

Chapter 9 reviews the historic development of the nursing process, then examines and summarizes the nursing process: basic components, the requirements and theoretical foundations for use, the functional health patterns approach, and future trends.

LEARNING OBJECTIVES

After mastering the content in this chapter, you should be able to do the following:

1. Identify the components of the nursing process.
2. Describe the significant historic developments in the evolution of the nursing process.
3. Discuss the requirements for effective use of the nursing process.
4. Explain the major theoretical foundations on which the nursing process is based.
5. Describe the functional health patterns approach to the nursing process.
6. Appraise future trends that will influence the nursing process.

■ Mastering the Information

MATCHING

Match the term in Column II with a definition, example, or related statement from Column I. Place the letter corresponding to the answer in the space provided. (Use each letter only once; some letters may not be used.)

COLUMN I

1. ______ Intervention strategies to reduce identified client problems are established, and a written summary of the care to be given is prepared.
2. ______ Subjective and objective data are collected systematically with the goal of making a clinical nursing judgment about a client or family.
3. ______ Assessment information is analyzed to determine actual or potential health problems.
4. ______ The nurse determines the client's reaction to nursing interventions and judges whether the goals of the management plan have been achieved.
5. ______ The plan is initiated, the response to the plan is evaluated, and the nursing actions and the client's response to those actions are recorded.

COLUMN II

a. Assessment
b. Diagnosis
c. Outcome identification
d. Planning
e. Implementation
f. Evaluation

COLUMN I

1. ______ A theory that uses inductive and deductive reasoning for gathering and processing information
2. ______ A theory that illustrates how the steps of the nursing process interact with each other using input, throughput, output, and feedback
3. ______ A theory with three phases: identifying the problem, determining alternatives, and selecting the most appropriate alternative

COLUMN II

a. System theory
b. Decision-making process
c. Information-processing theory
d. Problem-solving theory

TRUE–FALSE

Indicate if the following statements are true or false.

______ 1. The term "nursing process" was introduced by Lydia Hall in 1955.

______ 2. Induction is a reasoning process that proceeds from the general to the specific.

______ 3. The nursing process focuses on the client's unique problems and facilitates the development of individualized care.

______ 4. The decision-making process consists of three phases: input, throughput, and output.

______ 5. Writing and active listening are two skill requirements for effective use of the nursing process.

______ 6. The Western Interstate Commission on Higher Education identified the four steps of the nursing process as assessment, planning, implementation, and evaluation.

______ 7. Being an active listener involves focusing only on clients' verbal responses.

FILL IN THE BLANK

Supply the missing term or the information requested.

1. The six steps of the nursing process introduced by ANA (1991) are ________________, ________________, ________________, ________________, ________________, and ________________.

2. The ____________ is a problem-solving approach for discovering the healthcare needs of clients and their families.

3. The basic structural units that provide theoretical foundations of the nursing process are ________________, ________________, ________________, ________________, and ________________.

4. ________________ provide a framework for the collection of assessment data.

5. The evaluation phase of the nursing process involves a detailed reassessment of the entire plan of care, judgment about client goal ________________, and fulfillment of ________________ criteria.

■ Applying Your Knowledge

CASE STUDY

Cynthia Delmazom is a 39-year-old single mother. Her children are 13- and 16-year-old boys. Ms. Delmazom broke her right leg and sprained her right wrist in a fall at home. Her job will pay sick leave for 2 months, and the physician states she will be unable to work for 10 weeks. Ms. Delmazom and her sons live in a house with all bedrooms upstairs.

1. Discuss additional assessments needed to identify Ms. Delmazom's needs fully.
2. Identify individuals you would include in the process of developing the plan of care, and discuss your rationale for including these people.

3. Identify three actual or potential health problems related to Ms. Delmazom and her family, and determine an appropriate outcome for each problem stated.

CRITICAL INQUIRY EXERCISE

Develop a master chart outlining the nursing process and the five theoretical foundations on which it is based.

CRITICAL EXPLORATION

Reference online resources relative to information processing theory and develop a matrix demonstrating how cluster data can aid you in arriving at a nursing diagnosis for one of your clients.

■ Practicing for NCLEX

MULTIPLE CHOICE QUESTIONS

Circle the letter that corresponds to the best answer for each question.

1. Which one of the following statements accurately describes a nurse who is qualified to make a nursing diagnosis?
   a. Any baccalaureate-prepared registered nurse
   b. Any licensed registered nurse
   c. Any licensed nurse
   d. Only a master's-prepared registered nurse

2. Of the following characteristics of the nursing process, which one should *not* be included in the list?
   a. Orderly and systematic
   b. Interdependent
   c. Limited clinical application
   d. Client centered

3. Which of the following tools in the nursing diagnostic process is used to ensure accuracy in selecting the correct diagnosis?
   a. Observing, interviewing, and conducting a physical examination
   b. Measuring goal achievements
   c. Revising or modifying the client care plan to ensure accomplishment of client goals
   d. Cue clustering, cluster interpretation, and diagnostic validation

4. Of the following choices, which characteristic distinguishes the problem-solving process from the scientific problem-solving method?
   a. Controlled variables
   b. A focus on one identifiable problem
   c. Flexibility
   d. Isolated settings

5. According to the systems theory, throughput in relation to the nursing process occurs at which of the following points?
   a. During the assessment and planning steps of the nursing process
   b. After the diagnostic, planning, and implementation phases of the nursing process
   c. During the evaluation phase
   d. Before assessment and diagnoses

FILL IN THE BLANK

Supply the missing term or the information requested.

1. Writing skillfully requires the ability to ____________________ information.
2. The action phase of the nursing process is known as ____________________.
3. The systematic problem-solving approach toward giving individualized nursing care is summed up as the ______________________ ______________________.

4. One of the steps in the diagnostic reasoning process includes __________________ the database.

5. Healthcare records are considered __________________sources of patient information.

MULTIPLE-ANSWER MULTIPLE CHOICE

Circle the letter(s) corresponding to the appropriate answer(s). Circle all that apply.

1. The reasoning process used to make accurate clinical diagnoses about client problems is correctly identified as
   a. evaluative.
   b. communicative.
   c. diagnostic.
   d. interactive.

2. Of the following steps, which one is *not* a step outlined by Yura and Walsh as part of the nursing process?
   a. Assessing
   b. Identifying
   c. Implementing
   d. Evaluating

3. The reference point for all further nursing assessments after admission to a hospital or long-term care facility is best described as which of the following?
   a. Nursing history and physical assessment
   b. Physical assessment and nursing diagnosis
   c. Nursing history and nursing diagnosis
   d. Physical assessment and outcome identification

4. Which of the following is the primary source of information during a patient assessment?
   a. Client
   b. Health record
   c. Family member
   d. Family physician

5. The nursing process is used in settings with clients that include which of the following?
   a. Pediatric clients
   b. Geriatric clients
   c. Hospitalized clients
   d. All of the above

CHAPTER 10

Nursing Assessment

CHAPTER OVERVIEW

Chapter 10 defines assessment as the first phase of the nursing process and discusses how to prepare for assessment, assessment skills, and assessment activities.

LEARNING OBJECTIVES

After mastering the content in this chapter, you should be able to do the following:

1. Define the assessment phase of the nursing process.
2. Discuss the purpose of assessment in nursing practice.
3. Identify the skills required for nursing assessment.
4. Differentiate the three major activities involved in nursing assessment.
5. Describe and explain the process of data collection.
6. Explain the rationale for data validation.
7. Discuss the frameworks used to organize assessment data.
8. Perform a nursing assessment based on functional health patterns.

■ Mastering the Information

MATCHING

Match the terms in Column II with a definition, example, or related statement from Column I. Place the letter corresponding to the answer in the space provided.

COLUMN I

1. ______ Listening to body sounds using a stethoscope
2. ______ A visual examination of the client
3. ______ The specialized use of touch for data collection
4. ______ The striking of the body surface with one or both hands to produce sounds

COLUMN II

a. Percussion
b. Auscultation
c. Inspection
d. Palpation

COLUMN I

1. ______ The nurse explores his or her feeling or reaction to the client and reviews the literature pertinent to the client.
2. ______ The nurse and the client work toward achieving the specific task or goal.
3. ______ The nurse establishes rapport, clarifies roles, and alleviates anxiety.
4. ______ The nurse reviews goals or task attainment and summarizes the highlights of the interview.

COLUMN II

a. Preparatory phase
b. Introductory phase
c. Maintenance phase
d. Concluding phase

TRUE–FALSE

Indicate if the following statements are true or false.

______ 1. A synonym for subjective data is convert cues.

______ 2. An emergency assessment focuses on a few essential health patterns and is not comprehensive.

_____ 3. Intuition results when nurses make decisions based on the nursing process.

_____ 4. Assessment is best performed in a quiet, private setting.

_____ 5. Reassuring clichés may be used to facilitate communication.

_____ 6. The nurse assessment activities involve only data collection and data validation.

_____ 7. The process of listening to body sounds is termed percussion.

_____ 8. Time-lapse assessment and focus assessment center on the status of problems already identified.

_____ 9. Usually the most reliable source of information is the client.

_____ 10. Laboratory tests and diagnostic procedures are primary sources of data collection.

FILL IN THE BLANK

Supply the missing term or the information requested.

1. Name the four types of assessment.
   a.
   b.
   c.
   d.
2. List the four clinical skills used in assessment.
   a.
   b.
   c.
   d.
3. _______________ is a systematic data collection method that uses the senses of sight, hearing, smell, and touch to detect health problems.
4. Two types of data are _______________ and _______________.
5. When a nurse makes a clinical judgment based on insight, instinct, and clinical experience, this is termed _______________.
6. List two major types of sources for the collection of information about the client.

   ____

   ____
7. Identify five secondary sources that provide data that supplement, clarify, and validate information obtained from the client.

   ____

   ____

   ____

   ____

   ____
8. Name two of the three ways in which data may be organized.

   ____

   ____

SUBJECTIVE VS. OBJECTIVE DATA

Indicate if the following assessment data are subjective or objective. Mark "S" for subjective or "O" for objective in the space provided.

_____ 1. Burning and itching

_____ 2. Headache

_____ 3. Apical pulse rate of 82 beats per minute

_____ 4. Left foot swollen

_____ 5. Sharp leg pain

_____ 6. Skin rash

_____ 7. Nausea

_____ 8. Temperature of left upper arm

_____ 9. Bruises on left upper arm

_____ 10. Indigestion

■ Applying Your Knowledge

CASE STUDY

You are a nurse in a well-baby clinic. An 18-year-old unwed mother brings her 1-year-old daughter for a routine checkup. The child is bright-eyed and beautiful. She smiles freely but clings to her mother. During the physical examination you notice bluish areas on her back, buttocks, and thighs. There are also "scratches" on her arms. When these are shown to the mother, she mumbles something, then states, "My friend keeps her sometimes, and she usually gets those spots then." You observe that the child does not cry during the physical examination but attempts to withdraw and roll from the table. Consider the following in relation to a comprehensive appraisal of the situation.

1. Plan strategies for establishing rapport with the mother and child.
2. Formulate techniques or questions that you could use to obtain additional data.
3. List sources of data other than the mother and child that might clarify or support your guesses about the situation.
4. Determine how you will prioritize information.

CRITICAL INQUIRY EXERCISE

1. Arrange a visit to a local nursing home or healthcare facility. Obtain permission from a client to interview the client. Record your interview techniques, and record the client interview using a tape recorder. Your instructor should critique your interview skills and allow time for feedback.
2. Research organizations in your area that provide language and cultural support to clients from countries of origin other than the United States. Determine whether there are healthcare materials, translators, or support services you could use to improve your ability to collect accurate assessment information.

CRITICAL EXPLORATION EXERCISE

Obtain a nursing health history form (design your own or use one from a local healthcare agency). You and another student can complete the health history form on one another. Analyze one another's communication skills.

■ Practicing for NCLEX

MULTIPLE CHOICE QUESTIONS

Circle the letter that corresponds to the best answer for each question.

1. The registered nurse performs an admission assessment. Which of the following may be characterized as an admission assessment by the registered nurse?
   a. Emergency assessment
   b. Time-lapsed assessment
   c. Initial assessment
   d. Focus assessment

2. The primary purpose of the admission assessment is to
   a. achieve client-centered goals or tasks.
   b. evaluate the client's health status.
   c. develop a good rapport.
   d. identify changes in existing health.

3. Before the assessment begins, the client reports pain in the upper right quadrant of the abdomen. The nurse documents this type of data as which of the following?
   a. Evaluative
   b. Objective
   c. Overt
   d. Subjective

4. The nurse knows that the most reliable source of data collection for the client's nursing assessment is
   a. the client.
   b. the client's past medical records.
   c. the client's daughter.
   d. the client's spouse.

5. Of the following assessment skills, choose the one that is best described as laying the groundwork for collecting other kinds of data.
   a. Auscultation
   b. Interviewing
   c. Observation
   d. Physical examination

6. The *initial* nursing assessment of the client is the ultimate responsibility of which of the following healthcare professionals?
   a. Charge nurses and supervisors
   b. A professional registered nurse
   c. The admitting physician
   d. Any licensed healthcare person

FILL IN THE BLANK

Supply the missing term or the information requested.

1. Always consider the client's sociocultural background when using ________________.
2. Symptoms or covert clues are also known as ________________ data.
3. ____________________ involves recognizing and collecting cues.
4. The maintenance, or working phase, is the ________________ phase of an interview.
5. ____________________ is the specialized use of touch for data collection.
6. A nurse's use of insight, instinct, and clinical experience is considered ________________.
7. ______________________ factors can facilitate or hinder collection of assessment data.

MULTIPLE-ANSWER MULTIPLE CHOICE

Circle the letter(s) corresponding to the appropriate answer(s). Circle all that apply.

1. Secondary sources help provide necessary assessment information for clients who may
   a. have chronic physically debilitating conditions.
   b. speak English as a second language.
   c. have altered judgment and memory.
   d. have speech and hearing impairments.

2. The second phase of the nursing interview is known as which of the following?
   a. Maintenance
   b. Preparatory
   c. Orientation
   d. Preinteraction

3. Assessment cues that reveal foul smelling breath *may* signify which of the following?
   a. Ketosis
   b. Pulmonary infection
   c. Alcohol intake
   d. Oversecretion of sebaceous glands

4. Environmental factors that may be counterproductive to the collection of accurate and complete data assessment may include
   a. closing the curtain.
   b. turning down the heat.
   c. shutting the door.
   d. turning up the radio.
   e. leaving the curtain open.

5. The phase when the nurse and client meet is known as which of the following?
   a. Preparatory
   b. Introductory
   c. Maintenance
   d. Concluding
   e. Preinduction
   f. Working
   g. Orientation

ORDERING

Following are examples of a nurse's comments made during an interview. Place these comments in the correct sequence by numbering the items.

a. ______ "Mr. Jones, you have identified the following health concerns: intermittent numbness and tingling in your left leg, the need to control low back pain, and the desire to perform activities of daily living with minimal discomfort."

b. ______ "Now let us move to a nice, quiet place."

c. ______ "Hello, my name is Jan Fault. I am your nurse today."

d. ______ "Mr. Jones, is your low back pain associated with exercise or increased activity?"

CHAPTER 11

Nursing Diagnosis

CHAPTER OVERVIEW

Chapter 11 examines the second phase of the nursing process: nursing diagnosis. Emphasis is placed on the significance of nursing diagnosis to the practice of nursing and on the process of formulating nursing diagnoses.

LEARNING OBJECTIVES

After mastering the content in this chapter, you should be able to do the following:

1. Define diagnosis in relation to the nursing process.
2. State the meaning of nursing diagnosis.
3. Describe the components of a nursing diagnosis.
4. Discuss the significance of the nursing diagnosis for nursing practice.
5. Discuss the Nursing Diagnosis Extension and Classification (NDEC) project.
6. Differentiate between a nursing diagnosis and other healthcare problems.
7. Identify the clinical skills needed to make a nursing diagnosis.
8. Formulate nursing diagnoses for a client situation.
9. Discuss the categorization of nursing diagnoses by functional health patterns.

■ Mastering the Information

MATCHING

Match the terms in Column II with a definition, example, or related statement from Column I. Place the letter corresponding to the answer in the space provided.

COLUMN I

1. ______ Describes human responses to health conditions or life processes that may develop in a vulnerable individual, family, or community
2. ______ Describes a human response to a health problem that is being manifested
3. ______ Selecting a nursing diagnosis before analyzing pertinent data
4. ______ A statement made when there is not enough evidence to support the presence of the problem, but the nurse thinks it is highly probable
5. ______ A diagnostic statement that describes human response to levels of wellness in an individual, family, or community that have a potential for enhancement to a higher state

COLUMN II

a. Actual nursing diagnosis
b. Premature closure
c. A risk nursing diagnosis
d. A wellness nursing diagnosis
e. A possible nursing diagnosis

TRUE–FALSE

Indicate if the following statements are true or false.

______ 1. To cluster data means to give all details described by the client.

______ 2. The term "risk factor" is used to describe clinical cues in risk nursing diagnoses.

______ 3. The nurse is responsible and accountable for identifying and treating collaborative problems that focus on pathophysiologic responses, in conjunction with the physician.

______ 4. A cue is a piece of information—subjective or objective—collected during the nursing assessment.

______ 5. Diagnostic validation occurs in two stages: comparing the clusters to norms and evaluating the specific nursing diagnosis for its nursing-research base.

______ 6. The purpose of the NDEC project is to disseminate newly developed diagnoses among practicing nurses.

FILL IN THE BLANK

Supply the missing term or the information requested.

1. ________________validation occurs in ___________ stages.
2. Identify five of the seven axes used in NANDA's taxonomy I.
   a.
   b.
   c.
   d.
   e.
3. ________________of nursing diagnoses in ________________________systems allows ______________reimbursement for nurses.
4. List the three parts of an actual nursing diagnosis.
   a. ______________________________
   b. ______________________________
   c. ______________________________
5. Identify five of seven characteristics that support the significance of nursing diagnoses.
   a.
   b.
   c.
   d.
   e.

■ Applying Your Knowledge

CASE STUDY

Francine Black is 8 months pregnant. She is the mother of two preschool children. She has to work following the death of her husband 3 months ago in a plane crash. When she comes to the maternity clinic, she brings the two children with her. Throughout the waiting period, she is either screaming at the children or pulling on one or the other of them. Both of her feet are swollen, and she reports being constantly tired.

1. List four possible nursing diagnoses.
2. Cluster data under various nursing diagnoses, and justify your decision regarding data placement.
3. List additional data needed to validate each diagnostic statement.
4. Propose a plan for obtaining additional information about Mrs. Black, her children, the family, and community.
5. Consider bias that may influence your interpretation of data.

CRITICAL INQUIRY EXERCISE

1. In the clinical setting, develop a list of nursing diagnoses based on your assessment of an assigned client.
2. Analyze each diagnosis for the inclusion of a diagnostic label, related factors, and defining characteristics.

CRITICAL EXPLORATION EXERCISE

Using a nursing diagnosis reference book, compare your diagnostic statement to the defining characteristics and definition provided in the reference resource. Is your diagnosis supported or not? If not, what documentation is necessary for the diagnosis to be considered appropriate?

■ Practicing for NCLEX

MULTIPLE CHOICE QUESTIONS

Circle the letter that corresponds to the best answer for each question.

1. Nursing diagnosis is defined as
   a. the result of ordering complex information for the purpose of identifying pathologic processes.
   b. the process of clustering cues collected during the assessment phase of the nursing process.
   c. a clinical judgment about individual, family, or community responses to actual or potential health problems or life processes.
   d. an actual or potential health problem that focuses on the pathophysiologic responses of the body.

2. The NANDA taxonomy II is organized
   a. according to functional health patterns.
   b. according to basic human needs.
   c. alphabetically.
   d. using a multiaxial format.

3. Which of the following is not an approved NANDA nursing diagnosis?
   a. Decreased cardiac output
   b. Depression
   c. Impaired parenting
   d. Nutrition, less than body requirements

4. Which one of the following types of nursing diagnostic statements includes the diagnostic label, defining characteristics, and related factors?
   a. Actual nursing diagnosis
   b. Collaborative nursing diagnosis
   c. Risk nursing diagnosis
   d. Possible nursing diagnosis

5. Which of the following is a component of the nursing diagnosis phase of the nursing process?
   a. Data collection
   b. Priority setting
   c. Pattern identification
   d. Outcome identification

FILL IN THE BLANK

Supply the missing term or the information requested.

1. As of 2004, there are ________________ North American Nursing Diagnosis Association (NANDA)-approved nursing diagnoses.

2. A ________________ conveys information about a disease or pathology.

3. ____________ legitimizes the diagnosis and helps to discover its significance for the client.

4. Nursing diagnostic labels can serve as ____________________________ for specific client problems.

MULTIPLE-ANSWER MULTIPLE CHOICE

Circle the letter(s) corresponding to the appropriate answer(s). Circle all that apply.

1. By focusing attention on the actual or potential health needs of clients, nursing diagnoses increase which of the following factors regarding nursing intervention for each client?
   a. Quality
   b. Validity
   c. Quantity
   d. Specificity
   e. Accountability

2. Which of the following is/are *not* true of nursing diagnoses?
   a. Carry legal ramifications
   b. Cannot diagnose a medical condition
   c. Determine problems from assessment data
   d. Used to diagnose a medical condition
   e. Have no legal ramifications
   f. Convey information about the signs and symptoms of disease processes

3. Selecting a diagnosis before analyzing patient information to have adequate cues is known as
   a. cue clustering.
   b. premature closure.
   c. cluster interpretation.
   d. invalidation.
   e. risk diagnoses.

4. A taxonomy is best described as which of the following?
   a. A diagnostic system
   b. A validation system
   c. An evaluation system
   d. A classification system
   e. A cluster system
   f. A collection system

5. A diagnostic statement that describes the human response to levels of health with the potential to a higher state is best described as
   a. possible nursing diagnosis.
   b. wellness nursing diagnosis.
   c. risk nursing diagnosis.
   d. actual nursing diagnosis.

CHAPTER 12

Outcome Identification and Planning

CHAPTER OVERVIEW

Chapter 12 expands on the formulation of goals and measurable outcomes that provide the basis for evaluation for nursing diagnoses. Measurement criteria for outcome identification are listed along with examples of realistic goals. Activities performed in this phase of the nursing process are explained.

LEARNING OBJECTIVES

After mastering the content in this chapter, you should be able to do the following:

1. Define outcome identification and planning.
2. Explain the purposes of outcome identification and planning.
3. Discuss the Nursing Outcome Classification and the Nursing Intervention Classification projects.
4. Describe the components of the client plan of care.
5. Formulate a client plan of care for a client given a nursing assessment database.
6. Use a functional health approach to plan client care.

■ Mastering the Information

MATCHING

Match the terms in Column II with a definition, example, or related statement from Column I. Place the letter corresponding to the answer in the space provided.

COLUMN I

1. ______ The formulation of goals and measurable outcomes that provide the basis for evaluation for nursing diagnoses
2. ______ Something that takes precedence in position; is deemed the most important among several items
3. ______ An educated guess made as a broad statement about what the client's state will be after the nursing intervention
4. ______ A description of the parameter for achieving the goal
5. ______ The fourth phase of the nursing process; refers to the development of nursing strategies designed to ameliorate client problems
6. ______ The justification or reason for carrying out the intervention

COLUMN II

a. A priority
b. A client goal
c. Outcome identification
d. Scientific rationale
e. Qualifier
f. Planning

TRUE–FALSE

Indicate if the following statements are true or false.

______ 1. The client plan of care may be developed by any nurse or nursing assistant providing care to the client.

______ 2. Two important guidelines for developing a client plan of care are that the plan is nursing centered and is a step-by-step process.

______ 3. One goal may be stated for two to three nursing diagnoses.

______ 4. The client plan of care usually contains the nursing diagnosis, client goals, and nursing interventions as key elements.

______ 5. Components of instructional client plans of care outline only the subject matter (topics) for client teaching.

FILL IN THE BLANK

Supply the missing term or the information requested.

1. The purposes of outcome identification include:
   a.
   b.
   c.
   d.
2. High-priority nursing diagnoses are those that are potentially ________________ and require ________________.
3. A short-term goal can be met within ________________ or ________________, whereas a long-term goal requires more time, perhaps several ________________ or ________________.
4. Outcome criteria answer the questions ________________, ________________ ________________, ________________ ________________, ________________ ________________, and ________________.
5. List three of the four purposes of planning.
   a. ________________________________
   b. ________________________________
   c. ________________________________
6. Activities of the planning phase include:
   a.
   b.
7. Statements of appropriate nursing interventions are used to:
   a.
   b.
   c.
   d.
8. List five of the seven classifications of nursing interventions currently identified.
   a.
   b.
   c.
   d.
   e.

■ Applying Your Knowledge

CASE STUDY

Jason is a 15-year-old boy with diabetes (high blood glucose/sugar). He is admitted with a very high blood glucose level and states, "I had to have the milkshake and candy because the other kids would think I was strange otherwise." Jason received a diagnosis of diabetes a month ago, and this is his third hospitalization because of elevated blood glucose. He states that he doesn't know why this keeps happening to him. His mother states that she has been preparing his meals for him and sends lunches with him to school.

1. Using a functional approach, determine what dysfunctional areas Jason might have.
2. Formulate three nursing diagnoses from the above data and establish one goal and outcome criteria for each diagnosis.
3. How might Jason's dysfunctions differ if he were 5 years old, and how would this change the goals and outcome criteria you might establish?

CRITICAL INQUIRY EXERCISE

Choose three client goals from plans of care at your clinical setting. Evaluate the goals and criteria for accuracy of format.

CRITICAL EXPLORATION EXERCISE

Consider your plans for a career in nursing. Identify two short-term goals and two long-term goals you should meet. Critique the goals for appropriateness, including measurability and other components.

■ Practicing for NCLEX

MULTIPLE CHOICE QUESTIONS

Circle the letter that corresponds to the best answer for each question.

1. Jahel Marckee has a nursing diagnosis of feeding self-care deficit related to right-sided weakness manifested by inability to pick up a spoon and inability to open containers. An appropriate goal for Jahel related to this diagnosis is that he
   a. demonstrates a greater interest in eating.
   b. demonstrates an ability to feed himself with a spoon.
   c. has an assistant to open his food packages for him.
   d. is able to care for himself.

2. An appropriate client outcome criterion related to the goal of "client demonstrates correct skin care regimen" would be that the client
   a. uses sterile technique when replacing the soiled bandage on a wound with a saline-soaked dressing at the next dressing change.
   b. reveals increasing granulation of the wound, indicating effective healing, within 48 hours of beginning the skin care regimen.
   c. explains how the wound care should be done.
   d. observes the nurse as the skin care is provided each morning and assists the nurse in the process.

3. The statement "The client administers insulin correctly" provides a broad picture of a client's ability after effective client teaching. This statement is an example of which of the following?
   a. Client outcome criteria
   b. Client goal
   c. Defining characteristic
   d. Nursing diagnosis

4. A clinical plan of care prepared by an experienced nurse for a client which be of the following?
   a. Have more specific detail than the instructional plan of care done by student nurses
   b. Not include scientific rationale for each intervention
   c. Have client goals without outcome criteria
   d. Not be individualized to a specific client

5. When planning a critical path, any deviation from expected outcomes is called
   a. a qualifier.
   b. a variance.
   c. a priority.
   d. an outcome criterion.

FILL IN THE BLANK

Supply the missing term or the information requested.

1. Interventions can be initiated by the nurse, as well as ________________ or other healthcare providers.
2. The critical path is a cause-and-effect ________________ that describes a client's problems with ________________ outcomes.
3. Outcome criteria are ________________, measurable, and ________________.
4. Deviations from an expected outcome are considered ________________.
5. Life-threatening problems ________________ take precedence over routine care.

MULTIPLE-ANSWER MULTIPLE CHOICE

Circle the letter(s) corresponding to the appropriate answer(s). Select all that apply.

1. High priority nursing diagnoses are those that are which of the following?
   a. Likely to result in unhealthy consequences
   b. Potentially life threatening
   c. Require minimal intervention
   d. Are very important to people
   e. Require immediate action

2. Nurses use priorities to carry out which of the following?
   a. Plan care
   b. Classify client outcomes
   c. Determine outcome criteria
   d. Construct nursing interventions
   e. Determine the order of interventions

3. Taxonomy at the most abstract level includes how many domains?
   a. Four
   b. Seven
   c. One
   d. Three
   e. Five
   f. Two

4. The client's plan of care can be written in many ways, including which of the following?
   a. Metal card files
   b. Computerized care plans
   c. Internet blog sites
   d. Notebooks

5. Nursing actions specific to the needs of each client are documented as which of the following?
   a. Interventions
   b. Outcome identification
   c. Evaluation
   d. Assessment
   e. Data collection

CHAPTER 13

Implementation and Evaluation

CHAPTER OVERVIEW

Chapter 13 discusses the purposes of implementation and evaluation. It describes clinical skills needed to implement the client plan of care, methods for revising the client plan of care, and activities the nurse carries out during the evaluation phase of the nursing process. Quality assurance monitors used in nursing settings are presented.

LEARNING OBJECTIVES

After mastering the content in this chapter, you should be able to do the following:

1. Define implementation and evaluation.
2. Discuss the purpose of implementation and evaluation.
3. Describe clinical skills needed to implement the plan of care.
4. Explain methods for revising or modifying the plan of care.
5. Describe activities the nurse carries out during the evaluation phase of the nursing process.
6. Discuss the quality assurance monitors used in nursing settings.
7. Use a functional approach to implement and evaluate client care.

■ Mastering the Information

MATCHING

Match the terms in Column II with a definition, example, or related statement from Column I. Place the letter corresponding to the answer in the space provided. (Use each letter only once; some letters may not be used.)

COLUMN I

1. ______ Refers to the action phase of the nursing process in which nursing care is provided
2. ______ Statements of accountability that define requirements for quality nursing care and provide the basis for quality monitors
3. ______ The evaluation and judgment of a nurse's performance by other nurses
4. ______ Reviews by a nurse of the client's care or records to determine the extent to which the care or records meet established standards
5. ______ Mechanisms that ensure that quality client care is provided and standards are upheld

COLUMN II

a. Standards
b. Nursing monitors
c. Quality improvement programs
d. Implementation
e. Peer review

TRUE–FALSE

Indicate if the following statements are true or false.

______ 1. Technical competence means being able to communicate with clients to determine needs and to teach clients.

______ 2. Nurses manage collaborative problems using physician-prescribed and nursing-prescribed interventions to give nursing care.

______ 3. Supportive nursing interventions emphasize use of communication skills, relief of spiritual distress, and caring behaviors.

______ 4. Humor should never be used with clients experiencing emotional, psychological, or social problems.

______ 5. The goal of surveillance nursing interventions is to help the client retain a certain state of health.

______ 6. The nurse must know about current standards of care provided by nursing organizations, external review boards, and his or her own institution to evaluate nursing care.

______ 7. Evaluation can center on one of three areas: structure, process, or outcome.

FILL IN THE BLANK

Supply the missing term or the information requested.

1. The activities of implementation include the following: ________________, ________________, ________________, and ________________.
2. Intellectual skills used in implementation include ________________, ________________, and ________________.
3. List four of the five factors that determine the order of importance of nursing problems.
   a. ________________
   b. ________________
   c. ________________
   d. ________________
4. The ________________ assists in defining the role of the professional nurse by listing direct-care treatment performed within the nursing role.
5. Nursing interventions fall within three major categories: those using ________________ skills, those using ________________ skills, and those using ________________ skills.
6. ________________ nursing interventions include ensuring that other members of the nursing team carry out specified aspects of the plan of care, and those involved with the client or family return demonstration of skills.
7. Interpersonal interventions involve ________________ of client activities, ________________ nursing interventions, and ________________ interventions.
8. ________________ is defined as the judgment of the effectiveness of nursing care to meet client goals based on the client's behavioral responses.

■ Applying Your Knowledge

CASE STUDY

You are the unit manager for a 25-bed medical service. The director of nursing tells all unit managers to submit a quarterly report of the quality of care being given to the clients. Consider the following:

1. Determine the implementation activities that should be surveyed and reported to assess the quality of client care.
2. Summarize the evaluation activities that should be surveyed and reported in the quarterly report and information needed to determine how participants measured goal attainment.
3. Develop an outline for submitting the report.

CRITICAL INQUIRY EXERCISE

During a clinical experience, choose a client and prepare a nursing management plan.

- Identify two actual and potential nursing diagnoses if possible.
- Write three interventions for each nursing diagnosis.

CRITICAL EXPLORATION EXERCISE

Exchange management plans with a classmate and implement that student's plan. Critique the plan you implement for clarity of the interventions. Evaluate the effectiveness of the management plan toward meeting its goals.

■ Practicing for NCLEX

MULTIPLE CHOICE QUESTIONS

Circle the letter that corresponds to the best answer for each question.

1. Mr. Pill tells the nurse that he has difficulty sleeping at night during each period of hospitalization. Mr. Pill is in the terminal stage of lung cancer. Interventions should relate specifically to
   a. physician's orders.
   b. nursing diagnoses.
   c. teaching.
   d. technical skills.

2. The goal "maintains present weight of 165 pounds" can be evaluated best by which of the following measures?
   a. Monitoring dietary intake for each meal
   b. Restricting high-calorie foods
   c. Weighing the client on the same scale
   d. Determining the client's food preferences

3. Which of the following would indicate that the goal "Mr. T. will demonstrate improved circulation evidenced by strong radial pulses, ambulation without fatigue, and pink mucous membranes within 24 hours after admission" has been met?
   a. Mr. T. reports being tired after ambulating.
   b. Mr. T. has cyanotic mucous membranes within 12 hours of admission.
   c. Mr. T. has pale mucous membranes after ambulating.
   d. Mr. T. has strong bilateral radial pulses 8 hours after admission

The questions below refer to the following case study.

The following information is provided in the nursing plan of care for Mr. Creel, an 80-year-old man admitted from a nursing home after 5 days of not eating: Mr. Creel is lethargic and disoriented. He reports thirst and has cool, pale skin, along with regular respiration at 28/minute. His bowel sounds are active, and his urine output is 10 mL/hour. The urine is dark amber. One nursing diagnosis is fluid volume deficit related to inadequate fluid intake manifested by urinary output of 10 mL/hour. The goal statement to address the urine output is "demonstrate urine output greater than 30 mL/hour." The physician orders p.o. fluids to be increased to 1500 mL in 24 hours.

4. The most appropriate approach to interventions for Mr. Creel is
   a. nurse-prescribed interventions.
   b. nurse- and client-prescribed interventions.
   c. physician-prescribed interventions.
   d. nurse- and physician-prescribed interventions.

5. An appropriate nurse-physician intervention to address Mr. Creel's status would include
   a. offering approximately 500 mL of p.o. fluid each shift and monitoring urine output hourly.
   b. monitoring urine output hourly and reporting decreased output.
   c. limiting oral fluid intake and reporting hourly urine output.
   d. ambulating Mr. Creel hourly and monitoring pulse and respirations.

6. Careful assessment of a client reveals that he has limited knowledge about changing a dressing on his left gluteal area. He says that he is willing to change the dressing and will do exactly what the nurse tells him. Before initiating educational interventions, what else is needed on the part of the client?
   a. Willingness to follow the health regimen
   b. Physical and psychological ability to carry out the procedure
   c. An instruction method identical to that used to teach professional care
   d. Understanding of the pathologic process in wound healing

FILL IN THE BLANK

Supply the missing term or the information requested.

1. The ________________ assists in defining the role of the professional nurse by assisting direct-care treatments performed within the nursing role.
2. One of the purposes for carrying out evaluation is to collect ______________________ data.
3. ______________________ skills are used to carry out treatments and procedures.
4. The action phase of the nursing process in which nursing care is provided is referred to as ______________________________.

5. Measurement devices provide ____________________ information for the evaluation of nursing strategies.
6. Complete the following sequence explaining how the evaluation process could result in a revision to the plan of care.
   a. ___________, ___________, and___________ data for evaluation
   b. Compare data against ________
   c. Data show that the client goal is ________
   d. ________ the nursing diagnosis
   e. Formulate a plan, including __________ nursing diagnosis.
   f. Periodically ______________

MULTIPLE-ANSWER MULTIPLE CHOICE

Circle the letter(s) corresponding to the appropriate answer(s). Circle all that apply.

1. The foundation for the evaluation of the nursing process is considered the
   a. nursing diagnosis.
   b. outcome criteria.
   c. plan of care.
   d. client goal.
   e. nursing intervention.

2. Nurses may use measurement devices in the practice setting that include
   a. thermometers.
   b. blood glucose meters.
   c. intracranial pressure monitors.
   d. arterial lines.
   e. blood pressure cuff.

3. Objective data may be collected from sources that include
   a. laboratory reports.
   b. posture.
   c. health records.
   d. intuition.
   e. skin color.
   f. breath sounds.

4. All of the following are true of the quality improvement process, *except*
   a. also termed quality assurance monitors.
   b. focus on quantity of nursing services.
   c. measure the extent to which standards are achieved.
   d. have standards proposed by the American Nurses Association.
   e. one result of soaring healthcare costs.

5. When nurses use both nurse- and physician-prescribed interventions, the problems are considered
   a. cognitive.
   b. collective.
   c. maintenance.
   d. collaborative.
   e. qualitative.

CHAPTER 14

Critical Thinking

CHAPTER OVERVIEW

Chapter 14 discusses the definition of and elements involved in critical thinking. An overview of the conceptual development of critical thinking and implications for nursing is provided. A model of critical thinking is discussed, as are strategies for building critical thinking skills.

LEARNING OBJECTIVES

After mastering the content in this chapter, you should be able to do the following:

1. Explain the importance of critical thinking in nursing.
2. Discuss definitions of, characteristics of, and skills used in critical thinking.
3. Identify the three major factors that affect thinking.
4. Describe existing personal thinking skills.
5. Explore ways to enhance and develop critical thinking skills, especially as applied to nursing.
6. Set personal goals for developing critical thinking skills.

■ Mastering the Information

MATCHING

Match the terms in Column II with a definition, example, or related statement from Column I. Place the letter corresponding to the answer in the space provided. (Use each letter only once; some letters may not be used.)

COLUMN I

1. ______ Things seen only as good or bad, right or wrong
2. ______ Based on empathy, attempting to experience from another's point of view
3. ______ The process of gathering and clustering data to draw inferences
4. ______ Becoming aware of awareness and critiquing it
5. ______ Recognition that not all approaches are equally valid

COLUMN II

a. Critical reflectivity
b. Dualism
c. Relativism
d. Connected knowing
e. Diagnostic reasoning

TRUE–FALSE

Indicate if the following statements are true or false.

______ 1. Students should ignore their existing thinking skills to learn the new skill of critical thinking.

______ 2. Memorization-style thinking is key for the nursing tasks of sorting, organizing, and identifying relevant information.

______ 3. Critical thinking assumes a turning point because of a thought process.

______ 4. Inquisitiveness should be avoided by nurses while critically thinking.

______ 5. Nursing judgment is used in each step of the nursing process.

FILL IN THE BLANK

Supply the missing term or the information requested.

1. Critical thinking requires__________, ____________effort.
2. Students must build a knowledge base before beginning a ______________ experience.

3. Reasoning is based on data, ____________, and ____________.
4. List three of the eight parts of thinking and reasoning described by Paul (2004).
   a.
   b.
   c.
5. Discuss the activities in and purpose of reflection.

■ Applying Your Knowledge

CASE STUDY

Helga Sven is a 43-year-old senior nursing student. She has been assigned two clients: One client has a broken right arm and fractured fingers on his left hand. The other client has extreme fluctuations in his blood pressure and pulse and must have vital signs taken every 15 to 30 minutes. As Helga begins her morning shift, she notes the breakfast trays arriving. Her classmate says, "Wow, you'll never be able to take good care of both of those clients."

1. ______ Outline some of the first steps Helga should take in determining her best plan of care for each client.
2. ______ Discuss the factors that might affect Helga's thinking in the situation.
3. ______ Describe some strategies Helga might consider to provide effective care for her clients.

CRITICAL INQUIRY EXERCISE

1. Using the steps in Display 14-3, set goals for development of your thinking skills.
2. Consider what might interfere with your plan for development of your thinking skills.

CRITICAL EXPLORATION EXERCISE

Ask an older relative how he/she solved a difficult problem in his/her life. Consider how you might have approached the problem and which similar or different thinking skills you might have used.

■ Practicing for NCLEX

MULTIPLE-CHOICE QUESTIONS

Circle the letter that corresponds to the best answer for each question.

1. Malessa Malasanos, a student nurse, has an elderly client with a diagnosis of heart failure. Her client was treated in the emergency room and currently has no symptoms. Malessa's plan of care for her client should include
   a. all of the nursing measures on the standardized plan for clients with heart failure.
   b. those nursing measures needed to address her client's current and potential needs.
   c. only those nursing measures necessary to fulfill the orders delegated by the physician.
   d. the same nursing measures Malessa used for other elderly clients.

2. Kim Chin, a student nurse, wants to build her critical thinking skills. In an effort to learn how she thinks, she should
   a. ask her teacher to determine her thinking style.
   b. let her peers observe her to evaluate her thinking.
   c. observe a classmate in clinical and compare her behavior to the classmate's.
   d. keep a log of how she uses thinking skills on a regular basis.

3. The beginning shift vital signs of Malessa's client reveal a high blood pressure reading when her client previously had a normal pressure. Which of the following would indicate good thinking skills?
   a. Malessa calls the physician to report her client has experienced a serious complication.
   b. Malessa decides this reading is an error and discards it.
   c. Malessa records the elevated reading and plans to report it to the floor nurse at the end of the shift.
   d. Malessa retakes the blood pressure and considers possible causes if the second blood pressure reading is elevated.

4. A student nurse is reviewing a client's chart for laboratory data that might relate to the fever the client is demonstrating. The student is demonstrating what critical thinking behavior?
   a. Exploring ideas
   b. Identifying missing information
   c. Planning appropriate approaches
   d. Predicting consequences

5. Eugene Banks, a nursing student, is focused on nursing knowledge and skills steps. He is an example of a/an
   a. abstract thinker.
   b. concrete thinker.
   c. random thinker.
   d. sequential thinker.

FILL IN THE BLANK

Supply the missing term or the information requested.

1. ________________ reasoning means using critical thinking in healthcare.
2. Critical thinking occurs within an existing knowledge base and is ______________________ by clinical experience.
3. ____________________ learners are tactile and like to be actively involved.
4. Priority setting is an ___________________ nursing skill.
5. Critical thinking is important in all nurse-client ___________________.

MULTIPLE-ANSWER MULTIPLE CHOICE

Circle the letter(s) corresponding to the appropriate answer(s). Circle all that apply.

1. The nursing process *requires* all of the following *except*
   a. clinical reasoning.
   b. outcome identification.
   c. nursing assessment.
   d. nursing diagnosis.
   e. nursing research.
   f. implementation.
   g. planning.

2. The type of sensory learner who learns best by actively changing dressings and administering medications is considered which of the following:
   a. visual
   b. auditory
   c. kinesthetic
   d. abstract
   e. sequential

3. When students devise new rules and reasoning procedures, they are considered to be at which of the following stages, according to Benner, Tanner, and Chesla's model of skill acquisition?
   a. Novice
   b. Advanced beginner
   c. Proficient
   d. Competent
   e. Expert

4. Factors that may affect thinking can include which of the following?
   a. Attitude
   b. Learning style
   c. Level of preparation
   d. Gender issues
   e. Anxiety

5. Students who are social, preferring to study in groups, work together in skill labs, and share their knowledge and ideas, would most likely be considered
   a. collaborative.
   b. task oriented.
   c. competitive.
   d. people oriented.
   e. active experimenters.

CHAPTER 15

Communication of the Nursing Process: Documenting and Reporting

CHAPTER OVERVIEW

Chapter 15 identifies and discusses the principles involved in preparing and maintaining a concise and complete client record. Methods for effective organization of information into the various formats used to transfer or report it are reviewed.

LEARNING OBJECTIVES

After mastering the content in this chapter, you should be able to do the following:

1. Describe the purposes of the client record.
2. List the principles of charting.
3. Discuss the relevance of electronic media in documentation.
4. Explain how to use a nursing Kardex.
5. Properly record nursing progress notes by SOAP, PIE, FOCUS, or narrative format.
6. Identify flowsheets and critical pathways used in client records.
7. Complete a nursing history admission sheet and a nursing discharge summary.
8. Identify important data for the change-of-shift report.
9. Describe the procedure for telephone reporting.
10. Discuss the importance of confidentiality in documenting and reporting.

■ Mastering the Information

MATCHING

Match the terms in Column II with a definition, example, or related statement from Column I. Place the letter corresponding to the answer in the space provided. (Use each letter only once; some letters may not be used.)

COLUMN I

1. __g__ Record started at initiation of care indicating possible discharge needs and client teaching
2. __K__ Documentation that takes place as care occurs
3. __b__ Distinguishes between routine and prn medications
4. __a__ Series of flip cards in a portable file
5. __e__ Two or more people sharing information about client care
6. __j__ Review of records
7. __f__ Client record
8. __c__ Progress note relating to only one health problem
9. __i__ Written communication
10. __D__ One nurse reporting to oncoming staff about client status and care plan

COLUMN II

a. Kardex
b. Medication record
c. SOAP note
d. Change-of-shift report
e. Reporting
f. Legal document
g. Nursing discharge summary
h. Flowsheet
i. Documentation
j. Audit
k. POC (point-of-care) documentation

TRUE-FALSE

Indicate if the following statements are true or false.

_____ 1. Nursing discharge planning is done the day before discharge.

_____ 2. A charting error is corrected with a line drawn through it.

_____ 3. In SOAP, the S stands for subjective.

_____ 4. In "PIE," the "I" stands for implementation.

_____ 5. Nurses must have an order to initiate a consult.

FILL IN THE BLANK

Supply the missing term or the information requested.

1. Clearly documented information on the client record __________ the plan of care and ensures __________ of care.
2. Auditing is done for quality assurance by __________ selecting records to ascertain whether certain standards of care have been met and __________.
3. Any unusual happening in the healthcare agency is classified as an __________.
4. A charting error is never corrected by __________ it.
5. Discussions regarding electronically maintained records now focus on the "CPR" or "__________ record."

■ Applying Your Knowledge

CASE STUDY

Mr. W. F., an 80-year-old client, was admitted with multiple decubiti. He is now in contact isolation because of infection with methicillin-resistant *Staphylococcus aureus*. Upon making initial rounds, the nurse notices that Mr. W. F. is barely arousable. She immediately measures vital signs and performs an assessment and records the following data:

> 96.2; 52; 18; BP 104/60;
> Skin cool, dry, flushed;
> Radial pulses weak and irregular;
> Breath sounds equal and clear bilaterally;
> Bowel sounds hypoactive

The nurse telephones the physician to report the preceding findings. The physician orders a Foley catheter, Solu-Medrol 40 mg IVP, chest x-rays, CBC with differential, blood culture ¥ 2, urine for culture and sensitivity, ECG, and prothrombin time. The physician states that she will visit the client in about 45 minutes.

1. Document the above scenario using the SOAP format.
2. Construct a report to the physician about Mr. W. F.

CRITICAL INQUIRY EXERCISE

Write a source-oriented record and a problem-oriented record for the same client. Decide which form of charting you prefer and which form of charting you think yields the most information.

CRITICAL EXPLORATION EXERCISE

Identify a client for whom to write a change-of-shift report and trade information with a classmate. Determine whether each of you could adequately care for the client of the other based on the information provided.

■ Practicing for NCLEX

MULTIPLE CHOICE QUESTIONS

Circle the letter that corresponds to the best answer for each question.

1. The record on which nurses make entries in pencil is known as the
   a. discharge summary.
   b. flowsheet.
   c. Kardex.
   d. nursing care plan.

2. Dee Aldwin works to develop the computer system in her hospital. Using a combination of computer science, information science, and nursing science, she creates systems that assist in managing and processing nursing data. Dee's specialty area is referred to as
   a. computer specialist.
   b. nursing informatics.
   c. data processing.
   d. care management expert service.

3. Flowsheets are designed
   a. for planning and communicating purposes only.
   b. for relating only one healthcare problem.
   c. to free the nurse from writing out procedures done repeatedly.
   d. to reflect a nursing management plan that can guide client care.

4. A disadvantage of computerized documentation systems is
   a. legibility.
   b. accuracy.
   c. rapid communication.
   d. concern for confidentiality.

5. Which of the following best describes the components included in the SOAP note?
   a. "A" represents auditing of the note for clarity and completeness.
   b. A quote by the nurse about the client's condition is always placed in the subjective section.
   c. Objective findings include relevant data collected by the nurse.
   d. Quotes by the client concerning condition are placed in category "P."

FILL IN THE BLANK

Supply the missing term or the information requested.

1. A nursing care plan should be started when the client is ________________.

2. When a client refuses or the nurse does not give a drug for any reason, the ____________ must be circled on the medication record.

3. The ability to enhance consistency of data through _______ of language makes retrieval of information easier.

MULTIPLE-ANSWER MULTIPLE CHOICE

Circle the letter(s) corresponding to the appropriate answer(s). Circle all that apply.

1. Agencies require documentation using which of the following?
   a. 24 hour clock
   b. Atomic time clock
   c. Military time
   d. Digital clock
   e. Eastern Standard time

2. Point-of-care documentation occurs at which of the following points?
   a. Within 24 hours of care delivery
   b. As care occurs
   c. Before patient discharge
   d. At the client's bedside
   e. Before patient admission

3. If using the PIE charting system, the nurse knows the "P" is used to represent which of the following?
   a. Plan
   b. Protocol
   c. Problem
   d. Progress

4. Verbal orders should be cosigned by the ordering physician usually within this period of time.
   a. 8 hours
   b. 12 hours
   c. 24 hours
   d. 48 hours
   e. 72 hours

5. Which of the following could be considered a reportable "incident?"
   a. Falls
   b. Routine events
   c. Medication errors
   d. Injuries
   e. Needle sticks
   f. Equipment malfunctions

UNIT IV

Concepts Essential for Human Functioning and Nursing Management

CHAPTER 16

Health and Wellness

CHAPTER OVERVIEW

Chapter 16 discusses holistic healthcare modalities and identifies the connections among mind, body, and spirit in the manifestation of illness. The role of the holistic nurse as a caring colleague in assisting clients to improve their health is the principal focus of this chapter.

LEARNING OBJECTIVES

After mastering the content in this chapter, you should be able to do the following:

1. Define holism, holistic care, and wellness.
2. Compare and contrast the different methods of healthcare.
3. Discuss five models of the concept of health.
4. Identify the aspects of well-being that characterize health according to a holistic model.
5. Explain the concept of the health–illness continuum.
6. Use the nursing process to address potential problems related to health maintenance.

■ Mastering the Information

MATCHING

Match the terms in Column II with a definition, example, or related statement from Column I. Place the letter corresponding to the answer in the space provided. (Use each letter only once; some letters may not be used.)

COLUMN I

1. ______ Knowing and caring for oneself; a recognition of one's own strengths and limitations
2. ______ Deep personal thought and reflection
3. ______ A balance of the physical, psychological, social, and spiritual aspects of a person's life
4. ______ An action that does not meet expected norms
5. ______ The internal experience of a perceptual event in the absence of the actual external stimuli

COLUMN II

a. Wellness
b. Self-awareness
c. Dysfunction
d. Meditation
e. Imagery

COLUMN I

1. ______ Host—agent—environment
2. ______ Clinical model
3. ______ Health belief
4. ______ High-level wellness
5. ______ Holistic

COLUMN II

a. Health conceptualized as the absence of indications of illness
b. Characterized by the relationship between what a person believes and how the person acts
c. A causative model seeking a source or cause of illness
d. Acknowledges the unique interaction of an individual's mind, body, and spirit within the environment
e. Health as an ongoing process moving toward the person's highest potential of functioning

TRUE-FALSE

Indicate if the following statements are true or false.

______ 1. The intent of holistic health is to acknowledge and use the best elements of alternative and modern healthcare.

______ 2. The first dimension of a wellness lifestyle is the responsibility of the client.

______ 3. The concept of self as an active health agent spans all states of wellness or illness but is not useful for people at various developmental levels.

______ 4. In the clinical model, health is conceptualized in terms of seeking a specific source or cause of illness.

______ 5. Specific holistic healthcare interventions include such activities as prayer, meditation, and imagery, in addition to proven medical care.

______ 6. A healthcare provider cannot help or change others unless they want to be helped or changed.

______ 7. Health as defined by the World Health Organization is "a state of complete physical, mental, and social well-being, not merely the absence of disease or infirmity."

______ 8. Nursing diagnoses relating to health and wellness are formulated only by healthcare professionals with advanced degrees.

FILL IN THE BLANK

Supply the missing term or the information requested.

1. Each person defines health in relation to personal ________________ and ________________.

2. Four of the five models of the concept of health are ________________, ________________, ________________, and ________________.

NURSING ACTIONS

Below are actions by the nurse that represent the nurse functioning as a helper or rescuer. Place an "H" by those actions that are helper actions and an "R" by those actions that are rescuer actions.

1. ______ A client who has had a stroke that resulted in left arm paralysis is attempting to perform self-care. The nurse offers to assist the client with self-care.

2. ______ A new postoperative client states that she is not in pain, but she exhibits facial grimacing. The nurse administers pain medication to the client and tells the client that it is better to be medicated, instead of waiting for the pain to become severe.

3. ______ A client with diabetes is admitted to the hospital for the third time in a 6-week period with a diagnosis of uncontrolled diabetes. During a conversation with the client, the nurse asks the client to name some rewards of having diabetes and some consequences of having diabetes.

4. ______ A pediatric client tells the nurse that she likes taking her medicine from the syringe better than from the cup. When giving the change-of-shift report, the nurse informs the oncoming staff of the child's preference.

■ Applying Your Knowledge

CASE STUDY

Mr. Johnson, age 47 years, has received a diagnosis of hypertension. He has a wife and three children. The family is very active in the community and church. The physician-treatment regimen includes blood pressure medication taken twice daily, diet, and an exercise program. Mr. Johnson verbalizes to the nurse, "I have a very difficult time adhering to this plan. Are there any other options? They say once you begin blood pressure medication, it continues throughout life."

1. Using the holistic approach, identify how Mr. Johnson can gain a greater feeling of independence and control over his life.
2. The goal of holistic nursing is to use preventive, nurturing, and generative activities to assist the client toward achieving high-level wellness. Apply this goal to Mr. Johnson.
3. The nurse is an advocate of holistic healthcare modalities. Give examples of holistic healthcare modalities and how these modalities will benefit Mr. Johnson.

CRITICAL INQUIRY EXERCISE

Write a personal definition of health.

CRITICAL EXPLORATION EXERCISE

Watch television for 30 minutes. Identify concepts discussed during the program and commercials that relate to health and wellness.

■ Practicing for NCLEX

MULTIPLE-CHOICE QUESTIONS

Circle the letter that corresponds to the best answer for each question.

1. The nurse administers client history questionnaires, which gather information about nutrition, exercise, stress-reduction practices, spirituality, and home environment, to Mr. Jones. Through the use of these questionnaires, the nurse's primary aim is to
   a. gather information for Mr. Jones's medical records and insurance companies.
   b. increase Mr. Jones's awareness of lifestyle choices and their role in relation to his desire for wellness.
   c. assist the physician in establishing a medical diagnosis for Mr. Jones and in preventing illness.
   d. reduce the frequency of Mr. Jones's visit to the physician's office.

2. An intervention such as placing a rail on the bathtub to assist an elderly client with right side weakness is an example of
   a. therapeutic intervention for a dysfunction problem.
   b. rescuing intervention for a dysfunction problem.
   c. alternative therapy for a dysfunction problem.
   d. complementary therapy for a dysfunction problem.

3. The nurse allows Fran Wills' minister to visit her in the intensive care unit, although visiting hours are over for the evening. The nurse's action shows recognition of the importance of what in the healing process?
   a. Emotions
   b. Mental health
   c. Regulations
   d. Spirituality

4. Leon Pitts, an 18-year-old college football player who was injured on the football field, is instructed to apply and adjust his knee brace. Leon's involvement in his care regimen is designed to
   a. increase his sense of control and independence.
   b. reduce the workload of the healthcare personnel.
   c. remove the need for surgical intervention.
   d. direct his thoughts away from the disability.

5. Nora, a junior nursing student, sustained a compound fracture of her left tibia in an automobile accident. The nurse suggested Nora use Simonton's exercise to examine her period of hospitalization, which would help her to focus on
   a. the needs being met through illness.
   b. therapeutic effects of the medical plan.
   c. negative elements of acute debilitation.
   d. benefits of an education in nursing.

6. Fred Milton has diabetes. Because diabetes is a condition that can be controlled with the use of medication and diet, Mr. Milton is
   a. to be considered a disabled person who will require constant nursing intervention.
   b. not able to achieve a high level of wellness or function normally in a mobile society.
   c. in a chronically dysfunctional state and will require a great deal of healthcare.
   d. not necessarily a disabled person but should be able to adapt strengths toward being an able-bodied person.

FILL IN THE BLANK

Supply the missing term or the information requested.

1. A healthcare provider functioning as a _________________ neglects to determine if help being offered is wanted or needed.
2. _________________ sees people as ever-changing systems of energy.
3. _________________ is likely to be the initial step toward self-caring.
4. The first dimension of a wellness lifestyle is self-_________________.
5. Participating in self-care gives a greater feeling of independence and _________________.
6. _________________ is a state of disharmony among mind, body, emotions, and spirit.
7. Peer influence, personality characteristics, ethnicity, and socioeconomic factors may all affect a person's _________________ to illness.
8. _________________ is our body's way of signaling that we have exceeded our natural ability to mediate between our internal and external environments.

MULTIPLE-ANSWER MULTIPLE CHOICE

Circle the letter(s) corresponding to the appropriate answer(s). Circle all that apply.

1. The Rogerian or Therapeutic Model of Interaction lists three behaviors necessary for a positive, therapeutic relationship with clients. Which three of the following behaviors are included?
   a. Positive regard
   b. Holism
   c. Congruence
   d. Empathy
   e. Self-awareness
   f. Homeostasis
   g. Wellness
   h. Health promotion

2. A healthcare professional who focuses only on disease states or organ systems while caring for patients would be engaging in which of the following approaches?
   a. Rogerian
   b. Atomistic
   c. Holistic
   d. Dysfunctional
   e. Therapeutic

3. Because change occurs in stages and people can relapse at any point, what is the documented number of attempts that most people make before successfully maintaining a nonsmoking condition?
   a. Two
   b. Three
   c. Five
   d. Nine
   e. Ten

4. Using the health belief model, which of the following are important considerations?
   a. Age
   b. High-level wellness
   c. Disease state
   d. Empathy
   e. Developmental stage
   f. Congruence
   g. Positive regard

5. Therapeutic interventions for dysfunctional problems are directed at which one of the following choices?
   a. Altered function
   b. Preventing illness
   c. Contributing factors
   d. Socioeconomic factors
   e. High-level wellness
   f. Environmental conditions

CHAPTER 17

Complementary and Alternative Medicine

CHAPTER OVERVIEW

Chapter 17 discusses the role of holistic healthcare in nursing and explains the differences between allopathic and complementary and alternative medicines. Examples of commonly used holistic interventions are presented.

LEARNING OBJECTIVES

After mastering the content in this chapter, you should be able to do the following:

1. Explain the role of holistic healthcare in nursing.
2. Give examples of commonly used holistic interventions.
3. Explain the differences in allopathic, alternative, and complementary medicines.

▪ Mastering the Information

MATCHING

Match the terms in Column II with a definition, example, or related statement from Column I. Place the letter corresponding to the answer in the space provided. (Use each letter only once; some letters may not be used.)

COLUMN I

1. _____ Holistic healthcare
2. _____ Integrative healthcare
3. _____ Iatrogenic
4. _____ Psychomotor
5. _____ Allopathic medicine
6. _____ Integrative medicine

COLUMN II

a. Illness that results from treatment and may be traced to overuse and adverse responses to medications
b. Traditional Western medicine
c. Emphasizes humanism, choices, self-care activities
d. Healing-oriented medicine that occurs for the whole person
e. Considered a mental health problem
f. An evolving model that more accurately reflects the practice of medicine

TRUE-FALSE

Indicate if the following statements are true or false.

_____ 1. Therapeutic Touch is considered to be the cornerstone of lifestyle modification programs.

_____ 2. According to traditional Chinese medicine (TCM), Yang, which represents active, dynamic energy, is considered male and is superior to Yin, which is considered to be more foundational and female.

_____ 3. A 1998 study by Dalen supports the idea that most clients talk to their physicians about their interactions with nontraditional providers.

_____ 4. Studies show that more women than men tend to use complementary and alternative medicine therapies.

_____ 5. The first and most significant part of the Therapeutic Touch process is termed assessment.

______ 6. Holistic healthcare challenged Western medicine because clients wanted to be treated as whole persons, not as just a disease.

______ 7. Acupuncture, although popular, generally is ineffective and potentially unsafe.

______ 8. Nursing started to recognize the validity of holistic care in the early 1990s.

______ 9. One of the major goals of the Lewis and Clark expedition was to record herbs and their medicinal uses.

______ 10. After relaxation, pain relief is the second most reliable result of Therapeutic Touch.

FILL IN THE BLANK

Supply the missing term or the information requested.

1. Therapeutic Touch can be used in the following ways:
   a.
   b.
   c.
   d.
   e.
2. ______________ and acupuncturists may use ______________ therapies under their individual license.
3. Many consumers take herbs with some degree of risk because the ______________________ does not regulate them.
4. The Newtonian model in which the parts seem more important than the whole person is an approach considered to be ______________.
5. Meditation generally falls into four categories:
   a. ______________
   b. ______________
   c. ______________
   d. ______________

■ Applying Your Knowledge

CASE STUDY

You are the nurse interviewing a client on admission to 3 West, a busy medical unit. Your client, Ms. M., is a 45-year-old woman who has recently received a diagnosis of osteoarthritis. During your interview regarding current medications, you ask about the use of vitamins, minerals, and herbal supplements. She states that she does "take some Chinese herbs I get from my acupuncturist."

1. Do you document this information and, if so, how?
2. How does your knowledge or lack of knowledge regarding complementary and alternative medicine affect your response to Ms. M.?
3. Based on your knowledge of alternative and complementary medicine, what other modalities may Ms. M. be aware of or benefit from?

CRITICAL INQUIRY EXERCISE

Arrange an interview with an alternative or complementary medicine practitioner. Inquire as to the practitioner's area of expertise, training, client demographics, and reimbursement issues. Develop a list of complementary and alternative medicine practitioners in your area.

CRITICAL EXPLORATION EXERCISE

Research information regarding an herbal supplement of your choice using these online sources:

- American Botanical Council, www.herbalgram.org
- Herb Research Foundation, www.herbs.org
- Consumerlabs, www.consumerlabs.com

Compare information from each online source regarding "structure and function claims."

a. Are these claims consistent throughout each source?
b. What standardization issues are addressed regarding your herbal supplement. Do they vary according to your web source?

■ Practicing for NCLEX

MULTIPLE CHOICE QUESTIONS

Circle the letter that corresponds to the best answer for each question.

1. The meditation familiar to most people that focuses on a specific object using prayer, chants, or repetitive words is best described as which of the following?
   a. Receptive
   b. Expressive
   c. Concentrative
   d. Reflective
   e. Therapeutic

2. According to a 1993 *New England Journal of Medicine* article, visits to nontraditional providers exceeded visits to primary care physicians by which of the following percentages?
   a. 30%
   b. 45%
   c. 78%
   d. 94%
   e. 100%

3. Channels that allow energy or Qi to flow throughout the body are also expressed as which of the following?
   a. Mediums
   b. Meridians
   c. Meditations
   d. Modalities
   e. Mendacities

4. Currently, registered nurses can officially include some form of alternative/complementary medicine in their practice in this percentage of the United States.
   a. 10%
   b. 30%
   c. 40%
   d. 50%
   e. 80%
   f. 100%

5. The only peer-reviewed organization for professional herbalists specializing in herbal medicine in the United States is which one of the following?
   a. Food and Drug Administration
   b. U. S. Pharmacopoeia
   c. American Herbalist Guild
   d. American Botanical Council
   e. Herb Research Foundation

FILL IN THE BLANK

Supply the missing term or the information requested.

1. The term that truly captures the evolving model of healthcare is best described as ________________________.

2. Traditional Chinese medicine evolved more than 4000 years ago from ________________ philosophy.

3. Herbal products may make "structure and function" claims but cannot make ______________ and ______________ claims.

4. Therapeutic Touch involves making contact with the ____________ ____________ of the recipient.

5. Advances such as __________ and ______________ treatments present ethical and __________ dilemmas for nurses.

MULTIPLE-ANSWER MULTIPLE CHOICE

Circle the letter(s) corresponding to the appropriate answer(s). Circle all that apply.

1. Studies have shown that people most likely to use complementary and alternative medicine are which of the following?
   a. Men in the midwestern United States
   b. Women in the southern United States
   c. Women in France
   d. Men in China
   e. Men and Women in Japan
   f. Women in Alaska and Hawaii

2. Holistic interventions focus on the interrelated needs of
   a. mind and body.
   b. body and spirit.
   c. body image.
   d. mental health.
   e. mind, body, and spirit.

3. Traditional Chinese medicine is a complete healing system which includes which of the following?
   a. Massage
   b. Moxibustion
   c. Yin and Yang
   d. Acupuncture
   e. Allopathy
   f. Meditation
   g. Herbal treatments
   h. Qi gong
   i. Homeopathy

4. When discussing current dietary habits and preferences, the nurse should ask the client if he/she has been following which of the following nutritional plans?
   a. Atkins diet
   b. Vegetarian diet
   c. Macrobiotic diet
   d. South Beach diet
   e. 2000-calorie diet
   f. Low-cholesterol diet

5. Practitioners of acupuncture or traditional Chinese medicine are expected to meet which of the following criteria?
   a. Graduate from an accredited program
   b. Pass a state-certified examination
   c. Meet guidelines outlined by the state
   d. Complete a preceptorship and be "grandfathered" into licensing
   e. Pass a national certification examination

CHAPTER 18

Lifespan Development

CHAPTER OVERVIEW

Chapter 18 discusses the physical, cognitive, and psychosocial development of people across the lifespan. Developmental theories are reviewed. Functional health and the concept of anticipatory guidance related to the lifespan are discussed.

LEARNING OBJECTIVES

After mastering the content in this chapter, you should be able to do the following:

1. Relate genetics and environment to human development.
2. Explain the principles of development.
3. Identify the theorists and their theories of development.
4. Describe physical, psychosocial, and cognitive developmental patterns for different age groups.
5. Identify the major health needs of specific developmental age groups.

■ Mastering the Information

MATCHING

Match the terms in Column II with a definition, example, or related statement from Column I. Place the letter corresponding to the answer in the space provided. (Use each letter only once; some letters may not be used.)

COLUMN I

1. _____ His theory encompassed social and cultural influences-eight stages from birth to death presented as development crises.
2. _____ His theory is based on learning and learned behaviors called developmental tasks.
3. _____ He extended Piaget's work on moral reasoning to develop a theory of moral development.
4. _____ His theory characterizes psychosexual development across the lifespan; the theory includes the oral through genital phases and the id, ego, and superego.
5. _____ He was a humanistic theorist who organized human needs into a hierarchic framework.
6. _____ His theory discusses cognitive development based on the assumption that human nature is essentially rational.

COLUMN II

a. Piaget
b. Erikson
c. Freud
d. Havighurst
e. Kohlberg
f. Maslow

COLUMN I

1. _____ This is the neurosensory process that allows the environment to be experienced by each person.
2. _____ Physical–must learn new ways of taking in food and oxygen; cognitive–the person is at the sensorimotor stage; psychosocial–attachment or bonding develops at this time.
3. _____ Physical–baby fat decreases and lordosis has disappeared; cognitive–vocabulary increases with use of grammar and syntax, and concrete thinking is evident; psychosocial–industriousness and determination to master tasks are evident, and same-sex friendships are important.
4. _____ Physical–weight and height increase at rates faster than any other period; cognitive–systematic imitative behavior appears; psychosocial–fear of strangers or of separation from parents emerges.

5. ______ Physical–neuromuscular skills are refined, dresses self; cognitive–preoperational, asks meaning of words, magical thinking occurs; psychosocial–strives for individuality and explores own abilities. Associative play is noted.
6. ______ Physical–puberty is experienced with rapid growth; cognitive–formal thinking begins to emerge; psychosocial–identity search and self–discovery are noted.
7. ______ Physical–maturational development is complete with sexual function at a peak; cognitive–strong need to achieve intellectually and less egocentricity are noted; psychosocial–work, intimacy, and parenting emerge. Many hats are juggled while setting priorities to achieve success.
8. ______ Physical–growth begins to slow, and hair starts to gray; cognitive–reduction in speed of problem–solving or motor skills may interfere with some aspects of functioning; psychosocial–changes in roles occur, and a greater commitment to enjoying relationships may exist.
9. ______ Physical–all physiologic systems decline in overall function and efficiency; cognitive–learning a new task takes longer, and performance time is longer; psychosocial–the transition from working to retirement must be made.
10. ______ Physical–pot-bellied look is evident; cognitive-requests are received negatively; psychosocial-role expands to include peers or playmates and learns basic social skills.

COLUMN II

a. Adolescent
b. Infant
c. Toddler
d. Middle-aged adult
e. Neonate
f. Older adult
g. Perception
h. Preschooler
i. School-aged child
j. Young adult

■ Fill in the Blank

Supply the missing term or the information requested.

1. ________________ and ________________ are primary factors that drive development.
2. Growth and development are initiated at the ________________ of ________________.
3. The fetus responds to internal and external sounds during the ________________ trimester.
4. Long-term prenatal ______________ and periods of diminished ______________ can adversely affect later developmental functioning.
5. Toddlers and preschoolers have ________________ sleep patterns.
6. Identify the following descriptions related to self-concept or roles and relationships with the appropriate stage of development: newborn/infant, toddler/preschooler, adolescent, or young adult.
   a. _________ stage: Relationships with peers are egocentric.
   b. _________ stage: The many roles assumed include career, intimacy, marriage, and parenthood.
   c. ________ stage: The primary relationship is with the parents, and attachment is the foundation of its development.
   d. ________ stage: Sexual development and peer group are the two key influences. Role and relationship problems are exhibited by leaving home, difficulty relating with peers, and managing sexuality.

■ Applying Your Knowledge

CASE STUDY

Mrs. Fallopie is 36 years old, married, and has three children, ages 2, 7, and 13 years. Mr. and Mrs. Fallopie are both employed full time. Mrs. Fallopie is seen in the family health clinic by the nurse. She reports being tired and feeling emotionally drained. She also states, "My children and husband are so demanding, and I feel overwhelmed." A physical examination is completed on her first visit, and no health problem is found. The nurse sets up a second visit to follow up with a counseling session.

1. Discuss the developmental stage of each member of the Fallopie family in relationship to Erikson's and Freud's theories.
2. Identify major health needs specific for each member of the Fallopie family.
3. Determine the approach the nurse should use during the counseling session with Mrs. Fallopie. Focus on how lifespan development contributes to her feelings.

CRITICAL INQUIRY EXERCISE

1. Discuss how concepts of development can be used to understand the behavior of people of similar age.
2. Compare and contrast the values of an infant, toddler, school-age child, adolescent, and adult.

CRITICAL EXPLORATION EXERCISES

1. Assess your own physical, cognitive, and psychosocial developmental stage. Compare your findings with those traditionally characterized for an individual in your developmental age group.
2. Assess the factors contributing to problems with coping and stress tolerance for hospitalized clients in three different developmental age groups.

■ Practicing for NCLEX

MULTIPLE CHOICE QUESTIONS

Circle the letter that corresponds to the best answer for each question.

1. Which of the following is particularly prone to infections because of an immature immune system?
   a. An 18-year-old woman
   b. An 8-year-old girl
   c. A 5-year-old boy
   d. A 5-month-old boy

2. The nurse could prepare a teaching plan for a school-age child that addresses which of the following age-appropriate considerations?
   a. Decreased motor skills typical for this age of child
   b. Traffic accidents possible from independent excursions
   c. Risks for choking because of hand-to-mouth behaviors
   d. Tendency toward falls because of increasing mobility

3. A teaching plan for an adolescent should consider which of the following?
   a. Adolescents have unlimited ability to appreciate the cause-and-effect relationship between health behaviors and outcomes.
   b. Family relationships are of minimal importance at the adolescent stage of development.
   c. Suicide rarely occurs during adolescence because of the tendency toward egocentricity.
   d. The intense privacy needs of the adolescent may impede adequate healthcare.

4. Which of the following is true about health problems in the adult?
   a. Older adults are faced with specialized safety concerns determined by occupation.
   b. Older adults often must cope with chronic illnesses related to lifestyle patterns.
   c. Young adults are prone to falls because of changes in sensory and motor abilities.
   d. Young adults often find that the ability to manage health independently may be impaired by changes associated with aging.

5. Which of the following nursing measures would be most appropriate?
   a. Limiting fluid intake in infancy to account for the decreased metabolic rate and immature renal function
   b. Increasing the size of food portions during toddlerhood and the preschool years because of increased appetite
   c. Instructing teens that bulimia is the most effective weight-control measure available
   d. Teaching young adults to avoid health problems through exercise and optimal nutritional intake

6. Common health problems related to elimination may require which of the following nursing measures?
   a. Assisting older adults in managing incontinence or nocturia
   b. Instructing parents of an infant regarding methods to prevent bed-wetting
   c. Monitoring adolescents for complaints about the common problem of enuresis
   d. Teaching parents of preschoolers about ways to treat diaper rash

7. Activity and exercise across the lifespan may involve which of the following nursing interventions?
   a. Health teaching for adolescents regarding risks for heart and lung injury because of the flexibility of the rib cage
   b. Limiting a school-age child's movements in a hospital room to prevent accidents from exploring behaviors
   c. Monitoring newborns for decreased activity tolerance because of respiratory tract infection
   d. Encouraging a low-fiber, high-fat diet and decreased exercise for the adult and older adult

8. Infants may express pain in which of the following ways?
   a. Verbalizing the presence of pain
   b. Sleeping more often and longer than usual
   c. Pulling or rubbing the area of discomfort
   d. Continuing usual play activities

9. Which of the following is true about sexuality and reproduction in clients across the lifespan?
   a. Adolescents often have exhibitionistic-type behaviors.
   b. Body structure and function, sexual expression, and intimacy are primary aspects of human function in the toddler.
   c. STDs and AIDS are significant potential problems for the preschooler.
   d. The school-age child has increasing curiosity about sexual function, although same-sex friendships prevail.

10. Problems with coping and stress tolerance in the school-age child will most likely result from which of the following?
   a. Difficulty dealing with increasing autonomy
   b. Fears and characteristic fantasy, which cause related stress
   c. Performance expectations and academic pressures
   d. Severe separation anxiety from parental absence

FILL IN THE BLANK

Complete the following fill-in-the-blank exercises.

1. The process of ongoing change, reorganization, and integration occurring throughout life is called ________________.

2. Development includes periods of both relative stability and ________________.

■ Multiple-Answer Multiple Choice

Circle the letter(s) corresponding to the appropriate answer(s).

1. According the Freud's theory of psychosexual development a(n)
   a. infant seeks pleasure through oral gratification.
   b. toddler delays gratification by learning to control the anal sphincter.
   c. preschooler displays curiosity about genitals and gender differences.
   d. school-age child derives pleasure from accomplishments.

2. Which of the following are examples of the conventional level of Kohlberg's moral development theory?
   a. A child agrees to wash the dishes in order to go out with friends.
   b. A child comes home immediately after school to avoid being grounded.
   c. A child does not talk back to keep from getting a spanking.
   d. A child makes good grades to get a monetary reward.
   e. A child obeys a parent to avoid time out.

3. According to Havighurst, which of the following developmental task(s) is/are unique to the middle-age years?
   a. Achieving adult civic and social responsibility
   b. Achieving assurance of economic independence
   c. Adjusting to aging parents
   d. Assisting teenage children to become responsible and happy adults

ORDERING

Items A through H are identified as key development mental conflicts in Erikson's theory of psychosocial development. Read the list carefully. Place each conflict in the correct sequence by numbering the items.

a. ________ Autonomy vs. shame and doubt

b. ________ Ego integrity vs. despair

c. ________ Generativity vs. stagnation

d. ________ Identity vs. role confusion

e. ________ Industry vs. inferiority

f. ________ Initiative vs. guilt

g. ________ Intimacy vs. isolation

h. ________ Trust vs. mistrust

CHAPTER 19

The Older Adult

CHAPTER OVERVIEW

Chapter 19 examines health conditions that often occur together in older adults. A description of demographics for older adults is included, as is health promotion and health maintenance strategies that can assist the older adult to maintain quality of life.

LEARNING OBJECTIVES

After mastering the content in this chapter, you should be able to do the following:

1. Describe the demographics of older adults.
2. Discuss a comprehensive knowledge base that can help nurses display their commitment to providing humane and dignified care.
3. Explain physiologic changes and chronic illnesses that place older adults at greater risk for a decline in health and quality of life.
4. Identify health promotion and health maintenance strategies that can offer older adults advantages in maintaining optimal health.

■ Mastering the Information

MATCHING

Match the terms in Column II with a definition, example, or related statement from Column I. Place the letter corresponding to the answer in the space provided.

COLUMN I

1. ______ A psychotic illness, characterized by delusions and impairment in self-care, work, and relationships
2. ______ Characterized by excessive worry; occurs more days than not for at least 6 months; cannot be due to a medication or medical condition
3. ______ Characterized by mood swings that progress from symptoms of depression to symptoms of mania
4. ______ Relatively uncommon disorder; characterized by well-organized delusions, absence of hallucinations, less impairment in the person's functioning

COLUMN II

a. Bipolar disorder
b. Delusional disorder
c. Generalized anxiety
d. Major depression
e. Schizophrenia

TRUE–FALSE

Indicate if the following statements are true or false.

______ 1. The increase in life expectancy among both men and women is primarily due to a decrease in deaths related to heart disease and strokes.

______ 2. As of 1999, minorities make up the largest segment of people age 65 and older.

______ 3. Living arrangements are very similar among men and women of the older adult population.

______ 4. Older adults living alone are poorer than older adults living with family or nonrelatives.

______ 5. Antipsychotic medications should be used to treat depression and dementia only when behavioral and environmental strategies are ineffective.

______ 6. Older adults are often erroneously given diagnoses of depression.

______ 7. Nurses' efforts to assist older adults to meet self-care needs are hampered by limited community agencies available to provide necessary assistance.

______ 8. Normal sleep changes among older adults lead to less-frequent nighttime awakenings and more restful sleep.

______ 9. Despite many adverse consequences associated with aging, most older adults retain good function and quality of life.

FILL IN THE BLANK

Supply the missing term or the information requested.

1. Older adults experience impaired communication as a result of ____________, _____________, and ______________ deficits.

■ Applying Your Knowledge

CASE STUDY

Mr. Greer, who is 75 years old, has recently lost his wife of 50 years. He has moved in with his 45-year-old daughter, her husband, and their children. You have been assigned to provide home care for this client who has poorly controlled hypertension. During a recent visit, Mr. Greer's daughter seemed to be very upset. She shared with you that she was upset because her father went out on a date with a member of his church. She states that she doesn't think her father should be dating so soon after her mother's death and especially not at his age.

1. Develop a teaching plan to assist Mr. Greer's daughter to understand her father's need for companionship, as well as other psychosocial needs her father may have.
2. Reflecting on knowledge gained in this chapter, discuss other needs that Mr. Greer may have.
3. What are some issues that may arise in this family unit as a result of Mr. Greer moving in with the family?
4. Develop a list of strategies that may assist the family to adapt to the change in their family structure.
5. Identify community resources that may be beneficial to this family.

CRITICAL INQUIRY EXERCISE

Visit a long-term care facility for older adults. After obtaining permission, interview several older adult clients to determine whether they perceive their needs as being met. Identify the area of need that seems to be of greatest concern for the clients interviewed.

CRITICAL EXPLORATION

Visit an assistive living facility. Interview staff members at the facility. Ask staff members what they perceive to be the most important needs of the elderly. Also, obtain information about strategies used to meet the needs of their clients.

■ Practicing for NCLEX

MULTIPLE CHOICE QUESTIONS

Circle the letter that corresponds to the best answer for each question.

1. Which one of the following groups best represents the fastest growing segment of older adults?
   a. 65 to 74 years old
   b. 75 to 84 years old
   c. 85 years old and older
   d. 100 years old and older
2. Reality orientation is an appropriate intervention for which one of the following conditions?
   a. Alzheimer's
   b. Delirium
   c. Dementia
   d. Parkinson's
3. Which one of the following is a manifestation of depression in the older adult?
   a. Alcohol/substance abuse
   b. Chronic pain
   c. Poor cognitive performance
   d. Recent bereavement

4. The main provider(s) of care for older adults is/are
   a. families.
   b. home helpers.
   c. institutional staff.
   d. nurses.

5. Which of the following interventions can be used to assist older adults who are experiencing mobility impairments?
   a. Encouraging ambulation without assistive devices
   b. Limiting active range of motion
   c. Limiting passive range of motion
   d. Review of medications, especially hypotensive medications

6. The most common cause of chronic pain in the older adult is
   a. neuralgia.
   b. osteoarthritis.
   c. phantom limb.
   d. rheumatoid arthritis.

7. It would be appropriate for the nurse to recommend which one of the following activities to an older adult who is experiencing loneliness?
   a. Enroll in an aerobics exercise class.
   b. Have a glass of wine at bedtime
   c. Serve as a mentor to young kids or young adults.
   d. Limit interaction with others who are lonely.

8. Which one of the following statements is most accurate regarding sexuality and the older adult?
   a. Sexual activity and desire diminish as an individual gets older.
   b. Older men and women have similar perceptions of a satisfying sexual relationship.
   c. Nurses are more receptive to expressions of sexuality by older adults.
   d. Certain medical conditions make expression of sexuality difficult for the older adult.

FILL IN THE BLANK

Supply the missing term or the information requested.

1. As people age, the complex ________________ of their health conditions affects function and quality of life.
2. The proportion of older adults living in a family setting ______________ with age.
3. Poverty rates are ________________ among older women than among older men.
4. ______________ are the leading cause of accidental deaths in older adults.

MULTIPLE-ANSWER MULTIPLE CHOICE

Circle the letter(s) corresponding to the appropriate answer(s). Circle all that apply.

1. Which variable(s) is/are associated with a decrease in food intake among older adults?
   a. Decreased physical activity
   b. Increase in thirst
   c. Keen sense of smell
   d. Late onset of satiation
   e. Poor dentition

ORDERING

Below are variables that appear in the Braden scale for predicting pressure ulcer sore risk. Place an "H" by the variables that are associated with a high risk for ulcer development and an "L" by the variables that are associated with a low-risk for ulcer development.

1. ______ Unresponsive to painful stimuli
2. ______ Skin usually dry
3. ______ Frequently changes position without assistance
4. ______ Maintained on IV fluids for more than 5 days
5. ______ Frequently slides down in bed

CHAPTER 20

Individual, Family, and Community

CHAPTER OVERVIEW

Chapter 20 provides an overview of interactions between individuals and families and between families and communities. Conceptual frameworks for the study of families and communities are presented.

LEARNING OBJECTIVES

After mastering the content in this chapter, you should be able to do the following:

1. State interactions among individuals, family, and community.
2. Explain two different conceptual frameworks used to study the family.
3. Describe three methods nurses can use to assess a family.
4. Discuss family responsibilities for healthy function of all members.
5. Describe components that could be included in a definition of community.
6. Define family and community.
7. Compare various types of community.
8. Discuss the implications of different types of communities for nursing care.
9. Discuss community responsibilities for healthy function and the nurse's participation in community.

■ Mastering the Information

MATCHING

Match the terms in Column II with the definition, example, or related statement in Column I. Place the letter corresponding to the answer in the space provided. (Some letters may be used more than once; some letters may not be used.)

COLUMN I

1. ______ Children becoming adults, aging, and dying
2. ______ Having children, raising children
3. ______ Coping with the loss of a significant other, adjusting to altered living space
4. ______ Assisting children to move, readjusting the family unit
5. ______ An unattached adult

COLUMN II

a. Pre-expansion stage
b. Expansion stage
c. Dispersion stage
d. Replacement stage

TRUE–FALSE

Indicate if the following statements are true or false.

______ 1. Maslow's hierarchy of basic needs is useful to aid the nurse in prioritizing the needs of clients.

______ 2. Higgs and Gustafson believe that communities have one central need.

______ 3. Different types of communities offer different types of resources to their residents.

______ 4. Systems theory suggests that the community has responsibilities toward the family, but the family has only to depend on the community for help in meeting priority needs.

______ 5. The concept of "at-risk" target community groups refers to those most likely to encounter health-related problems.

_____ 6. No identified client is found in systems thinking. Individuals are seen as part of the family system.

_____ 7. Tasks not completed at one developmental stage produce chronic difficulties as the family struggles to master tasks at the next stage.

_____ 8. In a closed system, exchange occurs readily because of mutual trust, whereas in an open system, no exchange occurs.

_____ 9. Comprehensive nursing care must incorporate the interactions of clients with family members and with people at other institutions, such as places of employment, religious institutions, schools, or other social groups.

_____ 10. Healthcare workers participate in community feedback by volunteering for community activities, acting as resource people, and assessing community needs and services.

FILL IN THE BLANK

Supply the missing term or the information requested.

1. Write a brief definition of family.

   ____

2. Write a brief description of community.

   ____

3. Nursing care for the individual is best provided in the context of the client's ____________ and ____________.
4. ____________ frameworks provide useful guidelines for organizing family information.
5. Developmental frameworks focus on developmental ____________ and ____________ expectations of parents and children throughout the life cycle.
6. ____________ frameworks look at the interactions of the parts, such as individual family members that make up the whole.
7. A basic family assessment requires ____________, ____________, and ____________.
8. A community assessment focuses healthcare planning on two points: ____________ and ____________.
9. Four possible areas to be assessed in a family are ____________, ____________, ____________, and ____________.
10. Archer identified three general types of communities. These are ____________, ____________, and ____________.
11. Concepts important for the nurse to understand when viewing a family as a system are ____________, ____________, ____________, ____________, ____________, and ____________.
12. Warren identified six types of communities to provide a useful approach to examining communities. They are ____________, ____________, ____________, ____________, ____________, and ____________.

■ Applying Your Knowledge

CASE STUDY

Mrs. C. P. is a 65-year-old Hispanic woman who lives in the United States with her son, his wife, and their two children. Mrs. C. P. enjoys traveling to visit relatives and friends and caring for her grandchildren. She participates in the routine chores at her son's home, but arthritis causes severe pain and discomfort and limits activities. A hip replacement was done about 1 year ago to assist her with mobility. Her arthritis condition continues to worsen and limit her mobility. Recently she was hospitalized for back and knee pain. The nurse obtained the following information from Mrs. C. P. :

"My son's home does not have large doorways."
"My son and his wife work full time."
"I usually care for my grandchildren."

1. Discuss the four basic areas the nurse may assess for Mrs. C. P. and her family: developmental stage, wholeness, communication, and support.
2. Describe additional data that the nurse needs to obtain to apply the systems framework to Mrs. C. P.'s family.
3. Identify ways Mrs. C. P.'s family may benefit by using appropriate community resources.

CRITICAL INQUIRY EXERCISE

Ask classmates or friends to describe their communities.

CRITICAL EXPLORATION EXERCISE

Investigate the community resources available to the following persons in your community:

- Low-income elderly individuals
- Low-income families with infants and children

■ Practicing for NCLEX

Circle the letter that corresponds to the best answer for each question.

1. "At-risk" groups are identified in a community so that
   a. all residents can be alerted to possible problems.
   b. healthcare workers can be trained to deal with health and social problems.
   c. measures can be taken to prevent problems or to deal with them in the early stages.
   d. health and economic matters are given adequate funds for solution of those problems.

2. Mr. Clyde, a divorced 33-year-old former drug addict, is paralyzed from the waist down. During hospitalization, no family ties are evident; however, he reportedly has two teenage sons. How might the nurse assist him in meeting his needs as they relate to roles and relationships?
   a. Have get-well cards sent anonymously
   b. Provide paper and pen for letter writing to his sons
   c. Spend time with him after work hours
   d. Leave him alone to allow for meditation

3. A bilateral amputee is assisted by his wife and children from the wheelchair to the commode for bowel evacuation. This example best demonstrates the family's assistance to meet which needs?
   a. Nutrition and metabolism
   b. Activity
   c. Health perception and health maintenance
   d. Elimination

4. Mr. Cain had a stroke, but he has not accepted his present state of health. He is focused on himself and views things negatively. The nurse may intervene to assist the client with his health perception and health maintenance by
   a. refocusing attention to functions he can control.
   b. listening quietly to his complaints and reporting them to the physician.
   c. referring him to a psychiatrist.
   d. limiting visits by family members.

5. Mr. Pitts has been hospitalized for months following special spinal cord surgery. The Boys Club in his hometown is renamed The Pitts Boys Club, and a parade is planned to honor Mr. Pitts. Such community action should positively influence Mr. Pitts'
   a. coping and stress tolerance.
   b. self-perception and self-concept.
   c. cognition and perception.
   d. health perception and health maintenance.

6. An 80-year-old woman now lives with her daughter but sees herself as burdensome to the daughter's family. The nurse may assist her to build feelings of self-worth by focusing on which of the following?
   a. Her limitations and the future
   b. Her age and the past
   c. The things that she can do
   d. The things that others do for her

7. Melvin experienced a gunshot wound to the back and cannot use his lower extremities. His brother-in-law has agreed to install grab bars in the bathroom so Melvin can live with him and his family. This action is planned primarily to meet which of the following needs?
   a. Activity and exercise
   b. Cognition and perception
   c. Health perception and health maintenance
   d. Coping and stress tolerance

8. The nurse asks a client to describe his community. Such assessment focuses discharge planning on
   a. maximizing individual and family potentials and reducing healthcare costs.
   b. a method the client finds acceptable and a method using community resources maximally.
   c. an individual method of client education and a method of quick referral.
   d. minimizing the cost of hospitalization and reducing family stress.

9. Understanding family dynamics and the community context will assist the nurse in planning care that is
   a. compatible with the client's everyday life and therefore has the greatest chance of success.
   b. regimented according to predetermined medical and social regulations and policies.
   c. in harmony with the financial resources of the family and community.
   d. reasonable, inexpensive, current, and compatible with high technology.

FILL IN THE BLANK

Complete the following fill-in-the-blank exercises.

1. According to Duvall, families move through a cycle of ________________ stages.
2. Healthy functioning families exchange resources to a ________________ degree than do dysfunctional families.
3. An individual can meet some basic needs independently but often needs the family and the ________________ to meet other needs.
4. Nurses need to use community ________________ for their clients and to find means of participating in the community.
5. The community and environment affect the ________________ of the individual and the family.

MULTIPLE-ANSWER MULTIPLE CHOICE

Circle the letter(s) corresponding to the appropriate answer(s). Select all that apply.

1. According to Higgs and Gustafson, which of the following are community functions?
   a. Use of space
   b. Means of livelihood
   c. Production, distribution, and consumption of goods and services
   d. Limitation of its members
   e. Education
   f. Participation
   g. Isolation from other systems

2. Most social scientists agree that the family provides for which of the following needs of its members over time?
   a. Caring
   b. Economic
   c. Educational
   d. Nurturing
   e. Political
   f. Reproductive
   g. Sexual
   h. Socialization
   i. Spiritual
   j. Status

CHAPTER 21

Culture and Ethnicity

CHAPTER OVERVIEW

Chapter 21 presents theoretical interpretations of culture and related concepts. Techniques for grounding nursing assessments in the client's perspectives are discussed, along with methods for providing culturally sensitive nursing care.

LEARNING OBJECTIVES

After mastering the content in this chapter, you should be able to do the following:

1. Discuss characteristics of culture.
2. Define concepts related to culture.
3. Build an understanding of people by viewing human responses in a cultural context.
4. Identify patterns of one's own and others' behavior that reflect stereotypical thinking and ethnocentric assumptions.
5. Communicate effectively with people of diverse orientations.
6. Demonstrate an increased awareness of personal culturation and its influence on one's own nursing practice.
7. Conduct an ethnographic interview.

■ Mastering the Information

MATCHING

Match the terms in Column II with a definition, example, or related statement from Column I. Place the letter corresponding to the answer in the space provided. (Use each letter only once; some letters may not be used.

COLUMN I

1. ______ Reduces the extent to which we take environmental cues into account and allows one to respond almost without thinking
2. ______ The use of one's own culture as the only correct standard by which to view people of other cultures
3. ______ A principle that, at its extreme, assumes that nothing has meaning by itself and there is no absolute
4. ______ An appropriate and legal means by which a nurse may communicate with a client who does not speak his or her language

COLUMN II

a. A trained interpreter
b. Cultural relativity
c. Ethnocentrism
d. Cultural habituation

COLUMN I

1. _____ Preconceived and untested belief about people
2. _____ A self-conscious, past-oriented form of identity based on a notion of shared cultural or ancestral heritage
3. _____ Takes skin color as the primary indicator of social value
4. _____ Items or images that preserve and create a sense of special social identity
5. _____ Takes biologic characteristics as the markers of separate cultural identity
6. _____ A holistic belief system that is marginal and subordinate to the belief system of a culture

COLUMN II

a. Subculture
b. Stereotype
c. Ethnic emblems
d. Race
e. Racism
f. Ethnicity

TRUE–FALSE

Indicate if the following statements are true or false.

_____ 1. Culture is a belief system that is held by its members, consciously or unconsciously, as truth.

_____ 2. According to Douglas, construction and use of symbols as effective and powerful vehicles of human communication reflect the human capacity for culture.

_____ 3. Ethnicity may be made by the ethnic group itself or by the larger society to which it is subordinate.

_____ 4. Nurses must impose their attitudes about high-level wellness on clients to help them.

_____ 5. Nurses may expect that health information will readily change a client's attitude and values relating to health.

_____ 6. Understanding the culture and ethnicity of clients should help to improve the quality of care given.

_____ 7. Culture makes communication highly efficient among people who share the same culture, but it can seriously distort communication among people who do not understand each other's culture.

_____ 8. If the nurse and the client speak the same language but do not share the same culture, problems of communication will not arise.

_____ 9. Knowing cultural norms will not enable the nurse to predict the behavioral responses of individual clients.

_____ 10. The values and beliefs of an individual can best be assessed by inquiring about statements, gestures, and cultural.

FILL IN THE BLANK

Supply the missing term or the information requested.

1. List 10 of the 15 characteristics of culture.
   a. __________
   b. __________
   c. __________
   d. __________
   e. __________
   f. __________
   g. __________
   h. __________
   i. __________
   j. __________
2. Culture provides a __________ for reacting, feeling, behaving, and interacting socially.
3. The experience of not comprehending the culture in which one is situated is known as __________ __________.
4. __________ is a method in which the interviewer looks for, locates, and interviews people who have expert or a native's knowledge about a culture the interviewer needs to know.
5. __________ makes one's world familiar and predictable.
6. Cultural habituation is __________ and differentiates the __________ from the novice nurse.
7. Parameters used to define the term minority include __________, __________, and ethnicity.
8. Three components of the ethnographic interview are __________, __________, and __________.
9. The optimal key informant about a client is the __________.

10. The most effective methods for gaining information that reflects the client's perspective include open-ended questioning, the use of key informants, ________________, and ________________.

■ Applying Your Knowledge

CASE STUDY

Mr. Kim Chee, 46 years old, is an Asian American admitted to the hospital with back pain. Mr. Chee is scheduled for diagnostic procedures and possible surgery. Mr. Chee speaks English and communicates a feeling of uneasiness. He also refers to the hospital as a place of grief.

1. Discuss how the culturally sensitive nurse considers Mr. Chee's cultural background when planning care. Include the following in your discussion:
   - Assessment data the nurse obtains from Mr. Chee
   - How the assessment data are arranged to adapt to Mr. Chee's nursing and medical care
2. The nurse believes Mr. Chee is isolating himself. She assesses him staying in bed most of the day with his back turned and not socializing with members of his family. Describe how the nurse may communicate with Mr. Chee to determine his perception of his hospitalization and treatment.

CRITICAL INQUIRY EXERCISE

Keep a 3-day diary of problems that you perceive to be related to cultural variations.

- Document your reactions as soon as possible.
- Analyze your reactions in terms of the expectations of a culturally sensitive nurse.
- Submit a short written report to the instructor, the group leader, or a peer for critique.

CRITICAL EXPLORATION EXERCISE

1. Identify the ethnic groups in your hometown.
2. Prepare abstracts of five articles that describe at least two different cultures.
3. Conduct a cultural-assessment interview with a person of a culture or ethnic group different from your own.
4. Observe a nurse for at least 4 hours in a healthcare center that serves multicultural groups.

■ Practicing for NCLEX

MULTIPLE CHOICE QUESTIONS

Circle the letter that corresponds to the best answer for each question.

1. Mr. Wills will be regarded by his nursing peers as a culturally sensitive nurse if he
   a. tells funny stories about clients whose culture is different from his own and briefly documents subjective data.
   b. constantly voices his personal opinions about female nurses and their performance skills.
   c. records food preference, communication style, religion, ethnic background, and native language of clients in the nursing history.
   d. reports physical variations, such as race, home environment, height and weight, and body size of clients, during nursing rounds.

2. The goal of culturally informed case management is to
   a. introduce clients to the subculture of the hospital or healthcare agency.
   b. prevent or minimize culture shock for clients in the subculture of the hospital or healthcare agency.
   c. reinforce the belief systems held by the client population groups being served.
   d. incorporate nursing into the healthcare delivery system of the larger community.

3. Mara is a 17-year-old, single, pregnant girl. The nurse is trying to determine her perspective on prenatal care. The approach most likely to yield the desired information is to
   a. ask, "What do you believe about prenatal care?"
   b. observe Mara with a group of her friends.
   c. interview Mara's mother and her boyfriend.
   d. conduct an ethnographic interview with Mara.

4. Ms. King works in a clinic that serves a large Asian population. Following an introduction to a client, she should
   a. extend her hand for a handshake as a gracious social act.
   b. extend her hand to communicate a sense of friendliness and warmth.
   c. smile and nod her head repeatedly to indicate acceptance of all behavioral responses.
   d. recognize that a handshake may be viewed as socially unacceptable because it involves touching a stranger.

5. Mr. Hui is a middle-aged man from Laos. His wife died in the emergency room after sustaining injuries in an automobile accident. An autopsy is recommended, but Mr. Hui refuses. The nurse should immediately do which of the following?
   a. Explain the benefits of an autopsy for collecting insurance payments
   b. Tell Mr. Hui that he can contribute to medical research by permitting an autopsy
   c. Consider that Mr. Hui may view an autopsy as an attempt to separate the body and the spirit
   d. Request an interpreter to persuade Mr. Hui to sign the autopsy consent form

6. Stereotyping in nursing may result in
   a. wrong assessments and inappropriate interventions.
   b. more frustration on the part of the nurse than the client.
   c. less frustration on the part of the nurse and the client.
   d. fuller cooperation by clients and family members.

7. Clients and families have the right to receive care that is
   a. determined necessary by the health team.
   b. culturally acceptable to them.
   c. dictated as appropriate by medical research.
   d. technologically advanced and inexpensive.

8. Nurses will increase the quality and safety of care insofar as they
   a. take into account the impact of cultural influences on a client, family, or community.
   b. study advanced technologic procedures to promote physical healing.
   c. research cultural factors of dominant population groups.
   d. assign clients to categories according to ethnicity.

9. Fran Nix is a homeless woman with a 5-year-old son. She brings her son to the immunization clinic at the county health department. The nurse should expect that Ms. Nix
   a. will not keep the next clinic appointment because of her nomadic lifestyle.
   b. is not providing adequate nutrition for her son.
   c. should be instructed about follow-up care.
   d. needs information about low-income housing.

10. Cultural assessment data to be recorded in the nursing history include all of the following except
    a. characteristics of the client.
    b. discrepancies between the culture of the client and that of the nurse.
    c. discrepancies between the culture of the client and the client-care setting.
    d. discrepancies between medical and nursing diagnoses.

11. The United States Census Bureau asks each individual to identify his or her race, thus equating race with
    a. culture.
    b. ethnic identity.
    c. self-awareness.
    d. individuality.

12. Nurses are recognizable as a subgroup by which of the following characteristics?
    a. An authoritative stance toward clients, dress, and language
    b. Recognition by the public as a profession and technical skills
    c. Cohesiveness, dress, and earning power
    d. Social-support methods, dress, and earning power

13. Client assessments that give consideration to the client's perspective are most likely to yield
    a. more information than the nursing team can document.
    b. diagnoses and interventions appropriate to the client.
    c. information about biocultural variation, such as growth patterns and nutritional intolerances.
    d. inaccurate diagnoses and biased criteria for evaluating nursing services.

14. In the United States, Title VI of the Civil Rights Act mandates that hospitals receiving Medicare and Medicaid reimbursement admit clients without regard to
    a. medical diagnoses, physical condition, or ability to pay.
    b. diagnostic-related groups, ability to pay, and insurance coverage.
    c. cost of needed care, services available, or national origin of the client.
    d. race, color, or national origin of the client.

15. Mr. Powell is a community health nurse. When evaluating growth curves of Asian, African, Native American, and European children, he can accurately state
    a. children of the same age should measure within a very close range.
    b. shorter and smaller children show evidence of having a disease or malnutrition.
    c. variations may be found that are related to genetic and environmental factors.
    d. a health-education program is needed for all children who are shorter or smaller than the group norm.

FILL IN THE BLANK

Supply the missing term or the information requested.

1. Nursing derives the concept of culture from ________________.
2. In the domain of nursing, it is critical that the gathering and recording of subjective data be done without ________________ it.
3. For many Westerners, the color black signifies death and mourning, but ________________ does the same for the Chinese.
4. The main characteristic that distinguishes ethnic identity from culture is the ________________ selection of symbolic elements.
5. Culture links a wide variety of ________________ and events uniquely.

MULTIPLE-ANSWER MULTIPLE CHOICE

Circle the letter(s) corresponding to the appropriate answer(s). Select all that apply.

1. Accurate nursing assessments require that the nurse do which of the following?
    a. Maximize cultural sensitivity
    b. Maximize cultural relativity
    c. Minimize ethnocentric tendencies
    d. Accept absolute truths
    e. Minimize minority views

2. In North America, the nurse should view client unfamiliarity with Western ways as
    a. a challenge to health educators.
    b. a starting point for health education.
    c. an indication that health is not appreciated.
    d. a problem to be referred to social workers.

3. Discharge of a client from the hospital to the home environment may be viewed by the healthcare team as a self-explanatory demonstration of recuperation. The client may view it as the team giving up. This is an example of
    a. bias and prejudice.
    b. failure to assess the client's perspective.
    c. medical/nursing ethnocentrism.
    d. unavoidable miscommunication.

4. Subcultural identity can be which of the following?
    a. A source of social support
    b. A target for social elevation and depletion
    c. A target for stigma
    d. A target for exploitation
    e. A source for genocide

CHAPTER 22

Communication: The Nurse–Client Relationship

CHAPTER OVERVIEW

Chapter 22 discusses the elements of the communication process, the importance of language, the ingredients of therapeutic communication, and the relationship between communication and the nursing process. Techniques for developing effective communication skills to be used with people of different ages and languages are examined.

LEARNING OBJECTIVES

After mastering the content in this chapter, you should be able to do the following:

1. Define the four major types of communication.
2. Discuss the elements of the communication process and their relevance to nursing.
3. Describe how language and experience affect the communication process.
4. Explain the nature of the nurse–client relationship.
5. Distinguish between a professional and a social relationship.
6. Name the elements of an informal nurse–client contract.
7. Discuss four key ingredients of therapeutic communication.
8. Name two professional self-care safety nets.
9. Identify important assessment areas to address when communicating with clients.
10. Give an example for each type of therapeutic communication technique.
11. Identify three key nontherapeutic responses, explaining how each interferes with therapeutic communication.
12. Describe two special situations that affect communication.

■ Mastering the Information

MATCHING

Match the terms in Column II with a definition, example, or related statement from Column I. Place the letter corresponding to the answer in the space provided. (Use each letter only once; some letters may not be used.)

COLUMN I

1. ______ The process of getting the purpose into code
2. ______ A medium or carrier of a message
3. ______ A way of being helpful by facilitating interactions that focus on the client and the client's concern
4. ______ Warm, caring interest and concern for the person
5. ______ The ability to see into the experience of another and understand how a situation is viewed from the other person's perspective
6. ______ A message about a message that looks beyond just words
7. ______ The nurse listening and restating content back to the client to verify the nurse's understanding with the client
8. ______ Asking goal-directed questions to help the client focus on key concerns
9. ______ A pause in communication that allows the nurse and client time to think about what has taken place
10. ______ Elicits more than a "yes" or "no" answer

COLUMN II

a. Therapeutic communication
b. Positive regard
c. Encoding
d. Channel
e. Empathy
f. Metacommunication
g. Restatement
h. Silence
i. Focusing
j. Open-ended questions

TRUE–FALSE

Indicate if the following statements are true or false.

______ 1. Communication is a continuous, indispensable function of human beings.

______ 2. The nurse who speaks in a well-modulated voice, dresses in a professional manner, listens to clients, and gives information demonstrates congruence among verbal, nonverbal, and metacommunication.

______ 3. Effective communication within the nurse–client relationship is a natural process.

______ 4. The purpose of therapeutic communication is to help clients express and work through feelings and problems related to their condition, treatments, and nursing care.

______ 5. The main subject in the nurse–client relationship is the expected outcome of healthcare.

______ 6. A person with a limited vocabulary has more difficulty describing experiences than one with a rich, diverse vocabulary.

______ 7. Both the nurse and the client bring language and personal experiences into the communication that occurs between them.

______ 8. Development of common understanding is the aim of therapeutic communication.

______ 9. The main goal of communication between a nurse and a client is to obtain an informed consent for treatment.

______ 10. The nurse-client relationship is based on an informal contractual model.

______ 11. Active listening means that the nurse conveys back to the client an accurate picture of what the client is expressing.

______ 12. Restatement and reflection are two important techniques for accurately decoding a message and helping a client feel listened to and understood.

______ 13. The "therapeutic" nurse listens for exact words only.

______ 14. Open-ended questions and opening remarks are ways of getting a conversation started.

______ 15. The working phase is that part of the nurse–client relationship in which the nurse functions as the client's advocate.

FILL IN THE BLANK

Supply the missing term or the information requested.

1. Communication may be defined as a system of ______________ and ______________ messages that forms a connection between the sender and the receiver.

2. The main subject of communication in the nurse–client relationship is ______________, ______________, and ______________.

3. The elements of communication include ______________, ______________, ______________, ______________, ______________, and ______________.

4. The nurse–client relationship is focused on the ______________, is ______________, and has defined ______________.

5. The three phases in the nurse–client relationship are ______________, ______________, and ______________.

6. Verbal communication involves the use of __________________, spoken or written, whereas nonverbal communication uses __________________, __________________, __________________, __________________, __________________, and rate of speech or dress to convey messages.
7. The key ingredients of therapeutic communication are __________________, __________________, and __________________.
8. The __________________, __________________ relationship and __________________ communication are instruments used to implement the nursing process.

■ Applying Your Knowledge

CASE STUDY

Mr. Samuel, 46 years old, had an operation 3 days ago to repair a fractured leg. The nurse enters the room shortly after the physician's visit. Mr. Samuel is in Fowler's position with the head of the bed elevated 45 degrees and the overbed table across the bed; he is completing his menu. The nurse has cared for Mr. Samuel since his first day after surgery. He has verbalized the following concerns to the nurse:

"I have two children and a wife who depend on me."
"I can't believe that I'll be out of work for 3 months or more."
"Oh, what's going to happen in the meanwhile; bills are coming in."
"The doctor seemed so rushed. I had several questions to ask about insurance and rehabilitation, but I don't need rehabilitation."

Mr. Samuel is shaking his head from side to side, frowning, and at one point when he talks about the bills, he slams the pencil down hard on the table.

1. Identify verbal and nonverbal clues.
2. Discuss the use of advocacy with the statement, "I don't need rehabilitation."
3. The nurse–client relationship has been established. Discuss specific communication techniques the nurse should use to encourage expression of Mr. Samuel's feelings.

CRITICAL INQUIRY EXERCISE

Interview an elderly person regarding health beliefs.

- Tape the conversation (if permitted).
- Listen to the tape, and analyze your communication skills.
- Identify the techniques used.
- List the client's responses.
- List your thoughts and feelings.

CRITICAL EXPLORATION EXERCISE

1. Visit a nursery school and list the communication techniques used with small children.
2. View a short television program and identify examples of the following:
   - Nonverbal communication
   - Metacommunication
   - Barriers to communication

■ Practicing for NCLEX

MULTIPLE CHOICE QUESTIONS

Circle the letter that corresponds to the best answer for each question.

1. A client learns to trust the nurse during which phase of the nurse–client relationship?
   a. Working phase
   b. Visiting phase
   c. Orientation phase
   d. Terminal phase
2. The nurse is talking with a pregnant client who has not yet decided what type of pain control she will use during her labor experience. Which of the following statements by the nurse represents an advocacy approach toward the client?
   a. "You should let your physician decide what is best for you."
   b. "There is no right or wrong choice; all that counts is what you want."
   c. "If you do not want to hurt, you'd better get an epidural."
   d. "The choice is yours, but natural birth allows you to be more active in the process."

3. Mr. Jones tells the nurse that he is not receiving enough information about his condition from the physician. To facilitate open communication, the nurse should
   a. develop a teaching plan about the client's condition to be shared with the physician.
   b. assist the client in writing a list of questions to ask the physician.
   c. write the statement in the nurses' notes and highlight it in red.
   d. call and ask the physician to speak with the client immediately.
4. The "circle of confidentiality" within which the nurse may share information about a client includes which of the following?
   a. All people on the nursing staff
   b. All people in the nursing unit who are responsible for the client
   c. Any licensed healthcare provider in the system
   d. All family members who inquire about the client
5. Ms. Krell says to the nurse, "If I tell you something, will you promise to keep it a secret?" Before responding, it is important for the nurse to
   a. clarify the team concept when providing healthcare.
   b. gain a person's trust to serve as an advocate.
   c. understand the deep feelings and emotions of all clients.
   d. maintain confidentiality at all times to show professionalism.
6. A client admitted to the emergency room has been shot by police after killing a store manager. The nurses communicate freely with him. This is an example of regarding a person as "being of worth" because
   a. it is a legal requirement.
   b. he must be taught to respect the life of others.
   c. he is a prime suspect and a valuable witness.
   d. he is a human being.
7. A person with a comfortable sense of self is able to
   a. recall events of the distant past and relate them freely.
   b. forget unpleasant experiences and thus not talk of them.
   c. accurately evaluate illness and experiences and verbalize freely.
   d. take a more flexible view of life and communicate feelings.
8. One of the most important things a nurse can do to encourage a client to express real concerns is to
   a. stand near the client and maintain eye contact.
   b. sit down close to the client and provide privacy.
   c. avoid eye contact with the client and provide privacy.
   d. appear professional and confident.
9. Mr. Throm does not speak English. An interpreter is not available when he arrives in the emergency room. The nurse helps to decode his message by using pictures and gestures. This is an example of changing the
   a. message content.
   b. simplicity of content.
   c. channel of communication.
   d. source of communication.
10. Statements by the nurse such as "Go on . . ." and "I see . . ." help the client to keep on talking and expressing himself or herself. These are examples of
    a. focusing.
    b. encouraging elaboration.
    c. summarizing.
    d. looking for alternatives.
11. Melvin tells the nurse that he was involved in a motorcycle accident after he got off the school bus. The nurse asks, "What happened then?" The nurse is
    a. seeking clarification.
    b. focusing.
    c. reflecting.
    d. summarizing.
12. Ms. Phelps is recovering from a heart attack. After a teaching session about ways to promote healthful living, she says, "I understand my diet, how to take my medicines, and the things to avoid in order to get well." However, the nurse overhears her ask a family member to bring a package of cigarettes. Ms. Phelps's actions are an example of which type of communication?
    a. Incoherent communication
    b. Incongruent communication
    c. Congruent communication
    d. Confused communication

13. The nurse hears a frightened client whose thought processes are disturbed screaming, "I'm drowning." It is most likely that he may really mean which of the following?
    a. "I'm very frightened and out of control."
    b. "I have severe pulmonary congestion."
    c. "I know I have congestive heart failure."
    d. "My treatment is not helping me."

14. According to Brandler and Grinder, a person's view of the world is developed through several filters, which include
    a. neurologic receptor systems, language, and personal experiences.
    b. chemical receptor systems, language, and family lifestyle.
    c. brain waves, chemical receptor systems, and personal experiences.
    d. brain chemistry, genetic factors, and language.

15. Mr. Newton had a stroke, resulting in a prolonged period of oxygen deprivation to his cerebrum. He has not eaten for several days. When asked if he wants to eat, he mutters "No." The nurse could most appropriately conclude that Mr. Newton
    a. is not hungry and is unable to swallow.
    b. has brain damage, which prevents proper feedback.
    c. does not understand the spoken word.
    d. needs more time to respond.

FILL IN THE BLANK

Supply the missing term or the information requested.

1. ________________ responses are those that interfere with or block therapeutic communication.
2. ________________ includes the ability to respond receptively to the other person's experience while still maintaining objectivity and the ability to communicate clearly.

MULTIPLE-ANSWER MULTIPLE CHOICE

Circle the letter(s) corresponding to the appropriate answer(s). Select all that apply.

1. Which of the following is an example of an open-ended question?
    a. "Do you need anything from the nurse or doctor?"
    b. "How will you change your dressing at home?"
    c. "How are you doing today?"
    d. "What is it like being in the hospital?"

2. A 7-year-old girl is scheduled for a tonsillectomy. She asks the nurse if she will have pain. Desiring to reassure the child, the nurse may appropriately reply in which of the following ways?
    a. "There may be pain, but someone will be there to make you as comfortable as possible."
    b. "It will not hurt because of the medication."
    c. "You're a big girl, you can take a little pain."
    d. "Think about something else now, and let the doctor worry about the operation."

3. The metacommunication of a client who says one thing and does another may convey which message to the nurse?
    a. "I'm ready to accept responsibility for my health."
    b. "I don't care about my health."
    c. "I am angry that I have this condition and want it to go away."
    d. "I don't know what I should do about my diagnosis and treatment plan."
    e. "I'm not yet ready to accept my illness or condition."

4. Ms. Cripp stares out of the window and comments, "I know my children care about me." To promote continuity of communication, the nurse should
    a. repeat what Ms. Cripp said and encourage her to talk further.
    b. agree with Ms. Cripp.
    c. pick up on the cue as to what might be a problem for Ms. Cripp.
    d. change the subject to avoid upsetting Ms. Cripp.

5. An important advantage to the informal contractual relationship between a nurse and a client involves which of the following?
    a. Values
    b. Schedules and treatments
    c. Rights
    d. Treatments

CHAPTER 23

Caring for the Difficult Client

CHAPTER OVERVIEW

Chapter 23 examines and summarizes the role of the nurse when caring for a difficult client. Concepts related to nurse–client relationships, ethical issues, and potential aspects in client situations that may cause difficulty are discussed. An overview of strategies and approaches for addressing the difficult client is presented, as is a synopsis of the major issues associated with specific types of difficult clients. Application of the nursing process in the care of clients with alterations in respiratory function is emphasized.

LEARNING OBJECTIVES

After mastering the content in this chapter, you should be able to do the following:

1. Define *difficult client.*
2. Explain the concept of limit setting.
3. Discuss how the ethical principle of beneficence sometimes prevails over the ethical principle of autonomy.
4. List four ways to approach the angry client.
5. Discuss the concept of splitting.
6. Discuss an approach toward the drug-seeking client.

■ Mastering the Information

MATCHING

Match the terms in Column II with a definition, example, or related statement from Column I. Place the letter corresponding to the answer in the space provided. (Use each letter only once; some letters may not be used.)

COLUMN I

1. _____ The nurse may prohibit the weak client from getting out of bed without assistance.
2. _____ The nurse provides help to a confused client who wants to do everything alone.
3. _____ The client cooperates with nurse Amy but refuses to do anything nurse Abby asks.
4. _____ The client demonstrates behavior that is an obstacle to providing good nursing care.
5. _____ The client uses intimidation or flattery to achieve a desired end from the nurse.

COLUMN II

a. Beneficence
b. Difficult client
c. Limit setting
d. Manipulation
e. Splitting

TRUE–FALSE

Indicate if the following statements are true or false.

_____ 1. The nurse who feels an angry client may quickly escalate to violence should take measures to protect herself/himself and the client.

_____ 2. No nurse can provide appropriate nursing care unless he or she treats each client with the utmost respect and avoids generalizations.

_____ 3. The client who reports having a plan of action for committing suicide is unlikely to actually commit suicide.

_____ 4. A client with delirium may lie quietly in bed or may be angry and combative because of frightening delusions of persecution.

_____ 5. Direct confrontation should be avoided with a sexually provocative client.

FILL IN THE BLANK

Supply the missing term or the information requested.

1. Failure of the nurse to set limits in cases when the client may be harmed by a behavior or action considered ________________.
2. Delirium comes on acutely over __________ or days.
3. Identify the elements of the acronym HEAT that identify the steps the nurse should take to reduce client anger.
   a. H — ________________________
   b. E — ________________________
   c. A — ________________________
   d. T — ________________________
4. Identify five of nine rules for the verbal de-escalation of anger.
   a.
   b.
   c.
   d.
   e.

■ Applying Your Knowledge

CASE STUDY

Mr. Evans is a 25-year-old man with sickle cell anemia, which was diagnosed when he was 4 years old. He has been hospitalized on numerous occasions for sickle cell crises and usually requires 2 to 3 days of intravenous fluid and pain medication. Mr. Evans has a history of drug abuse and use of recreational drugs such as heroin and cocaine. He has been in the hospital for 5 days after demanding to be admitted for sickle cell crisis when no symptoms were noted. The doctor has changed his medication to prn Tylenol and is preparing to discharge him. Mr. Evans demands intravenous Demerol, stating he is in agony. Mr. Evan's mother arrives and asks why her son is allowed to suffer and is not being given medication for his pain.

1. How would you address Mr. Evan's request for Demerol?
2. Describe the physical assessments you might make to determine if Mr. Evans might be experiencing pain.
3. Discuss how you would respond to Mr. Evan's mother.
4. Discuss ways that the nurse can help Mr. Evans address his medication addiction after discharge.

CRITICAL INQUIRY EXERCISE

1. Develop a list of community resources that may be used by a client who has a history of suicide attempts who is being discharged home with no family support system.
2. Search the Internet for articles related to caring for clients who display sexually provocative behavior.

CRITICAL EXPLORATION EXERCISE

Discuss with a nurse on the floor and two non-nurse healthcare providers strategies for dealing with the difficult client.

a. Identify one example from each of a difficult client situation each had to deal with and the strategies used to address each situation.
b. Identify ways in which the nurse and other healthcare providers may collaborate to address dealing with difficult clients.

■ Practicing for NCLEX

MULTIPLE CHOICE QUESTIONS

Circle the letter that corresponds to the best answer for each question.

1. Gina Barnes, an intoxicated client, is exhibiting strong anger behavior nearing violence. Which behavior by the nurse would be appropriate to de-escalate the client's behavior?
   a. Pat the client on the shoulder and stare into her eyes
   b. Sympathetically agree with everything the client says
   c. Firmly tell the client she is wrong to behave in this manner
   d. Use short phrases and sentences with simple vocabulary

2. Mr. Pells has oxygen in his room that must remain on at all times. He tells the nurse that he will smoke in his room no matter what anyone says. The nurse removes all cigarettes and matches from the room and informs Mr. Pell that he cannot smoke in the room. What is the nurse exercising in this situation?
   a. Autonomy
   b. Authority
   c. Empathy
   d. Malfeasance
3. Which action would take priority when setting limits with a delusional client?
   a. Identifying how far the client may travel from the room without an escort
   b. Instructing the client to use the urinal and not urinate on the floor
   c. Limiting the use of television at night so that the client gets adequate rest
   d. Asking the client not to rearrange the furniture to look like it does at home
4. Which action would be appropriate when caring for a client with delirium?
   a. Administer a central nervous system depressant to calm the client
   b. Move the client to a quiet room far away from the nurses' station
   c. Restrict visitors and family to allow the client quiet time alone
   d. Check the client's room and assess status regularly every 2 hours
5. Mr. Todd presents in the emergency room with alcohol intoxication and angry abusive language and behavior. The most immediate concern in this situation would be
   a. asking Mr. Todd to watch his language because other patients are present.
   b. emoving Mr. Todd from the emergency room.
   c. calming Mr. Todd by listening and determining his major concern.
   d. sedating Mr. Todd to prevent him from harming himself or others.

FILL IN THE BLANK

Supply the missing term or the information requested.

1. The primary action the nurse should take if a client appears depressed and withdrawn is to determine if ____________ ____________ is present.
2. The single most important factor in addressing the angry client who appears to be getting violent is to use verbal ____________ skills to reduce the client's anger level.
3. ________________ is an acute impairment of thinking, memory, and perception caused by medical conditions, medications, surgery, or trauma.

MULTIPLE-ANSWER MULTIPLE CHOICE

Circle the letter(s) corresponding to the appropriate answer(s). Circle all that apply.

1. With which client should the nurse use strategies designed to approach the angry client.
   a. The client who has become frightened or upset because of something specific
   b. The chronically angry or easy-to-anger client who is otherwise cognitively intact
   c. The delirious, agitated client; although a specific incident may lead to the anger, fear and anger are inherent in many types of delirium
   d. The client who touches the nurse's buttocks and comments on how firm the muscles are
   e. The intoxicated client or client in alcohol or drug withdrawal
   f. The client with a major psychiatric disorder (e.g., bipolar disorder, schizophrenia, Alzheimer's disease, antisocial personality disorder)
2. When providing care to a client who appears depressed and withdrawn, the nurse should consider what interventions to take the highest priority?
   a. Teaching the client the many causes of depression
   b. Identifying if the client has had thoughts of committing suicide
   c. Teaching the client to relax with a hobby
   d. Placing the client who reports a suicide plan of action on suicide precautions
   e. Obtaining a television and radio for the client's room

CHAPTER 24

Client Education

CHAPTER OVERVIEW

Chapter 24 examines the basic principles underlying client teaching. The teaching and learning process and the use of the nursing process as a framework for client teaching are discussed. Emphasis is placed on the importance of individualized client teaching.

LEARNING OBJECTIVES

After mastering the content in this chapter, you should be able to do the following:

1. Describe important qualities of a teaching–learning relationship.
2. Explain the domains of knowledge and how learning relates to each.
3. Identify four purposes of client education.
4. Define factors that inhibit and facilitate learning.
5. Discuss important assessment data used to individualize client teaching.
6. Describe teaching methods and evaluation strategies.
7. Explain the abilities, needs, and motivations of different age groups as they pertain to learning.

■ Applying Your Knowledge

MATCHING

Match the terms in Column II with a definition, example, or related statement from Column I. Place the letter corresponding to the answer in the space provided. (Some letters may be used more than once.)

COLUMN I

1. __c__ Client will correctly give self-injection.
2. __b__ Client will state the four basic food groups.
3. __b__ Client will identify three situations illustrating when the doctor should be notified.
4. __a__ Client will verbalize feelings about having acquired immunodeficiency syndrome.
5. __c__ Client will walk the length of the hall one time.

COLUMN II

a. Affective domain
b. Cognitive domain
c. Psychomotor domain

TRUE–FALSE

Indicate if the following statements are true or false.

__F__ 1. A client's blood relatives always provide more support and are more willing to participate in the client's care than are friends.

__F__ 2. The nurse should always complete teaching within the time frame outlined in the teaching plan.

__F__ 3. A person's use of spoken language is a good indicator of his or her literacy level.

__T__ 4. People have varying learning styles, and people in different age groups require different approaches.

__T__ 5. The nurse can influence, but not control, the process in client education.

FILL IN THE BLANK

Supply the missing term or the information requested.

1. Define pedagogy and andragogy.
   a. instruction of children
   b. instruction of adults
2. Learning is the acquisition of skills or knowledge by practice, study, or instruction.
3. The nurse should make sure that the room is not too hot or cold because environment has an effect on learning.
4. List four positive qualities that characterize the teaching relationship.
   a. Client focus
   b. Holism
   c. Negotiation
   d. Interaction
5. motivation provides drive and incentive and is a powerful determinant of success in client education.

■ Applying Your Knowledge

CASE STUDY

Ms. C. L., a 24-year-old African American woman, has received a diagnosis of new-onset diabetes mellitus. She presented to the hospital experiencing dizziness, headache, polyuria, polydipsia, and numbness in arms and legs for several weeks. She is attending business school. Ms. C. L. reports that she administered insulin injections to her grandmother with diabetes. Ms. C. L. voices that she wants to learn everything and do everything that she is supposed to because she has two children who need her. Physician orders include:

Humulin N 6 units + Humulin R 4 units sc q a. m.
Humulin N 4 units + Humulin R 4 units sc q p. m.
1800 kcal diet
Blood glucose monitoring q 4 h
Diabetic teaching

1. Construct a teaching plan for Ms. C. L. Include the following:
   a. Topic of presentation
   b. Three client-centered goals with measurable outcomes
   c. An outline of the content
   d. Teaching strategies
   e. Method of evaluations
2. Discuss the abilities and motivations of Ms. C. L.'s age group as they pertain to learning.

CRITICAL INQUIRY EXERCISE

Talk with the staff development nurse about the teaching plans at your clinical facility for a select client illness.

CRITICAL EXPLORATION EXERCISE

1. Assess the presence of pedagogic and andragogic approaches to learning in the teaching plan.
2. Assess the domains of knowledge addressed in the plan.

■ Practicing for NCLEX

MULTIPLE CHOICE QUESTIONS

Circle the letter that corresponds to the best answer for each question.

1. Which of the following teaching methods would be most effective when trying to modify the client's attitude or emotional responses?
   a. Lecture
   b. Independent study
   c. Skill demonstration
   d. Role playing
2. Which of the following factors should the nurse consider when planning client education?
   a. Economic status
   b. Health beliefs
   c. Surgical history
   d. Ambulatory status

3. A written plan of care should be developed before client teaching for which of the following reasons?
   a. It will provide the nurse with an opportunity to assess the client's literacy level.
   b. It eliminates the need for evaluation.
   c. It will foster communication with other professionals so that they may take part in the teaching.
   d. It ensures that insurance claims will be reimbursed.

4. Which of the following activities would be most appropriate for initiating a teaching session with a client?
   a. Give the client the written materials first and allow him or her to read over the materials quickly.
   b. Verbally give the client information on the subject and then allow him to ask questions.
   c. Assess the client's current level of knowledge of the subject.
   d. Show the client audiovisuals about the subject, followed by an informal quiz.

5. When using return demonstrations during client teaching, the nurse should
   a. give feedback, acknowledging competency and suggesting areas for improvement.
   b. offer a scenario to the client and ask him or her what would be the response.
   c. focus on identifying deficits.
   d. explain the skill while slowly demonstrating it to the client.

6. The use of an interpreter/translator
   a. is recommended for all federally run programs.
   b. should be a family member whenever possible.
   c. requires that the interpreter/translator needs only a general knowledge of the language.
   d. will increase the teaching time needed per session.

FILL IN THE BLANK

Supply the missing term or the information requested.

1. ____________ is an effective teaching strategy for teaching affective behavior to children and adults.
2. ____________ may point out deficits in learning that may not be evident in a single session.

MULTIPLE-ANSWER MULTIPLE CHOICE

Circle the letter(s) corresponding to the appropriate answer(s). Select all that apply.

1. Developing a realistic approach for learning includes assessing which of the following?
   a. The client's energy level
   b. The client's age
   c. The client's emotional state
   d. The client's admission date

2. Indicate the evaluation method(s) that would be beneficial to evaluate psychomotor learning.
   a. Return demonstration
   b. Simulations
   c. Oral tests
   d. Written tests
   e. Check-off lists

CHAPTER 25

Care Management

CHAPTER OVERVIEW

Chapter 25 discusses prospective payments in home healthcare. Key assessments and a model for home care are presented. Common nursing diagnoses, goals, and nursing interventions for addressing altered home care management are discussed.

LEARNING OBJECTIVES

After mastering the content in this chapter, you should be able to do the following:

1. Describe management of healthcare needs in the home from a systems perspective.
2. Identify factors that influence the client's ability to manage healthcare within the home.
3. Explain the major areas requiring assessment by a home care nurse.
4. Describe nursing roles and responsibilities in home care.
5. Identify the importance of community resources in the care of clients receiving home care services.

■ Mastering the Information

MATCHING

Match the terms in Column II with a definition, example, or related statement from Column I. Place the letter corresponding to the answer in the space provided.

COLUMN I

1. ______ Public or private agency designed to care for terminally ill clients and their families
2. ______ A professional approach to providing care that focuses on the whole person, not just health-related issues
3. ______ Engagement in activities for the purpose of protecting the rights of others while supporting the patient's responsibility for self-determination
4. ______ A collaborative/interactive process between the nurse and client to progress toward the client's goal
5. ______ Described as entering into the "caring moment"

COLUMN II

a. Advocacy
b. Hospice
c. Case management
d. Aesthetic/spiritual communication
e. Patient education

COLUMN I

1. ______ The nurse evaluates the visit's purpose and reviews pertinent records and information.
2. ______ The nurse and family summarize accomplishments and plan for future visits.
3. ______ The nurse reviews with the client the overall purpose and source of referral.
4. ______ The nurse records findings and plans for the next visit.
5. ______ The nurse establishes the professional therapeutic relationship and implements the nursing process.

COLUMN II

a. Postvisit phase
b. Previsit phase
c. In-home phase
d. Initiation phase
e. Termination phase

TRUE–FALSE

Indicate if the following statements are true or false.

_____ 1. Harris advises home health nurses to resist the increasing use of technology and rely on basic nursing skills.

_____ 2. Nurses ought to be familiar with emergency-care services, equipment rental stores, visiting nurses services, homemaker services, and the location of welfare and Medicare/Medicaid offices in the community.

_____ 3. The use of alternative and complementary health modalities is facilitated through aesthetic expression.

_____ 4. Telenursing is a highly effective strategy to provide an alternative to home visits.

_____ 5. A complex medical treatment regimen with multiple medications is a common risk factor associated with the need for home care.

_____ 6. All clients recover and are rehabilitated more rapidly in the home environment.

FILL IN THE BLANK

Supply the missing term or the information requested.

1. As a client moves from one environment to another, nurses must consider the client's ability to carry out ________________ of ________________.
2. The current basis for most ________________ home health services is an ________________ or a ______________ problem requiring skilled care.
3. Three of five phases of the home visit suggested by Stanhope and Lancaster are ________________, ________________, and ________________.
4. For care management to be balanced, the nurse's approach must include strategies that engage the whole person: ________________, ________________, and ________________.
5. Alterations in the ability to maintain oneself in a home environment may occur as a result of decreased functional abilities, insufficient family or social ________________, or insufficient community ________________.

■ Applying Your Knowledge

CASE STUDY

Mrs. Franklin, 55 years old, is hospitalized for a chronic respiratory condition. She has been treated and is scheduled to go home with a regimen of four oral medications. One of her medications is an inhaler she will use for the first time. Mrs. Franklin is the primary source of income for her family since her husband recently lost his job and her 19-year-old son does not work. Her doctor has stated she should work no more than 20 hours per week because of her respiratory condition. Both her husband and her son smoke heavily.

1. Consider the health care needs Mrs. Franklin may have after discharge.
2. Explain the areas requiring assessment by a home care nurse.
3. Discuss community resources that might be beneficial for Mrs. Franklin after discharge.

CRITICAL INQUIRY EXERCISE

1. Perform a functional assessment for your own family.
   a. Identify family structure for caregiving.
   b. Identify family strengths for home-health maintenance.
   c. Describe family communication patterns with healthcare agencies.
   d. List social factors that affect home health maintenance.

2. Review a family health record with a nurse at the local health department or home healthcare agency to identify levels of care being received.

CRITICAL EXPLORATION EXERCISE

1. Accompany a community-health nurse during a home visit.
2. Locate a community-service directory for your community by calling the newspaper office, library, radio station, television station, or official health department.
3. Form two or more groups. Using community-service directories from different communities, complete the following:
   a. Identify agencies to assist with home maintenance management.
   b. Discuss availability, accessibility, and acceptability of technical or professional resources for home maintenance management.

■ Practicing for NCLEX

MULTIPLE CHOICE QUESTIONS

Circle the letter that corresponds to the best answer for each question.

1. Sara is a 16-year-old single parent of an 8-month-old daughter. She states, "I want to raise my own child." The most important consideration in planning care for Sara relates to which of the following?
   a. Her financial deficits related to grooming and providing quality food for herself and her infant
   b. Her ability to organize work and child care, manage financial responsibilities, and provide a safe, nurturing environment for herself and her infant
   c. Her ability to transport herself and her infant, cook, clean, wash clothing, and study for school
   d. Her ability to find affordable shelter, participate in social activities, and continue in school
2. If a family makes a decision regarding the care of a client that appears to the nurse to be unloving, irresponsible, overprotective, or self-sacrificing, the nurse should
   a. report the decision to the social worker for referral to the courts.
   b. refrain from additional interactions with the family because they are not responding to nursing interventions.
   c. report the decision to the physician and the social worker and request referral to higher authorities.
   d. refrain from making judgments about the decision and take action to work with the client and family to meet outcome goals.
3. Ms. Johns, 82 years old, is a childless widow who lives alone, has diabetes, and has been admitted to the hospital with diabetic ketoacidosis. Her chart states that she has been admitted for complications of her diabetes in February, April, and June of this calendar year. You realize that she has ___________ risk factors associated with the need for home care.
   a. three
   b. five
   c. two
   d. four
4. Mr. Toms, a 77-year-old widower who lives alone, has hypertension that is well-controlled by medications and diet. It has been determined that Mr. Toms' blood pressure goes up when he is unable to get a low-sodium diet. Mr. Toms should be referred to which of the following?
   a. The hospital dietitian
   b. Area agency on aging
   c. American Heart Association
   d. Meals on Wheels
5. An 80-year-old man forgets about financial affairs such as paying utility bills and insurance premiums. His eyesight is too poor for balancing his checkbook and reading necessary instructions. An appropriate intervention might be to suggest which of the following?
   a. Suggest that the home health aide assist with such matters
   b. Suggest placement in an extended care facility to provide for safety
   c. Suggest that a relative or friend be given power of attorney to handle financial affairs
   d. Suggest placement in a nursing home to promote self-growth and good nutrition
6. Mr. and Mrs. Hampton are preparing to take their infant daughter home after 3 weeks in the hospital. The parents receive training on the use of the apnea monitor that will be part of home care for their infant. As the home health nurse, you will be alert for
   a. signs of normal socialization and peer relationships.
   b. signs of parental closeness and bonding with their infant.
   c. signs of adequate financial resources.
   d. signs of altered health maintenance because of spiritual beliefs.

7. ________ is a nursing responsibility in all areas of practice.
   a. Consultation
   b. Claim processing
   c. Case management
   d. Case finding

8. Which of the following patients would be the best candidate for home care?
   a. Jennifer has an open leg wound and will rely on her brother to help her in her plan of care. She lives in a one-story apartment with elevator access.
   b. Abrilla, a client recovering from stroke with right-side weakness, has a two-story home and no friend or relatives to assist her.
   c. Aziz, 21 years old, was recently accidentally blinded and has no family. He must leave the dorm because he cannot resume study this school term.
   d. Marlon, a psychotic client whose condition is controlled by medication, lives with his mother in a rat-infested building with no running water.

9. Ms. Bishop, 65 years old, lives with her terminally ill husband for whom she is the primary caregiver. The role of the hospice nurse for Ms. Bishop will include
   a. managing pain and treating symptoms.
   b. developing and implementing a teaching plan discussing alternative medicines.
   c. assisting in bereavement and reorganizing her life.
   d. clarifying the source of referral and the purpose of the visits.

10. Sue, a home health nurse, will provide client teaching to a family with a child who has brain damage. She will prepare the father and mother to perform care; in addition, she will prepare extended family and a close neighbor who will assist as needed. Which of the following steps is listed in the correct order in which Sue will proceed when providing this client teaching?
    a. Step 1: Sue will negotiate learning goals.
    b. Step 2: Sue will evaluate client education.
    c. Step 3: Sue and the client develop and implement a teaching plan.
    d. Step 4: Sue assesses and gathers information.

FILL IN THE BLANK

Supply the missing term or the information requested.

1. ________________ is the acronym that describes the system for reporting and collecting standardized information.
2. The ________________ acts as a facilitator of the patient/caregiver system.
3. The model for home care that includes motivational factors of the person and family that is discussed in the chapter is the ________________ model.

MULTIPLE-ANSWER MULTIPLE CHOICE

Circle the letter(s) corresponding to the appropriate answer(s). Circle all that apply.

1. Select the components of the case management process the nurse will implement.
   a. Assessment
   b. Planning
   c. Coordinating
   d. Making referrals
   e. Monitoring medical progress
   f. Prescribing appropriate medications and treatments
   g. Monitoring outcomes and the plan's effectiveness
   h. Determining case closure
   i. Continuing on the case until the client dies
   j. Filing and completing paperwork

UNIT V

Essential Assessment Components

CHAPTER 26

Health Assessment of Human Function

CHAPTER OVERVIEW

In Chapter 26, the use of the functional health assessment to establish a thorough client database is discussed. Techniques and equipment used in the assessment process are reviewed, and an overview of lifespan considerations related to the individualized functional nursing assessment is provided.

LEARNING OBJECTIVES

After mastering the content in this chapter, you should be able to do the following:

1. Organize a nursing assessment.
2. Discuss preparation of the client and the environment to foster data collection.
3. Differentiate between objective and subjective data.
4. Discuss methods to obtain subjective information during the client interview.
5. Describe techniques of inspection, palpation, percussion, and auscultation used in the physical assessment.
6. Describe methods to obtain objective data during the physical examination.
7. Individualize the functional nursing assessment based on lifespan considerations.

■ Mastering the Information

MATCHING

Match the terms in Column I with a definition, example, or related statement from Column II. Place the letter corresponding to the answer in the space provided. (Use each letter only once; some letters may not be used.)

COLUMN I

1. ____ Auscultation
2. ____ Bruit
3. ____ Chief complaint
4. ____ Clubbing of nails
5. ____ Heave
6. ____ Gait
7. ____ Diaphragm
8. ____ Resonance
9. ____ Tangential lighting
10. ____ Thrills

COLUMN II

a. A manner of walking
b. A sign of chronic hypoxia
c. The art of listening for sounds of movement within the body
d. The degree to which sound propagates; percussion over air produces sound
e. Abnormal arterial sounds caused by increased turbulence of blood flow
f. Abnormal movement over precordium that is forceful at the area of the PMI
g. Provided by indirectly shining a lamp so that a shadow is over the area being examined
h. Vibrations or pulsations that may be noted over the precordial area
i. A flat piece of the stethoscope that responds best to high-frequency sounds
j. The first subject usually discussed in a client interview; the client's specific reason for seeking care

TRUE–FALSE

Indicate if the following data are appropriate or inappropriate for use in assessing the cardiovascular system. Mark "True" if the data are appropriate or "False" if the data are inappropriate.

__T__ 1. History of chest pain or discomfort

__T__ 2. Palpation of vibrations on pulsation in any precordial area

__F__ 3. A 24-hour dietary history

__T__ 4. Inspection of the point of maximal impulse

__F__ 5. Percussion of the lower abdominal area

FILL IN THE BLANK

Supply the missing term or the information requested.

1. The purpose of a health assessment is to establish a __database__ for the client concerning normal __abilities__, __risk factors__ that can contribute to dysfunction, and actual __alteration__ in normal function.

2. Objective data are collected through four basic techniques of physical examination: __inspection__, __ascultation__, __percussion__, and __palpation__

3. Assessment of a person's health perception and health maintenance reveals knowledge, behavior, and attitudes toward __prevention__ and __healthy living disease__

4. Assessment of activity and exercise should focus on three systems: __posture__, __gait__, and __movement__

5. Three of the six factors that contribute to cognition are: __memory__ __awareness__, and __language__

6. Assessment of roles and relationships describes the quality of a person's __family__, __work__, and __social__ roles.

7. A __Comprehensive assess__ encompasses the physical, psychological, social, and spiritual dimensions of living.

8. Nursing assessment of the newborn is made shortly __after birth__ and at __24__ hours of age.

9. Six pieces of equipment you might use when assessing the neurologic system are __Snellen__, __Tuning fork__, __Penlight__, __Hot + cold__, __hammer__ and __vanilla__.

■ Applying Your Knowledge

CASE STUDY

Mr. C. J., 58 years old, is admitted to the hospital with a medical diagnosis of congestive heart failure. Mrs. C. J. states, "He has been short of breath for several days but is worse today." Mr. C. J. states, "I missed a couple of days taking my medication because I went to visit my son and forgot to bring my medication. Oh, my feet started to swell about 3 days ago." The nurse's initial assessment findings include:

Height: 5 feet 7 inches; weight: 178 lb

Vital signs: oral temperature, 100.8°F; apical pulse, 108; respiration, 34; blood pressure, 130/88

Wheezing with scattered rhonchi lower lobes noted; productive cough; thick, yellow secretions; chest symmetrical

Glasgow, 13, conversation confused, hand grip equal, follows commands, PERLA, moves all extremities

Skin warm, moist, and pink; red area over heel and coccyx

Pulse irregular; S1 and S2 noted; peripheral pulses, 3+; ankle edema, 2+

Abdomen soft with bowel sounds in all quadrants

1. Determine subjective and objective data from the assessment data given.
2. Discuss the interview method the nurse will use to obtain additional subjective data from Mr. C. J.
3. Discuss the techniques—palpation, percussion, auscultation, inspection—and equipment the nurse used to obtain each piece of objective data.
4. Organize the assessment data using the functional health pattern. Include lifespan considerations for Mr. C. J.

CRITICAL INQUIRY EXERCISE

Interview a friend and ask health history questions. Which questions were difficult to clarify? How could you become more comfortable approaching a client about sensitive subjects?

CRITICAL EXPLORATION EXERCISE

1. Perform a respiratory assessment of an infant or newborn and an adult older than 70 years. Compare and contrast the findings.
2. Listen to your own breath sounds or those of a classmate at a time when a respiratory tract infection is present.
3. Conduct a full functional assessment of a client on the clinical unit. Identify any abnormalities found through inspection, auscultation, palpation, and percussion.

■ Practicing for NCLEX

MULTIPLE CHOICE QUESTIONS

Circle the letter that corresponds to the best answer for each question.

1. Data in which of the following areas would be most helpful to the nurse when assessing Mr. Tye's musculoskeletal function?
   a. Ambulation and coordination
   b. Capillary refill in extremities
   c. Respiratory rate, depth, and pattern
   d. Skin color, temperature, and turgor
2. Which of the following is the most direct indication of Mr. Tye's nutritional status?
   a. Respiratory rate and pattern
   b. Skin color and temperature
   c. Joint mobility and range of motion
   d. Weight and height measurements
3. Mr. Tye would be evaluated as possibly having an elimination problem if which of the following were noted?
   a. A flat abdomen with a hollow sound on percussion
   b. Active bowel sounds auscultated in all quadrants
   c. The last bowel movement passed was 1 week ago
   d. Urine is pale yellow and without sediment
4. Deep palpation is most appropriate in which of the following situations?
   a. When checking skin temperature
   b. To locate tender or painful areas
   c. For determination of organ size
   d. Assessment of the skin's moisture
5. To determine if an abdominal mass is solid or filled with air, the nurse should
   a. auscultate.
   b. inspect.
   c. palpate.
   d. percuss.
6. Functional health assessment should involve
   a. auscultating the radial and brachial pulses.
   b. interviewing the client to obtain objective data.
   c. monitoring the client's vesicular breath sounds.
   d. performing the physical assessment before the history.

7. Normal breath sounds include
   a. adventitious breath sounds over the main bronchial areas.
   b. bronchial breath sounds in the lower lung lobes.
   c. bronchovesicular breath sounds posteriorly between the scapulae.
   d. vesicular breath sounds over the major airways.

8. Which of the following would be appropriate when assessing a newborn?
   a. Ask the parents to leave the room to protect the child's modesty.
   b. Let the child listen with the stethoscope to allay fear of the equipment.
   c. Test the child's reflexes and weigh the child.
   d. Uncover the child completely during the entire examination.

FILL IN THE BLANK

Supply the missing term or the information requested.

1. The best approach to obtaining a sexual history is to introduce subjects of least sensitivity first.
2. The assessment of values and beliefs includes the significance of religious affiliation and religious practices.

MULTIPLE-ANSWER MULTIPLE CHOICE

Circle the letter(s) corresponding to the appropriate assessment technique(s). Select all that apply.

1. Which assessment procedure is appropriate?
   a. Performing indirect percussion by tapping on the area with the fingertip of the middle finger or thumb
   b. Evaluating body temperature using the back of the hand
   c. Removing all coverings from the client's body while palpating specific areas
   d. Asking the client to breathe through the mouth when auscultating breath sounds
   e. Turning off nasogastric suction before auscultating bowel sounds
   f. Questioning significant others regarding memory loss or changes in behavior of client when assessing the neurologic system
   g. Placing all tubings and drains on the scale when obtaining a weight using a bed scale
   h. Performing invasive procedures with the toddler or preschooler before auscultating heart sounds
   i. Assessing level of consciousness by questioning the client about the current date and place
   j. Weighing a client before voiding

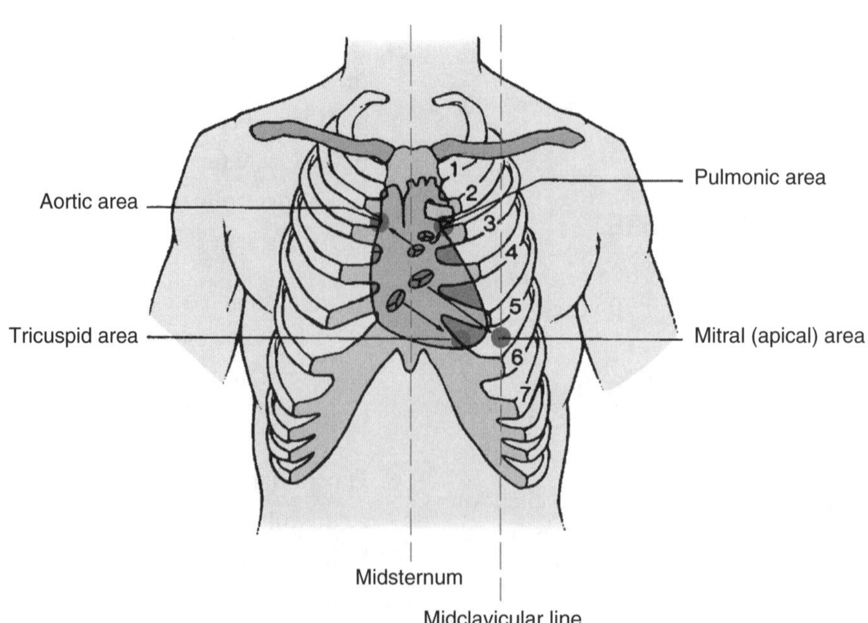

2. To better assess low-frequency sounds, the nurse should take which action(s)?
   a. Lower the head of the client's bed to amplify sounds.
   b. Listen to the sounds without the use of the equipment.
   c. Use the bell of the stethoscope.
   d. Use the diaphragm of the stethoscope.

3. When assessing the abdomen, which technique(s) is/are appropriate?
   a. Auscultating for bowel sounds first
   b. Palpating for abdominal masses first
   c. Percussing for gas or bladder distention first
   d. Positioning the client in lateral Sims position first

HOT SPOT QUESTIONS

Indicate by placing the appropriate letter over the area you would auscultate to locate the requested heart sounds

a. Tricuspid
b. Mitral
c. Aortic
d. Pulmonic

CHAPTER 27

Vital Sign Assessment

CHAPTER OVERVIEW

Chapter 27 examines and summarizes the significance of vital sign assessment to the process of clinical decision making. Factors influencing vital sign findings and techniques for accurate assessment are also presented.

LEARNING OBJECTIVES

After mastering the content in this chapter, you should be able to do the following:

1. Describe the procedures used to assess the vital signs: temperature, pulse, respirations, and blood pressure.
2. Describe factors that can influence each vital sign.
3. Identify equipment routinely used to assess vital signs.
4. Identify rationales for using different routes for temperature assessment.
5. Identify the location of commonly assessed pulse sites.
6. Describe how to assess orthostatic hypotension.
7. Recognize normal vital sign values associated with various age groups.

■ Mastering the Information

MATCHING

Match the terms in Column II with a definition, example, or related statement from Column I. Place the letter corresponding to the answer in the space provided.

COLUMN I

1. ______ The body's built-in thermostat
2. ______ Affects both the pulse rate and blood pressure
3. ______ Pulse rate below 60
4. ______ The amount of air moving in and out with each breath
5. ______ Pulse rate above 100
6. ______ Fluctuations in pulse that correlate with inspirations and expirations
7. ______ Absence of respirations
8. ______ Abnormal breath sounds associated with partially obstructed lower airways
9. ______ Breathing pattern characterized by increased rate and depth
10. ______ Difficulty breathing

COLUMN II

a. Apnea
b. Tachycardia
c. Dyspnea
d. Bradycardia
e. Hypothalamus
f. Autonomic nervous system
g. Sinus arrhythmia
h. Tidal volume
i. Kussmaul respirations
j. Wheezing

TRUE–FALSE

Indicate if the following statements are true or false.

_____ 1. An irregular pulse should be counted for a full minute, preferably at the apical site.

_____ 2. A pulse deficit is the mathematical difference between the systolic and diastolic pressure readings.

_____ 3. The rectal glass thermometer tip is blunt to decrease trauma to the rectal mucosa.

_____ 4. When checking for orthostatic hypotension, if the client appears unsteady, you should check the blood pressure and then return the client to the supine position.

_____ 5. Simultaneous bilateral palpation of the carotid pulses can seriously impair blood flow to the brain.

_____ 6. When assessing a young child's vital signs, the respirations and pulse should be taken first because they are the least invasive.

_____ 7. Stressed or anxious clients may have an elevated temperature without an underlying pathology.

_____ 8. In people with healthy respiratory systems, the normal stimulus to breathe is hypoxia, a decreased O_2 level.

_____ 9. People living at high altitudes, such as in the mountains, compensate for changes in O_2 needs by decreasing their respiratory rate.

_____ 10. Infants' respiratory rates are slower than those of adults because the need for O_2 is not as great.

FILL IN THE BLANK

Supply the missing term or the information requested.

1. _______________, _______________, and _______________ are three external factors that are believed to affect body temperature measurement.
2. A person's temperature is usually lowest around _______________ and highest from _______________ to _______________.
3. Identify four of nine sites where the pulse is commonly assessed. Also describe how each pulse is located.

   a.

   b.

   c.

   d.
4. Identify four of eight factors that can affect respiratory rate, rhythm, and depth.

   a.

   b.

   c.

   d.

■ Applying Your Knowledge

CASE STUDY

Mrs. Franklin, 55 years old, is hospitalized for a chronic respiratory condition. The assessment data are collected at 4:00 PM.

Respiratory
Objective
Increased anterior and posterior diameter of the chest with barrel-shaped appearance
Respiration 28 per minute
Oxygen at 1 L/minute nasal cannula
Sitting in upright position to breathe
Adventitious breath sounds
Subjective
"When I get up from the chair I get really short of breath."
Cardiovascular
Objective
Pulse 110 apical
Radial pulse 102
Pulse is irregular; 2+ quality
Blood pressure 140/90 mm Hg lying, 136/80 mm Hg standing
Subjective
"I am very anxious this evening."
"I feel dizzy when moving from the bed to the chair."

1. The nurse obtains a temperature reading of 38°C.
   a. Explain the most appropriate technique to obtain Mrs. Franklin's temperature.
   b. Convert the temperature reading to °F.

2. Discuss how Mrs. Franklin's subjective assessment data will affect vital signs.

3. Discuss Mrs. Franklin's abnormal assessment finding in relation to the following terms:
   a. Orthostatic hypotension
   b. Tachycardia
   c. Dyspnea
   d. Pulse deficit

4. State appropriate nursing strategies as indicated.

5. Discuss all additional factors that will affect Mrs. Franklin's vital signs. Include lifespan development.

CRITICAL INQUIRY EXERCISE

1. Design a teaching plan for a family member of a client being discharged home who will be required to have vital signs assessed on a daily basis. Highlight the following points:
   a. Correct use of equipment
   b. Correct measurement of vital signs
   c. Care of equipment
   d. Situations requiring notification of the physician

CRITICAL EXPLORATION EXERCISE

Assess vital signs for a client in each of the following groups: infant, athlete, and elderly. Compare your findings among the clients. Identify similarities and differences. Provide rationales for the differences identified.

■ Practicing for NCLEX

MULTIPLE CHOICE QUESTIONS

Circle the letter that corresponds to the best answer for each question.

1. Mr. Sykes, in room 252, had nasal surgery yesterday and has nasal packings in both nostrils that cannot be removed. Based on this information, you know
   a. Mr. Sykes should not have his temperature assessed until the nasal packings are removed.
   b. Mr. Sykes should have his temperature assessed at the axillary site.
   c. assessment of an oral temperature is contraindicated for Mr. Sykes.
   d. the oral route for temperature assessment is acceptable; however, Mr. Sykes should take several deep breaths before the nurse checks his temperature.

2. Irregularities in the heart rhythm may be related to which of the following?
   a. An overstimulation of the parasympathetic nervous system
   b. Heart disease, medications, and electrolyte imbalances
   c. Oxygen administration by mask or cannula
   d. Inadequate reflex compensation to position change

3. The client who has received a narcotic is most likely to experience which of the following?
   a. Decreased respiratory rate
   b. Kussmaul respirations
   c. Tachycardia
   d. Pulmonary congestion

4. False high blood pressure measurements may be the result of all the following except
   a. the arm positioned below the level of the heart.
   b. a blood pressure cuff that is too small.
   c. the client in the supine position.
   d. a client whose arm is not supported during assessment while sitting or standing.

5. Which is believed to be the most reliable route of temperature assessment?
   a. Oral
   b. Axillary
   c. Rectal
   d. There is no significant difference in reliability among the three routes.

6. The amount of blood ejected from each ventricle with each heartbeat is referred to as
   a. stroke volume.
   b. cardiac output.
   c. perfusion volume.
   d. effective circulating volume.

7. A cyclic breathing pattern characterized by shallow breathing alternating with periods of apnea is referred to as
   a. Biot's.
   b. Cheyne-Stokes.
   c. Kussmaul.
   d. respiratory failure.

8. The tip of the oral thermometer is ________ and may be color coded ________.
   a. blunt, blue
   b. blunt, red
   c. slender, blue
   d. slender, red

9. When assessing for a pulse deficit, the nurse should
   a. simultaneously count the apical and radial pulse.
   b. count pulsations at or after completion of the selected time interval.
   c. count the pulse for 15 seconds and multiply by 4, if the pulse is regular.
   d. ask another nurse to help and count for 1 full minute.

10. When assessing the respiratory rate of an adult, the nurse should
    a. instruct the client to breathe in and out of his or her mouth.
    b. count for 30 seconds and multiply by 2, if the respirations are irregular.
    c. tell the client that you are preparing to measure his or her breathing rate.
    d. observe the sternal notch in clients whose respirations are shallow.

FILL IN THE BLANK

Supply the missing term or the information requested.

1. Ms. Lee has just finished her daily cup of coffee. How long should you wait before taking her temperature? ________________
2. How much time should elapse before sequential cuff inflation on any one limb during blood pressure measurement? __________________
3. Mr. Beasley is admitted to your unit with a diagnosis of congestive heart failure. When assessing his pulse, you note that it is thready, weak, and easily obliterated with pressure. The quality of this pulse is _____t.
4. The Celsius conversion for a temperature of 99°F is _________.
5. The normal range of respiratory rate for an adult at rest is _______.

MULTIPLE-ANSWER MULTIPLE CHOICE

Circle the letter(s) corresponding to the appropriate answer(s). Circle all that apply.

1. When assessing the blood pressure, the nurse should do which of the following?
   a. Use the bell of the stethoscope
   b. Inflate the cuff 30 mm Hg higher than the point at which the pulse disappears
   c. Palpate the radial or brachial pulse during inflation of the cuff
   d. Inflate the cuff to between 180 and 200 mm Hg

ORDERING

Items A through J are key steps to follow when assessing the client's blood pressure. Read the list carefully. Place each step in the correct sequence by numbering the items.

a. ______ Wrap the deflated cuff snugly around the upper arm.

b. ______ Inflate the cuff until the brachial pulse is no longer palpable, then inflate the cuff 30 mm Hg more.

c. ______ Record the blood pressure.

d. ______ Identify the systolic and diastolic pressure readings.

e. ______ Slowly release valve and note reading when pulse reappears.

f. ______ Fully deflate the cuff and wait 1 to 2 minutes.

g. ______ Deflate the cuff and remove it from the client's arm.

g. ______ Repalpate the brachial pulse, and place the stethoscope bell over the site.

i. ______ Slowly release the valve so the pressure drops 2 to 3 mm Hg.

j. ______ Reinflate the cuff 30 mm Hg above the reading where the brachial pulse disappeared.

UNIT VI

Selected Clinical Nursing Therapeutics

CHAPTER 28

Asepsis and Infection Control

CHAPTER OVERVIEW

Chapter 28 discusses nursing practices aimed at providing a safe and therapeutic environment designed to protect clients, family members, and healthcare providers from acquiring infections.

LEARNING OBJECTIVES

After mastering the content in this chapter, you should be able to do the following:

1. Identify the six components of the chain of infection.
2. Explain examples of ways that infection may occur.
3. Describe factors that increase the risk of infection in various settings.
4. Discuss the role of healthcare personnel and health agencies in infection control.
5. Identify ways that caregivers can increase their protection against infectious exposure.
6. Explain ways that caregivers can decrease the exposure of clients to infection.
7. Differentiate between medical and surgical asepsis.
8. Demonstrate good handwashing technique and incorporate it as an integral part of practice.
9. Describe appropriate situations for using cleaning, disinfection, and sterilization.
10. Discuss the two-tiered system of isolation.
11. Identify age-related considerations in preventing the transmission of infectious diseases.

■ Mastering the Information

MATCHING

Match the terms in Column I with a definition or related statement from Column II. Place the letter corresponding to the answer in the space provided.

COLUMN I

1. __e__ Medical asepsis
2. __d__ Antiseptic
3. __a__ Disinfection
4. __c__ Infectious disease
5. __b__ Nosocomial infections

COLUMN II

a. The process used to reduce the number of potential pathogens from the surface of an object, usually by chemical or physical means

b. Infections associated with healthcare delivery settings

c. The pathology or pathologic events that result from the invasion and multiplication of microorganisms in a host

d. A chemical used on living objects

e. Also known as "clean technique"

COLUMN I

1. f Retards bacterial growth on living organism
2. b An agent that prevents bacterial multiplication but does not kill all forms of the organism
3. a A chemical agent that kills microorganisms
4. d Microorganisms that are capable of harming people
5. e Poisoning of tissue
6. c A chemical used on lifeless objects

COLUMN II

a. Bactericidal agent
b. Bacteriostatic agent
c. Disinfectant
d. Pathogens
e. Sepsis
f. Antiseptic

COLUMN I

1. d Refers to measures to control and reduce the number of pathogenic organisms present
2. a The complete destruction of all microorganisms, leaving no viable form of organisms, including spores
3. b Used when microorganisms are transmitted by small particle droplets
4. e An object must be free of all microorganisms, and a person must be as free as possible of microorganisms
5. c Used when microorganisms are transmitted by large particle droplets

COLUMN II

a. Sterilization
b. Airborne precautions
c. Droplet precautions
d. Medical asepsis
e. Surgical asepsis

TRUE–FALSE

Indicate if the following statements are true or false.

F 1. Infectious exposure and risk of contracting infectious disease remain the same throughout a person's lifespan.

T 2. Sources of organisms, also called reservoirs, are elements in the environment.

T 3. Infections always are passed from one person to another more easily in a hospital than in the community.

T 4. Clean, nonsterile gloves should be worn when direct contact with moist body substances from any client is anticipated.

T 5. A child is being cared for under protective isolation. This means that he/she cannot have fresh fruits and vegetables.

T 6. Never recap a needle or sharp object after use on a client because such an action increases possible exposure to infection.

T 7. Hazardous wastes come from healthcare facilities.

T 8. Waterproof, disposable bagging is used for contaminated linen to contain pathogens and protect hospital personnel from contamination.

T 9. Isolation procedures and barrier practices are important in preventing the spread of infection.

T 10. Institutional waste disposal methods are important factors in infection control.

FILL IN THE BLANK

Supply the missing term or the information requested.

1. Regulatory agencies at Local/State, regional, provincial, and national levels are involved in the control of infection and institutional waste to protect clients, staff, and the community.

2. Each department in the hospital must have written policies and procedures for the control of infection.

3. Employee health programs that monitor and counsel personnel are important components of institutional and community infection-control programs.

4. Handwashing techniques should be learned by all healthcare persoinel, the client, and care provider.

5. Cleaning, disinfection, and sterilization can be accomplished by various methods and agents.

6. The psychological effects of isolation may include clients feeling dirty or untouchable.

7. The chain of infection includes the infectious agent, the source, the portal of exit, the mode of transmission, the portal of entry, and a susceptable host.

8. The risk factors that contribute to the development of nosocomial infections are grouped into three categories: those in the environment, those related to the theraputic regimen, and those related to the resistance of the client.

9. Six of the seven types of infectious institutional waste are blood, lab cultures, body parts from surgery, contaminated equipment, food, and diapers.

10. Common chemical disinfectants include chlorine, formaldehyde, and glutaraldehyde.

■ Applying Your Knowledge

CASE STUDY

Client A: A client is on isolation precaution because of wound infection. Wounds are draining large amounts of white drainage with foul odor. Dressing changes are done three times a day and prn.

Client B: A client on the fourth day after abdominal surgery has a temperature of 102.8°F. The abdominal incision is free of redness and intact with approximate edges. A Foley catheter was inserted during surgery and discontinued 3 days after surgery.

Client C: A client with cancer who is receiving chemotherapy and radiation treatments is admitted with low WBC and an open skin area on the coccyx (stage 2 ulcer).

1. Discuss how the chain of infection may occur in each of the above clients.
2. Isolation may be ordered for the above clients. Determine which client(s) may require isolation and the type of isolation needed.
3. Identify ways to use medical asepsis, surgical asepsis, or both when caring for each client.
4. Discuss the risk of nosocomial infections for all three clients.
5. Identify ways the nurse can decrease infection exposure for each client.

CRITICAL INQUIRY EXERCISE

1. Interview an infection-control nurse regarding the role and responsibilities of the job.
2. Interview an Environmental Protection Agency worker.

CRITICAL EXPLORATION

1. Obtain and review a finger-stick incident report from your instructor or a local healthcare facility.
2. Follow a client from the ward to the surgical waiting area and then to the operating room table. Note the measures taken to minimize postoperative infections.
3. Accompany a client in the labor and delivery suite. Note the measures taken to protect the mother and newborn from infection.

■ Practicing for NCLEX

MULTIPLE CHOICE QUESTIONS

Circle the letter that corresponds to the best answer for each question.

1. The most effective way to prevent the spread of infection is
   a. autoclaving.
   b. disinfecting.
   c. immunizing.
   d. handwashing.

2. The most frequent mode of transmission in healthcare facilities is contact transmission of infectious organisms on
   a. hands of personnel or clients.
   b. linens and towels.
   c. personal articles.
   d. equipment and supplies.

3. When all organisms and their spores are destroyed on an object, it is said to be
   a. aseptic.
   b. sterile.
   c. disinfected.
   d. decontaminated.

4. The physician requests a pair of sterile scissors. A pair of scissors found at the bedside is in an original factory wrapping that has been opened but taped closed again. Which of the following should the nurse do?
   a. Check the hospital policy manual regarding use of opened supplies.
   b. Obtain a pair of sterile scissors that have not been opened.
   c. Provide the scissors to the physician because they are available and probably have not been used.
   d. Question another nurse regarding the sterility of the scissors found at the bedside.

5. A visiting nurse is in a home where there is no running water. Which of the following may be used as an alternative to handwashing?
   a. Wipe hands slowly with newspaper or tissue
   b. Wipe hands thoroughly with dry paper towels
   c. Wipe hands with a wipe or alcohol swabs
   d. Wipe hands with a dry washcloth or sterile gauze

6. The Joint Committee on Accreditation of Healthcare Organizations and the Centers for Disease Control published guidelines for storage, cleaning, and disinfection and for
   a. layouts of client rooms in the healthcare setting.
   b. lighting that is considered adequate.
   c. use of equipment and supplies in healthcare.
   d. handling of healthcare equipment.

7. Which of the following nurses may not be allowed to work with clients who have diseases such as rubella, hepatitis B, or AIDS?
   a. Recently graduated nurse
   b. Licensed practical nurse
   c. Associate-degree nurse
   d. Pregnant nurse

8. Healthcare workers with exudative lesions or weeping dermatitis should refrain from direct care and handling of client care equipment until
   a. all redness has disappeared.
   b. the lesions and condition resolve.
   c. the supervisor sees the lesions.
   d. the amount of exudate diminishes.

9. Employees who work in high-risk areas, such as pediatric wards, dialysis units, or transplant units, can be required to
   a. demonstrate skill in donning gown and gloves as a condition of employment.
   b. identify common disinfectants and antiseptics as a condition of employment.
   c. prove immunization currency as a condition of employment.
   d. show knowledge of barrier nursing as a condition of employment.

10. The effectiveness of a surgical scrub is determined by which of the following?
   a. The length of time a person scrubs, type of antiseptic used, and length of fingernails
   b. Adequacy of friction, thoroughness of surfaces cleansed, and minimum duration of use of antiseptic
   c. Amount of water used, the type of cleansing agent, and the interest of the healthcare worker
   d. The length of time a person scrubs, the type of antiseptic used, and the educational status of the caregiver

FILL IN THE BLANK

Supply the missing term or the information requested.

1. Any item entering a sterile tissue or the vascular system must be Sterile
2. Sterile technique is used to prevent the introduction of microorganisms from the environment into the client.
3. Most long-term flora reside in the nailbed and under the fingernails.
4. antiseptic agents are used in skin preparation and surgical scrubs to reduce the number of transient microorganisms.
5. Medical and surgical asepsis vary in the technique for proper handwashing.
6. Infectous disease refers to pathology or pathologic events that result from the invasion and multiplication of a microorganism in a host.
7. Multicellular organisms that live on other organisms and are potentially pathogenic to humans are parasites.
8. Needlesticks are one of the most frequently occurring, potentially serious exposures for healthcare personnel and account for one third of healthcare accidents.
9. Any item that may come in contact with the mucous membrane or broken skin must be free of all microorganisms with the exception of Spores
10. Items that come in contact with the skin, such as bed linens or blood pressure cuffs, can be cleaned and reused.

MULTIPLE-ANSWER MULTIPLE CHOICE

Circle the letter(s) corresponding to the appropriate answer(s). Circle all that apply.

1. Indicate the substances that are common antiseptics.
   a. Povidone-iodine
   b. Sodium hydrochloride (Dakin's)
   c. Chlorhexidine gluconate (Hibiclens)
   d. Acetic acid
   e. Ammonia
   f. Hydrogen peroxide
   g. Hexachlorophene
   h. Alcohol

2. Which statement(s) is/are accurate?
   a. Room placement is not a major concern for clients with altered mental status or children younger than 5 years.
   b. Protective isolation is used to prevent a high-risk person from exposure to pathogens.
   c. A client on droplet precautions should wear a mask when outside the room.
   d. The nursing goals for clients in isolation should be directed at preventing the spread of microorganisms while maintaining the client's social support system.

CHAPTER 29

Medication Administration

CHAPTER OVERVIEW

Chapter 29 examines and summarizes the basic principles of medication administration. Use of the nursing process as a mechanism for facilitating safe medication administration is discussed. Particular emphasis is placed on the assessment process.

LEARNING OBJECTIVES

After mastering the content in this chapter, you should be able to do the following:

1. Describe essential components of a medication order.
2. Discuss pharmacokinetic principles of drug action.
3. List the five rights of proper medication administration.
4. Calculate proper drug dosage using different systems of drug measurement.
5. Discuss the importance of designing systems within healthcare institutions for medication administration that emphasize client safety.
6. Discuss important assessment data to obtain from the client during the initial interview and before medication administration.
7. Develop an individualized teaching plan to improve client knowledge of medications.
8. Describe recommended guidelines and procedures for medication administration by each route.
9. Incorporate evaluation of medication effectiveness and documentation into medication administration practices.

■ Mastering the Information

MATCHING

Match the terms in Column II with a definition, example, or related statement from Column I. Place the letter corresponding to the answer in the space provided.

COLUMN I

1. ______ The process of chemically changing the drug in the body
2. ______ A registered name assigned by the manufacturer
3. ______ A drug administered for therapeutic effects
4. ______ The delivery of medication to target cells and tissue
5. ______ Placing the pill under the tongue and allowing it to dissolve
6. ______ Medications given by injection or infusion
7. ______ Medication designed to absorb through the skin for a systemic effect

COLUMN II

a. Medication
b. Parenteral
c. Trade name
d. Metabolism
e. Sublingual
f. Distribution
g. Transdermal

TRUE–FALSE

Indicate if the following statements are true or false.

______ 1. A drug is a medication administered for its therapeutic effect.

______ 2. Telephone and verbal medication orders must be signed by the physician before the medication is actually given.

______ 3. Nurses have the right and responsibility to decline administering a medication if they feel it jeopardizes client safety.

_____ 4. When administering parenteral medication, strict asepsis must be implemented.

_____ 5. The ophthalmic medications are placed directly on the pupil in the eye for best absorption.

_____ 6. Liquid medication should never be placed in the rectum, only suppository forms.

_____ 7. Ampules are thin-walled glass containers that hold a single dose of a liquid medication.

_____ 8. IV medication should be prepared and packaged in a sterile manner and should not be prepared in an oil or aqueous suspension.

_____ 9. The intermittent infusion technique is used to infuse medication for continuous periods of time.

_____ 10. In community-based care, the client's physical condition may influence his or her ability to take medication as prescribed.

_____ 11. Medication toxicity occurs when a client develops a decreased response to a medication, requiring an increased dosage to achieve therapeutic effect.

_____ 12. Mild allergic reactions commonly manifested by hives (urticaria), pruritus, and rhinitis can occur within minutes to 2 weeks after administration.

FILL IN THE BLANK

Supply the missing term or the information requested.

1. List three ways in which medications may be classified.
   a. Clinical composition
   b. Clinical action
   c. Theraputic effect on body
2. Give the meaning of the following abbreviations:
   a. qid 4 x a day
   b. prn as needed
   c. SQ Subqutaneous
   d. OD right eye
   e. ac before meals
3. Describe the procedure for counting narcotics at the end of the shift. Count meds as Shift change
4. Metric, Apothecary and household are the three systems used to calculate drug dosages.
5. Identify the four steps the nurse should take to ensure safe administration of medications.
   a. interpret instructions
   b. 5 rights
   c. Calculate dosage
   d. document
6. Identify the information that is required by federal law to be included on narcotic control sheets.
   a. Name
   b. Date & hour given
   c. Doc's name
   d. Amt given
   e. Nurses name
7. Identify the five rights of medication administration.
   a. Dose
   b. Route
   c. Time
   d. Pt
   e. Med
8. Identify the two landmarks that are used when locating the dorsogluteal site.
   a. Post. illiac Spine
   b. Greater trochanter
9. All stated client allergies should be written on the Pt record, cover of record and ect.
10. Barcode, unit dose, auto med machine, and self-admin supply are the four systems used to ensure the safe storage and administration of medications.

■ Applying Your Knowledge

CASE STUDY

Mr. K. J. is discharged on the following medication:

Digoxin 25 mg p.o. every day
Lasix 20 mg p.o. every other day
Potassium 20 mEq twice a day
Verapamil 120 mg p.o. twice a day
Insulin: Humulin R 8 units and Humulin N 16 units before breakfast
Humulin R 8 units and Humulin N 8 units

The physician instructed Mr. K. J. to continue the following medications at home as needed:

Saline nose drops as needed every 3 to 4 hours
Lotrisone cream 2 to 3 times a day to affected area of skin
Polytrim ophthalmic solution 2 gtts into right eye 3 times a day

1. Determine if all of the above medications for Mr. K. J. have essential components before his discharge.
2. Discuss community-based care for Mr. K. J. to include psychosocial, physical, and financial conditions that may influence the client's compliance with medication regimens.
3. Discuss assessment data to obtain from Mr. K. J. if you were readmitting him to the hospital for diagnostic tests requiring him to remain NPO.
    a. Which of the above medications will require monitoring of drug levels?
    b. Discuss the physical assessment finding that should be considered before medication administration.
4. Describe guidelines for safely administering the above medications to Mr. K. J.-oral, topical, nasal, SQ, ophthalmic.

CRITICAL INQUIRY EXERCISE

During a clinical experience, observe the process used for checking narcotics at the change of shift. Document your observations. Is the process effective? Why or why not?

CRITICAL EXPLORATION EXERCISE

Develop an individualized teaching plan for the client who is to be discharged on home medications. Provide rationales for strategies and interventions used.

■ Practicing for NCLEX

MULTIPLE CHOICE QUESTIONS

Circle the letter that corresponds to the best answer for each question.

1. A system of medication distribution in which the medication is prelabeled and prepackaged in individual doses by the pharmacy is referred to as
    a. self-administered medication.
    b. stock supply.
    c. unit dose.
    d. Safe-T-Dose.
2. Which of the following dangers is associated with the use of over-the-counter medications?
    a. Considered unsafe when used as directed
    b. Illegal use of the drug
    c. Serious drug interactions
    d. Should be used under the supervision of a nurse
3. What component of the following drug order is missing? Order: Ampicillin 500 mg every 12 h.
    a. Frequency of administration
    b. Route of administration
    c. Stop date
    d. Strength of dose
4. A single order for a medication that is to be given immediately is referred to as a
    a. one-time order.
    b. prn order.
    c. standing order.
    d. stat order.
5. In the hospital setting, narcotics are kept where as a safety measure?
    a. Nursing service
    b. Hospital pharmacy
    c. Medication drawer at the client's bedside
    d. Locked drawer or box

6. A second nurse is required to witness and countersign the narcotic sheet when
   a. any narcotic is given.
   b. the primary nurse is suspected of drug abuse.
   c. all or part of a narcotic is to be discarded.
   d. a nonprescription pain medication is administered.

7. The primary site of medication metabolism is the
   a. intestines.
   b. liver.
   c. lungs.
   d. kidneys.

8. The primary site of drug excretion is the
   a. intestines.
   b. liver.
   c. lungs.
   d. kidneys.

9. Mrs. Lewis, age 70 years, is admitted with a diagnosis of acute renal failure. Based on this information, you know that Mrs. Lewis should be monitored closely for signs of
   a. drug intolerance.
   b. gastric irritation.
   c. drug toxicity.
   d. polyuria.

10. Which of the following medications require that you assess the pulse before administering it?
    a. Ampicillin
    b. Digoxin
    c. Insulin
    d. Nitroglycerin

11. When pouring a liquid medication, you should measure from which of the following?
    a. From the top of the medication cup
    b. From the top of the meniscus
    c. From the bottom of the meniscus
    d. From the middle of the medication cup

12. Medication absorption is most rapid when given by which route?
    a. By mouth
    b. Intravenously
    c. Intramuscularly
    d. Subcutaneously

13. Mr. Haddock is to receive 250 mg of erythromycin "po tid c- meals." This means which of the following?
    a. By mouth with meals every third day
    b. Before meals three times a day
    c. By mouth with meals three times a day
    d. By mouth after meals three times per week

14. When receiving oral medications through a nasogastric tube, the client should be assisted to which of the following positions?
    a. Fowler's
    b. Dorsal recumbent
    c. Supine
    d. Sims

FILL IN THE BLANK

Supply the missing term or the information requested.

1. Ms. Lucky is to receive Demerol 75 mg IM. On hand you have Demerol 100 mg/mL. How many milliliters should Ms. Lucky receive? __________
2. ________________ refers to the physiologic and biochemical effects of a drug on the body.
3. ________________ is the desired effects of a medication.
4. ________________ is the process by which the drug moves through the body and is eliminated.
5. ________________ result from an immunologic response to a medication to which the client has been sensitized.
6. A ________________, or nonproprietary, name is simpler than the chemical name from which it is often derived.

MULTIPLE-ANSWER MULTIPLE CHOICE

Circle the letter(s) corresponding to the appropriate answer(s). Circle all that apply.

1. After administering an injection, the nurse should
   a. dispose of the syringe and needle in a needle disposal box.
   b. recap the needle before disposal.
   c. break the needle before disposal.
   d. throw the needle in a disposal box and the syringe in the trash.

ORDERING

Items A through E are key steps to follow when drawing up two medications in one syringe. Read the list carefully. Place each step in the correct sequence by numbering the items.

a. ______ Aspirate a volume of air equal to the medication dose from the first medication (vial A). Inject air into the vial.

b. ______ Aspirate a volume of air equal to the medication dose from the second medication (vial B). Inject air into vial B.

c. ______ Clean the tops of the vials.

d. ______ Insert the needle into vial A, invert the vial, and withdraw the required volume of medication.

e. ______ Invert vial B and withdraw the required volume.

CHAPTER 30

Intravenous Therapy

CHAPTER OVERVIEW

Chapter 30 discusses the basic concepts of intravenous therapy. The equipment and procedure needed for initiation and maintenance of fluid therapy are outlined, as is the procedure for the discontinuation of infusion therapy. A discussion of central line transfusions and blood administration issues and procedures is also provided.

LEARNING OBJECTIVES

After mastering the content in this chapter, you should be able to do the following:

1. Explain the purpose of intravenous infusion therapy.
2. Identify the two major types of solutions administered intravenously.
3. List equipment necessary to administer peripheral and central intravenous therapy.
4. State guidelines for site selection in venipuncture.
5. Outline the nurse's role in initiating, monitoring, maintaining, and discontinuing intravenous therapy.
6. Describe potential complications of intravenous therapy, total parenteral nutrition, and blood transfusions.
7. Identify principles of client and family education associated with intravenous therapy.

■ Mastering the Information

MATCHING

Match the terms in Column II with a definition, example, or related statement from Column I. Place the letter corresponding to the answer in the space provided.

COLUMN I

1. e Peripheral insertion device
2. a Delivers 60 drops per mL
3. f Plasma protein that contains factor VIII
4. b Isotonic fluid that is compatible with blood and blood products
5. d Plasma protein found in the plasma
6. g Hickman or Broviac are examples of these
7. c Hypotonic fluid

COLUMN II

a. Minidrip
b. Normal saline
c. D5W
d. Albumin
e. Over-the-needle catheter
f. Cryoprecipitate
g. Central venous catheter

TRUE–FALSE

Indicate if the following statements are true or false.

F 1. Febrile reactions can occur because of the recipient's hypersensitivity to the donor's white blood cells and should be considered life threatening.

F 2. To prepare an IV site, 70% alcohol should be used, instead of povidone-iodine, because it is a better bactericide.

F 3. Implanted vascular access devices allow long-term access, and because the catheter protrudes from the skin, they allow ease of medication administration.

T 4. A 22-gauge needle is smaller in diameter than an 18-gauge needle.

T 5. When choosing a venipuncture site, the distal portion of a vein is punctured first, leaving the more proximal sites for later.

F 6. Hypertonic solutions are administered when a client requires cellular hydration.

F 7. Alarms on intravenous infusion pumps may be turned off until the underlying problem is discovered.

F 8. Absence of a backflow of blood into the tubing when the IV bag is lowered below the level of infusion is diagnostic of IV infiltration.

FILL IN THE BLANK

Supply the missing term or the information requested.

1. Identify the three different crystalloid solutions and give an example of each.

   a. Isotonic
   b. Hypotonic
   c. Hypertonic

2. Identify three of the six access devices used for intravenous (IV) infusion.

   a. peripheral insertion device
   b. intermittent infusion &
   c. central venous catheter

3. Identify three of the six reasons for initiating IV therapy.

   a. adequate fluid intake
   b. electrolyte balance
   c. glucose for energy

4. Identify four of six factors, besides the drip factor, that can affect the rate of an IV infusion.

   a. clossed air vent
   b. position of extremety
   c. kink in tubing
   d. height of IV bottle

■ Applying Your Knowledge

CASE STUDY

Jamal Reed is a 6-year-old boy with sickle cell anemia. He is admitted with pain in his joints caused by blood clotting in the small blood vessels in the knees and elbows. He is placed on IV fluids at 250 mL/hour. He is ordered to have a complete blood count.

1. Design a teaching plan to explain to Jamal his IV therapy and the activity limitations needed to avoid and detect complications.
2. Describe each blood component in the body, and indicate why each component may be administered.
3. Determine the information you would need to calculate the drip rate for Jamal's IV, and outline measures that might be taken to ensure accurate delivery of fluid volume and prevent fluid overload.

CRITICAL INQUIRY EXERCISE

Interview a colleague, relative, or friend who has experienced an IV infusion for at least 42 hours. List their subjective and objective responses.

CRITICAL EXPLORATION EXERCISE

1. Examine two of your assigned clients in the clinical area and determine:
   a. two possible locations for an IV catheter insertion.
   b. the best size catheter needed for each client.
2. Ask a classmate to assess the same clients and compare results.

■ Practicing for NCLEX

MULTIPLE CHOICE QUESTIONS

Circle the letter that corresponds to the best answer for each question.

1. Phlebitis can be reduced if which of the following is done?
   a. Large veins rather than small veins are used.
   b. Catheters rather than needles are used for starting IV infusions.
   c. The IV site is not disturbed until permanently discontinued.
   d. The IV rate is increased 10 mL/hour greater than the prescribed rate.

2. Which of the following interventions is appropriate for the client exhibiting signs and symptoms of an air embolism?
   a. Have the client stand up and take deep breaths.
   b. Place the client on his or her left side with head down.
   c. Place the client on his or her back with the head of the bed elevated.
   d. Place the client in the prone position.

3. A factor that does not affect flow rate is
   a. position of the extremity.
   b. tonicity of IV fluid.
   c. patency of the catheter.
   d. the solution container.

4. Ms. Lucky has an IV of 0.9% NaCl ordered to infuse at 125 mL/hour. The nurse, during the initial assessment, discovers that Ms. Lucky's IV is 125 mL behind. The most appropriate intervention would be
   a. to regulate the IV rate to 250 mL/hour for 1 hour then adjust the rate to 125 mL/hour and notify the physician.
   b. to regulate the IV to 140 mL/hour for the next 8 hours and notify the physician.
   c. to regulate the IV to 125 mL/hour and refer to hospital policy for further actions.
   d. not to alter the IV in any way.

5. A 500-mL bag of IV fluids would be most appropriate for administering fluids to
   a. Stephanie, who is to receive 5% dextrose in water at a rate of 20 mL/hour.
   b. Lewis, who is to receive a blood transfusion.
   c. Dominique, who is to receive 1000 mL of one-half normal saline.
   d. Kyle, who is to receive 0.9% NaCl at 125 mL/hour.

FILL IN THE BLANK

Supply the missing term or the information requested.

1. The colloid solutions include blood products and parenteral nutrition
2. When peripheral vein access is not available or when long-term venous therapy is anticipated, medication may be given through a Central venous access device.

MULTIPLE-ANSWER MULTIPLE CHOICE

Circle the letter(s) corresponding to the appropriate answer(s). Circle all that apply.

1. Which of the following are signs of fluid volume overload?
   a. Warm, moist skin
   b. Flat neck veins
   c. Dyspnea
   d. Crackles in lung bases

2. Before an infusion is discontinued, the nurse should
   a. apply a warm compress to the site.
   b. put on disposable gloves.
   c. check for catheter breakage or damage.
   d. document the time the IV will be discontinued.

3. Ten minutes after the beginning of a blood transfusion, the client reports a headache and chills. The client also has an elevated temperature. This client shows symptoms of which condition?
   a. A febrile reaction
   b. An allergic reaction
   c. A hemolytic reaction
   d. Circulatory overload

ORDERING

Items a through l are key steps to follow when changing IV solutions and tubing. Read the list carefully. Place each step in the correct sequence by numbering the items.

a. ______ Spike the tubing into the blood component container.

b. ______ Close the roller clamp on the existing tubing.

c. ______ Compare the solution with the physician's order.

d. ______ Prime the drip chamber with blood component.

e. ______ Spike the saline container keeping the roller clamp shut.

f. ______ Regulate the infusion according to the physician's orders.

g. ______ Flush the tubing with blood component.

h. ______ Close the roller clamp on the new tubing.

i. ______ Disconnect the old tubing from the needle hub.

j. ______ Secure the tubing with tape.

k. ______ Document the procedure.

l. ______ Insert the new tubing into the needle hub.

CHAPTER 31

Perioperative Nursing

CHAPTER OVERVIEW

Chapter 31 describes key concepts in providing care for the surgical client preoperatively, intraoperatively, and postoperatively. Auxiliary aspects of perioperative nursing are discussed, including client preparation, equipment and supplies, physiologic considerations, and possible complications.

LEARNING OBJECTIVES

After mastering the content in this chapter, you should be able to do the following:

1. Describe the three phases of perioperative client management.
2. Discuss the effects of surgery on health and function.
3. Identify lifespan considerations for the client undergoing a surgical procedure.
4. Describe appropriate perioperative client teaching.
5. Discuss emotional support, safety, and asepsis during the intraoperative phase.
6. Identify appropriate nursing assessments in the recovery facility and during the postoperative period.
7. List common postoperative complications and appropriate nursing care to promote normal function.
8. Develop an appropriate discharge plan for the surgical client.

■ Mastering the Information

MATCHING

Match the terms in Column II with a definition, description, or related statement from Column I. Place the letter corresponding to the answer in the space provided.

COLUMN I

1. ______ Type of surgery that confirms the type and extent of a disease
2. ______ Rhinoplasty, mammography, skin grafting
3. ______ Amnesic, excited, surgical, and toxic
4. ______ Repair of fracture
5. ______ Injection of a local anesthetic agent into the subarachnoid space
6. ______ Period extending from the time the decision is made to have surgery to the client's recovery from the surgical intervention
7. ______ Inserted close to the incision and made of stainless steel
8. ______ Common type of anesthesia for a simple biopsy or cataract extraction
9. ______ Operative consent form completed during this period
10. ______ Example of type of surgery that includes appendectomy, hysterectomy, and fracture fixation

COLUMN II

a. Skin staples
b. Spinal anesthesia
c. Urgent
d. Reconstructive
e. Nerve bundle block (local)
f. Explorative
g. Preoperative
h. Curative
i. Stages of anesthesia
j. Perioperative

FILL IN THE BLANK

Supply the missing term or the information requested.

1. Perioperative nursing involves three distinct phases: ________________, ________________, and ________________.
2. Although the scrub and circulating nurses have different specific tasks, they share the responsibility for accounting for all ________________ and ________________ at the close of surgery.
3. Identify five of the nine factors that may contribute to hypothermia in the surgical theater/operating room (OR).
   a.
   b.
   c.
   d.
   e.
4. Adequate intravascular volume and blood pressure are indicated by an output of ________ to __________ mL/hour.
5. Preoperative preparation of the client includes starting _________ access, ensuring _________ status, administering ____________________ medications, and initiating bowel and ______________ preps.
6. ________________ are especially helpful during the intraoperative phase when wound closure is occurring.
7. Identify five of the six elements of information the recovery room (RR) nurse will need to know to plan care effectively.
   a.
   b.
   c.
   d.
   e.
8. Identify the six requirements that must be met before a client is discharged from an ambulatory surgical unit.
   a.
   b.
   c.
   d.
   e.
   f.
9. Normally, a bowel movement should occur ________________ days after resuming a normal diet.
10. The nurse may employ nonpharmacologic techniques in pain management that may include ________________ and ________________.

■ Applying Your Knowledge

CASE STUDY

Ms. Jones, age 28 years, is pregnant with her first child. She is admitted to the hospital because she has gone into labor. During labor, the monitor reveals that the fetus is in distress. An emergency cesarean section is scheduled. Ms. Jones arrives in the operating room with tears in her eyes. She is shivering and states, "I am scared."

1. As the circulating nurse in the operating room, describe how you can best meet the emotional needs of Ms. Jones.
2. Discuss the outcome criteria that will indicate that Ms. Jones' emotional needs are being met.

CRITICAL EXPLORATION EXERCISE

1. Accompany a client perioperatively, noting the role of the nurse at each phase of the process. Identify the varying needs of the client at each level, and provide rationales for the targeted solutions.
2. Design a discharge care plan for an abdominal surgery client whose background is culturally or ethnically different from your own.

■ Practicing for NCLEX

MULTIPLE CHOICE QUESTIONS

Circle the letter that corresponds to the best answer for each question.

1. Optimal nutrition benefits the surgical client by
   a. encouraging carbohydrate anabolism.
   b. encouraging protein anabolism.
   c. promoting gastrointestinal motility.
   d. promoting wound healing.

2. Brittany Henderson, 3 years old, is scheduled for an open lung biopsy at 8:00 AM. When the circulating nurse arrives to take her to the OR, Brittany grabs her mother's neck and begins screaming hysterically. The nurse realizes that Brittany is
   a. having a temper tantrum.
   b. probably experiencing a normal separation anxiety.
   c. overstimulated and tired.
   d. attempting to manipulate her mother.

3. Clients who are candidates for an emergency surgical procedure whose NPO status is unknown usually receive
   a. bowel prep.
   b. laxative.
   c. nasogastric tube.
   d. rectal tube.

4. Morris West has arrived in OR 8 for an exploratory laparotomy. The circulating nurse has a primary duty to
   a. evaluate tubes for patency.
   b. locate laboratory studies.
   c. review the client's chart for history of the illness.
   d. protect the client's health and safety needs.

5. Regional anesthetics have the advantage of minimizing the complications that sometimes occur with general anesthesia, in particular, ________ complications.
   a. pulmonary and gastrointestinal
   b. metabolic and musculoskeletal
   c. endocrine and genitourinary
   d. cardiac and endocrine

6. Janet DuBois is scheduled for an endoscopy at 9:00 AM. This type of surgery is classified as
   a. curative.
   b. exploratory.
   c. diagnostic.
   d. palliative.

7. The amnesia stage of analgesia occurs when?
   a. First
   b. Fourth
   c. Second
   d. Third

8. As the scrub nurse, you know that ________ helps to minimize the time the client is under anesthesia and the wound is open.
   a. awareness
   b. creativity
   c. anticipation
   d. communication

9. Dr. Benjamin prefers to use absorbable skin-closure methods. The scrub nurse plans to have available which of the following?
   a. Staples
   b. 3-0 Chromic
   c. Clips
   d. 4-0 Silk

10. Malignant hyperthermia is thought to have a ________ component.
    a. communicable
    b. cultural
    c. genetic
    d. viral

FILL IN THE BLANK

Supply the missing term or the information requested.

1. Malignant hyperthermia manifests as a sudden, rapid increase in body temperature, possibly as rapid as ______ degrees centigrade per 5 minutes.
2. When Joy Pruitt is admitted to the RR after a cholecystectomy, you expect her initial vital signs to be monitored every ________ minutes.

3. Mr. Alexander has returned from an uncomplicated rhinoplasty. He does not have a urinary catheter. You expect him to void within _________ hour(s) of his return from surgery.

MULTIPLE-ANSWER MULTIPLE CHOICE

Circle the letter(s) corresponding to the appropriate answer(s). Circle all that apply.

1. Kathy Owens, 3 months old, is transferred to the OR for a 6-hour emergency surgery. As the nurse caring for her, you realize the critical importance of monitoring the loss of which of the following?
   a. Heat
   b. Blood
   c. Sleep
   d. Urine

2. As a general rule, normal bowel tones should be present before
   a. ambulation is begun.
   b. intravenous fluids are discontinued.
   c. deep breathing is encouraged.
   d. pain medication is administered.
   e. food or fluids are consumed.

3. Miss Waters developed a transient hypothermia secondary to changes in environmental temperature while in surgery. The nurse in the immediate postoperative period may use what treatments to address Miss Waters' hypothermia?
   a. Blankets
   b. Electric warming devices
   c. Cold intravenous fluids
   d. Ice packs
   e. Tepid baths

SECTION II

Human Function and Clinical Nursing Therapeutics

UNIT VII

Health Perception and Health Management

CHAPTER 32

Safety

CHAPTER OVERVIEW

Chapter 32 discusses the importance of safety in normal health function. Intrinsic and extrinsic factors that affect safety in healthcare facilities, the home, and the workplace are examined and summarized.

LEARNING OBJECTIVES

After mastering the content in this chapter, you should be able to do the following:

1. Identify national organizations that focus on safety concerns of clients and healthcare workers.
2. Recognize the importance of safety in the home and healthcare environments.
3. Relate special safety considerations to specific developmental stages.
4. Identify factors that affect safety and common manifestations of altered safety.
5. Identify individual safety patterns through assessment.
6. Using assessment, identify people at risk for safety dysfunction.
7. Characterize the appropriate nursing diagnoses for altered safety.
8. Discuss teaching topics and nursing interventions to promote safe homes and healthcare environments.
9. Identify nursing interventions for altered safety.

■ Mastering the Information

MATCHING

Match the terms in Column II with a definition, example, or related statement from Column I. Place the letter corresponding to the answer in the space provided.

COLUMN I

1. ______ Occurs when an electric current travels through the body rather than through electrical wiring or when static electricity builds up on the surface of the body
2. ______ Inability to obtain adequate oxygen due to being trapped in a confined place
3. ______ A protective device, material, or equipment attached or adjacent to the person's body that restricts freedom of movement or normal access to one's body
4. ______ Inability to inhale air into the lungs due to airway obstruction
5. ______ Thermal or chemical injury to body tissue

COLUMN II

a. Burns
b. Electric shock
c. Suffocation
d. Restraints
e. Asphyxiation

COLUMN I

a. ______ Beware of automobiles, strangers, and stray animals. Identification bracelets, fingerprinting, and frequent photographs may prove beneficial.

b. ______ Establish a buddy system for outdoor sports; wear helmets when bicycling, riding, or for contact sports; avoid alcohol.

c. ______ Use car seats and sturdy toys that are free from sharp or small removable objects.

d. ______ Dress in nonrestrictive, nonflammable, but adequate clothing. Use warm bath water and provide clean air.

e. ______ Provide adequate lighting, grab bars, and nonskid surfaces on stairs, in the kitchen, and in the bathroom.

COLUMN II

a. Newborns or infants
b. Toddlers
c. Preschoolers
d. School-age children
e. Older adults

TRUE–FALSE

Indicate if the following statements are true or false.

______ 1. Safety is a basic human need that is essential in the healthcare environment, the home, and the community.

______ 2. Pervasiveness, perception, and management are characteristics of safety.

______ 3. Nursing intervention to promote safety is very limited because of the broad scope of the problem.

______ 4. Safety allows other basic human needs, such as love, belonging, and self-esteem, to be met and personal goals to be accomplished.

______ 5. Factors that contribute to risks of motor vehicle accidents include lack of defensive driving techniques, failure to use helmets by bicycle riders and skateboarders, and use of alcohol and other substances.

______ 6. Safety from infection is a high priority in the healthcare environment.

______ 7. Poison prevention in the healthcare environment can be accomplished primarily through safe medication preparation.

______ 8. Three cardinal rules of radiation protection are to minimize the time of exposure, maximize distance from the source, and use appropriate shielding.

______ 9. The Occupational Safety and Health Administration is an agency that only records statistical data regarding occupational accidents.

______ 10. The primary focus of community safety programs is crime prevention.

______ 11. Nurses should be especially careful when bathing clients because any open or fluid-filled lesion is a potential source of pathogenic organisms.

______ 12. Correct filing of an incident report includes documenting, in the client's medical record, that the report has been filed.

FILL IN THE BLANK

Supply the missing term or the information requested.

1. ________________ have recognizable patterns of occurrence with corresponding controls.
2. ________________ is a major characteristic of safety.
3. ________________ and ________________ alter one's ability to perceive hazards, express concerns, and follow safety precautions.
4. Falls, fires, burns, poisonings, suffocation, electrical shock, radiation injuries, infection, street-related illnesses, and motor-vehicle accidents are manifestations of ________________.
5. Falls in healthcare facilities are frequently associated with walking to the ________________.

6. Nursing interventions to promote health and safety function involve providing a safe healthcare environment and client _______________.
7. It is important for nurses to educate parents about the developmental capabilities of infants and children and the specific _______________ needed for their care.
8. Nurses must be familiar with emergency interventions for disasters. These include _______________ and filing incident reports.

■ Applying Your Knowledge

CASE STUDY

Mr. Franks, 70 years old, lives alone. He expresses concern that he may fall at home or become ill and not be able to get to the phone.

1. Discuss the other information, besides the above-stated client concerns, that you as his nurse would consider important to the assessment process.
2. Discuss your rationale for why you believe Mr. Franks can continue to live at home or why you believe Mr. Franks will need to have other living arrangements made for him.

CRITICAL INQUIRY EXERCISE

Interview key people in the community who are responsible for community safety—for example, an occupational health nurse, a fire marshall, or a police chief.

CRITICAL EXPLORATION EXERCISE

1. Plan your own fire or disaster evacuation route from home and the workplace or school.
2. List at least two topics for discussion of safety with the following groups:
   a. School-age children
   b. parent-teacher organization group
   c. senior citizens group
   d. A group of community leaders
   e. A group of nursery-school or day-care personnel

■ Practicing for NCLEX

MULTIPLE CHOICE QUESTIONS

Circle the letter that corresponds to the best answer for each question.

1. When hazards exist, there is the potential for
   a. client teaching.
   b. altered safety function.
   c. altered personal function.
   d. altered self-care activities.
2. Features of a home safety plan include
   a. adequate ventilation, reliable heating system, fire escape routes, nonskid bathtub surface, and carefully stored toxic substances.
   b. pollution of air and water sources, safe medication distribution routes, nonskid floors, and client education.
   c. adequate ventilation, stairway lighting, street lighting, crime prevention, traffic control, and client education.
   d. client education, caregiver education, self-help devices, restraints, and proper medication administration.
3. Careless smoking habits, faulty electrical equipment, and failure to attend to food cooking on the stove are common causes of
   a. altered physiologic function.
   b. altered safety function.
   c. fires in the workplace.
   d. fires in the home.
4. A young child has an intravenous infusion in progress. To prevent him or her from pulling it out, the physician wrote an order for restraints. Which type of restraint is most appropriate?
   a. Jacket or vest restraint
   b. Mummy restraint
   c. Wrist restraints
   d. Belt restraints
5. The nurse in a healthcare facility is extremely careful about medication preparation and administration. This is primarily an attempt to ensure
   a. personal protection.
   b. accident prevention.
   c. poison prevention.
   d. infection control.

6. The nurse plays an important role in maintaining a safe healthcare environment and also plays an important role in
   a. educating clients and families about safety in the home, workplace, and community.
   b. identifying hazards in the home and healthcare facility.
   c. personal protection from hospital-acquired infections or radiation hazards.
   d. conducting health fairs, lecturing regarding pollution problems, and identifying potential radiation leaks.

7. Which subjective data should the nurse document to validate the safety function of an individual?
   a. Statements of concern for the welfare of offspring
   b. Questions about treatment modalities
   c. Questions about heating and lighting
   d. Statements regarding concerns or perceptions of hazards

8. Questions such as, "Does the person use appropriate restraints when riding in a car?" "Can the person read traffic signs or longer warnings?" and "Does the person have up-to-date immunizations?" may reveal data about
   a. normal pattern identification.
   b. dysfunctional identification.
   c. risk for injury.
   d. history of accidental injuries in one's life.

9. Initial nursing actions to promote safety and security for the client who is admitted to a healthcare facility include
   a. introduction of the staff to the client and orientation of the client to the immediate environment.
   b. notification of the client and family members about room assignments and the facility's policies and procedures.
   c. scheduling medication and treatments to facilitate rest and comfort.
   d. placing side rails on the bed and placing a night light in the bathroom.

10. Jerry, 30 years old, has a violent temper. He has been evicted from his apartment for fighting with the manager. A likely nursing diagnosis for Jerry is risk for injury related to
    a. homelessness and coping mechanism.
    b. change in income and lifestyle.
    c. lifestyle changes and altered nutrition.
    d. homelessness and physiologic changes.

11. The nurse visits in a home environment with beautiful shrubbery and houseplants. Which of the following family members may be at risk for altered safety?
    a. Newborn twins
    b. Preschoolers
    c. Teenagers
    d. Parents

12. A community health nurse notices throw rugs, stacked newspapers, frayed electrical cords, and old rags in the home of an elderly person who uses a walker to assist with ambulation. Which of the following is the most appropriate nursing action?
    a. Ignore the situation because it is evident that the person cannot clean the house.
    b. Clean the house and instruct family members of the reason.
    c. Discuss the situation with the caregiver, and identify sources of help.
    d. Refer the family to the local welfare department.

FILL IN THE BLANK

Supply the missing term or the information requested.

1. Infants, older adults, and people impaired by illness or drugs are at high risk for injury resulting from ________________.
2. When a person reports a serious preventable injury or a recent change in ability to participate safely in activities of daily living or if unsafe behavior is observed, the nurse may determine that ________________ patterns of safety exist.

3. The client's decision-making capabilities can best be assessed by asking ________________ questions appropriate to the client's age and life experiences.
4. The inability of a person to complete activities of daily living safely is an indication of the need for ________________.

MULTIPLE-ANSWER MULTIPLE CHOICE

Circle the letter(s) corresponding to the appropriate answer(s). Circle all that apply.

1. Which of the statements is accurate?
   a. Regular or multipurpose dry chemical fire is used to extinguished class B fires of flammable liquids.
   b. Special dry powder is needed to extinguish a class C electrical fire.
   c. Multipurpose dry chemical, carbon dioxide, or liquified gas is needed to extinguish a class A fire involving paper, wool, or cloth.
   d. Water, multipurpose dry chemical, loaded steam, or carbon dioxide may be used to extinguish a class A fire involving wool or cloth.
   e. Special dry powder is needed to extinguish a class C electrical fire.
2. Nursing interventions in a healthcare facility for altered safety function when preventive measures fail may include which measures?
   a. Educating the clients and staff regarding the most frequently occurring accidents
   b. Filing incident reports
   c. Filing and documenting nosocomial infections
   d. Fire evacuation
   e. Emergency first aid for poisoning
   f. Cardiopulmonary resuscitation
   g. Orientation of clients to the use of the call light and bed controls
   h. Administration of obstructed airway techniques
3. Which safety restraint practice(s) is/are appropriate?
   a. Adolescents should wear safety restraints and avoid riding with friends impaired by alcohol or other substances.
   b. Toddlers and preschoolers (20-60 pounds) should be secured in a rear-facing car seat, semireclined with head supported.
   c. Infants (10-20 pounds) should be secured in a forward-facing booster car seat.
   d. Children weighing more than 60 pounds should be secured with a properly applied lap and shoulder harness.

ORDERING

1. The following are the leading categories of accidents resulting in death in the United States. Number the list in order of frequency of accidents (from most frequent to least frequent).
   a. ________ Poisonings
   b. ________ Drownings
   c. ________ Falls
   d. ________ Motor vehicle accidents
2. Order the predispositions to altered safety based on developmental age group in which it occurs (from the youngest to the oldest at-risk age group—newborn to older adult).
   a. ______ Beginning age for learning safety rules; should learn to avoid playing with matches, electric cords, plugs
   b. ______ Can reach up to new sources of items; delights in opening and closing doors, turning knobs, climbing on furniture, and all sorts of active play
   c. ______ Immature thermoregulation and limited neurologic and musculoskeletal development
   d. ______ Autonomy develops; explores sexuality and learns new skills, such as driving a car, horseback riding, bicycling, and swimming
   e. ______ Increased involvement in work situations and in new recreational pursuits, such as hiking, hunting, and mountain climbing
   f. ______ Failing eyesight, hearing loss, and decreased proprioception

CHAPTER 33

Health Maintenance

CHAPTER OVERVIEW

Chapter 33 examines and summarizes the basic concept of health maintenance. Use of the nursing process as a mechanism for facilitating health maintenance is discussed. Particular emphasis is placed on the assessment process.

LEARNING OBJECTIVES

After mastering the content in this chapter, you should be able to do the following:

1. Describe characteristics essential for normal health.
2. Give examples of health-promotion and disease-prevention behaviors.
3. Describe important lifespan development considerations related to health maintenance.
4. Recognize major factors that affect motivation and health maintenance.
5. Describe factors that place an individual's health at risk
6. Characterize manifestations of altered health maintenance.
7. Obtain subjective data through a nursing history to assess health maintenance.
8. Provide appropriate information about common illnesses that may result from altered health maintenance.
9. List resources for client-teaching information on health maintenance.
10. Value health promotion concepts and act as a role model for clients.

■ Mastering the Information

MATCHING

Match the terms in Column II with a definition, example, or related statement from Column I. Place the letter corresponding to the answer in the space provided.

COLUMN I

1. ______ Includes identifying abnormalities within a population through screening and self-examination
2. ______ Includes lifestyle factors directed toward high-level wellness and prevention of disease
3. ______ Seeks to minimize individual disability from disease or dysfunction

COLUMN II

a. Primary prevention
b. Secondary prevention
c. Tertiary prevention

TRUE–FALSE

Indicate if the following statements are true or false.

______ 1. Health-maintenance activities are behaviors that the person in a stable state of health uses to maintain or improve that state of health.

______ 2. People with a low perceived barrier to health are less likely to pursue healthy behaviors than are those with high perceived barriers.

______ 3. Individuals have the option to accept or reject the healthy behaviors nurses promote.

______ 4. Health promotion is characterized by both approach behaviors and avoidance behaviors.

______ 5. Coping behaviors that people use to handle everyday situations may help or harm their health.

______ 6. Addiction is both a psychological problem and a physical illness.

FILL IN THE BLANK

Supply the missing term or the information requested.

1. Briefly describe the four characteristics of normal health maintenance.
   a.
   b.
   c.
   d.
2. Identify two of four nursing diagnoses that are closely related to health maintenance.
   a.
   b.
3. Identify one health-maintenance behavior that should be emphasized during each of the following developmental periods:
   a. ________ Infancy
   b. ________ Toddlerhood
   c. ________ Adolescence

■ Applying Your Knowledge

CASE STUDY

Ms. McTyre is 101 years old and has lived at a local nursing home for 2 years. Before that time, she lived in another state. She moved here because her husband died, and her daughter, who is 75 years old, wanted her to be close to her in case she became ill. Ms. McTyre states that people think that it is wonderful to live to be 101 years old, but it is also hard. She states that she is accustomed to being independent, but now she is on a fixed and limited income, she is confined to the nursing home facility for the most part (she visits with her daughter about every other week), and all of her friends are "back home." Ms. McTyre gets up every morning and dresses herself, including putting on make-up and her jewelry. She can walk with a walker, but most of the time she travels through the nursing home by wheelchair because of pain related to a previous hip fracture. She attends scheduled activities at the facility and delivers the mail to other residents on her unit. She has no acute health problems at this time.

1. Discuss factors that are affecting or have the potential to affect Ms. McTyre's health maintenance in both positive and negative ways.
2. Identify nursing interventions to address Ms. McTyre's health-maintenance needs.

CRITICAL INQUIRY EXERCISE

Perform a self-assessment of your health-maintenance behavior. Answer the following questions.

1. What is your personal definition of health?
2. How has your family influenced your perception of health?
3. Do any of the following factors affect your health-maintenance behaviors? If so, how?
   a. Environment
   b. Economic status
   c. Lifestyle and habits

CRITICAL EXPLORATION

Tour your community and identify any of the following factors that might affect health-maintenance behaviors:

a. Traffic
b. Employment opportunities
c. Food availability—food markets, fast food or other restaurants

■ Practicing for NCLEX

MULTIPLE CHOICE QUESTIONS:

Circle the letter that corresponds to the best answer for each question.

1. When assessing a client's health-maintenance status, the nurse should do which of the following?
   a. Compare the client's status to the nurse's health status as a baseline
   b. Ignore the client's opinion of his or her capabilities; consider facts only
   c. Perform a health history interview
   d. Use high-level wellness as normal

2. Which of the following factors could be perceived as a barrier to pursuing healthy behaviors?
   a. Genetics
   b. Access
   c. Culture
   d. Wealth

3. Which of the following is a manifestation of altered health maintenance?
   a. Hypertension
   b. Breast self-examination
   c. Pregnancy
   d. Immunization

4. Which of the following possible risk factors can be modified?
   a. Genetic background
   b. Family history
   c. Race
   d. Stress

5. Which of the following would be considered a defining characteristic for the nursing diagnosis of altered health maintenance?
   a. History of lack of health-seeking behavior
   b. High risk for infection
   c. Altered communication skills
   d. Report of client exercising two to three times weekly

6. Which of the following would be an appropriate intervention to promote health maintenance?
   a. Educating the client about curing chronic illness
   b. Encouraging the client to comply with routine healthcare visits
   c. Teaching the client to examine self and eliminate the need for physicals
   d. Instructing the client to take antibiotics when cold symptoms are noted

7. The cardinal symptom of myocardial infarction is
   a. persistent chest pain.
   b. dizziness.
   c. shortness of breath.
   d. sweating.

8. An appropriate outcome criteria for the goal "The client will adopt appropriate health-seeking behaviors related to testicular self-examination" would be that:
   a. the nurse provides written material on examination techniques.
   b. the client reads a book on low-cholesterol diets within the next week.
   c. the client distinguishes normal from abnormal findings during a testicular self-examination.
   d. the nurse will call the client annually to remind him to see the physician.

FILL IN THE BLANK

Supply the missing term or the information requested.

1. What behavior has been linked most often to the occurrence of cancer? __________
2. The primary risk factors for cardiovascular disease that cannot be changed include race and __________________.

MULTIPLE-ANSWER MULTIPLE CHOICE

Circle the letter(s) corresponding to the appropriate answer(s). Circle all that apply.

1. Warning signs of cancer include which of the following?
   a. Indigestion or difficulty swallowing
   b. Nagging cough or hoarseness
   c. Headache that radiates to the eyes
   d. Change in bowel or bladder habits

UNIT VIII

ACTIVITY AND EXERCISE

CHAPTER 34

Self-Care and Hygiene

CHAPTER OVERVIEW

Chapter 34 examines and summarizes the basic concepts of self-care and hygiene. Various factors that influence self-care abilities and basic principles of hygiene are presented. Particular emphasis is placed on helping clients to achieve as much independence in self-care as possible.

LEARNING OBJECTIVES

After mastering the content in this chapter, you should be able to do the following:

1. Discuss the importance of self-care and hygiene in health and illness.
2. Describe the effects of health and illness on the ability to perform self-care.
3. Discuss important subjective and objective areas of assessment in identifying self-care deficits and individualizing a plan for self-care.
4. Demonstrate basic hygiene skills, such as bathing, shampooing hair, perineal care, foot care, back massage, toileting, and bedmaking.
5. Demonstrate proper care of eyes, ears, and teeth, including care of dentures, glasses, contact lenses, and hearing aids.
6. List beneficial client teaching for each of the four areas of self-care.

■ Mastering the Information

MATCHING

Match the terms in Column II with a definition, example, or related statement from Column I. Place the letter corresponding to the answer in the space provided.

COLUMN I

1. __a__ Head and trunk elevated 80 to 90 degrees
2. __c__ Head of bed elevated 15 to 45 degrees
3. __b__ Entire bed tilted with feet downward
4. __d__ Entire bed tilted with head downward

COLUMN II

a. High Fowler's
b. Reverse Trendelenburg
c. Low Fowler's
d. Trendelenburg

COLUMN I

1. __b__ Support network
2. __a__ Skills
3. __c__ Communication
4. __b__ Financial resources
5. __a__ Cognitive abilities
6. __b__ Water

COLUMN II

a. Internal resources
b. External resources

 Study Guide to Accompany Craven and Hirnle's Fundamentals of Nursing: Human Health and Function, 5th edition, by Joyce Young Johnson, Bennita W. Vaughans, and Phyllis Prather-Hicks.

TRUE–FALSE

Indicate if the following statements are true or false.

F 1. Regression is an abnormal defense mechanism exhibited by some children that should be identified early and discouraged.

T 2. Food consistency is important for clients who have difficulty swallowing.

T 3. The inability to perceive reality appropriately may cause inattentiveness to the need for personal care.

F 4. Filing the toenails of clients with diabetes or other clients with poor circulation is contraindicated because of the increased likelihood of injury.

F 5. When cleansing the eyes, a different part of the washcloth should be used if an infection is suspected.

T 6. When performing oral care, the client should be taught to brush, then floss.

F 7. The client who has dentures should remove them only for cleaning and should replace the dentures after cleaning is completed.

T 8. Blind clients can be oriented to the location of food on a plate by referring to the numbers on a clock.

F 9. Asepsis is not necessary when making a bed because linens for bedmaking are not considered sterile.

FILL IN THE BLANK

Supply the missing term or the information requested.

1. Identify five factors that affect normal self-care.
   a. Pain
   b. motivation
   c. Motor Skills
   d. Energy
   e. Surgery

2. Identify the five types of therapeutic baths.
   a. Sitz
   b. Hot H2O
   c. Warm ''
   d. Cool ''
   e. Soaks

3. Identify three of seven steps that may be taken to help the client who is having difficulty voiding.
   a. warm bedpan
   b. Run H2O
   c. analgesics

4. Identify four of the nine nursing diagnoses that frequently exist along with self-care deficits.
   a. Skin integrity
   b. anxiety
   c. altered nutrition
   d. Impared oral mucus membrane

■ Applying Your Knowledge

CASE STUDY

Mr. Luigio, 82 years old, fell down the stairs of his home and fractured his left hip. At the present time, he is a resident in a nursing home facility. He needs assistance with bathing and dressing. He is continent of urine and feces and uses a urinal and bedpan for elimination. He is confined to bed but feeds himself. He states that he plans to return to his home eventually.

1. Assess each variable presented in the Index of Activities of Daily Living (Table 34-2). Decide in which variables Mr. Luigio expresses independence and in which ones he expresses dependence.
2. Select an identified area of dependence, and develop a plan of care to meet the client's needs in that area. Foster as much independence as possible in the plan of care.
3. Identify Mr. Luigio's overall level of self-care using the information in Table 34-1. Provide data to support your evaluation.

CRITICAL INQUIRY EXERCISE

During a clinical experience, perform an assessment of an assigned client's self-care abilities.

a. Assess each variable presented in the Index of Activities of Daily Living (Table 34-2). Decide if the individual is independent or dependent.
b. Select an identified area of dependence, and develop a plan of care to meet the client's needs in that area and to foster as much independence as possible.

CRITICAL EXPLORATION

Identify the client's overall level of self-care using the information in Table 32-1. Provide data to support your evaluation.

■ Practicing for NCLEX

MULTIPLE CHOICE QUESTIONS

Circle the letter that corresponds to the best answer for each question.

1. Ms. Spencer is to remain on bed rest until her second postoperative day. During this period, what method of bedmaking would be most appropriate?
   a. Making an unoccupied bed
   b. Making an occupied bed
   c. Making an opened bed
   d. Making a closed bed

2. A client who is at risk for developing foot drop should be provided with a
   a. foot brace.
   b. trapeze bar.
   c. foot board.
   d. bed cradle.

3. The preferred position for the client receiving a backrub is
   a. prone.
   b. supine.
   c. Fowler's.
   d. side lying.

4. When giving the client a bed bath, which of the following sequences is preferred?
   a. Face, arms, legs, chest, back, and buttocks
   b. Face, chest, arms, legs, back, and buttocks
   c. Face, chest, arms, back, buttocks, and legs
   d. Face, arms, chest, legs, back, and buttocks

5. When providing oral care for the unconscious client, the nurse should
   a. open the client's mouth by placing the thumb in the corner of the mouth to break the seal.
   b. place the client in a side-lying position with a towel or pad under the chin.
   c. swab the lips with lemon glycerin at least every hour.
   d. not attempt to brush the teeth because the client may aspirate.

6. When collecting data related to self-care abilities, the nurse should observe and interview the client for
   a. gender.
   b. height.
   c. pain.
   d. race.

7. When shaving the male client, the nurse should
   a. soften the beard with a warmed towel before beginning.
   b. pinch up the area to be shaved.
   c. shave in the opposite direction of hair growth.
   d. use a safety razor to avoid cuts if the client is at risk for excessive bleeding.

8. Symptoms of contact lens overwear include
   a. excessive tearing.
   b. swelling of the eyelids.
   c. pale conjunctiva.
   d. dull throbbing.

9. To foster optimal hearing for the client who has a hearing aid, the nurse should
   a. increase the voice volume.
   b. repeat what is said, using the same words.
   c. speak slowly and clearly.
   d. stand close to the client's ear.

10. Ms. Snider is a 70-year-old woman who is experiencing altered fine-motor functioning secondary to the medical diagnosis of Parkinson's disease. Based on the information provided, which of the following articles of clothing would be best suited for Ms. Snider?
    a. Pajamas
    b. Sweat suits
    c. Dresses with large buttons down the front
    d. Dresses with a zipper down the front

FILL IN THE BLANK

Supply the missing term or the information requested.

1. The safe temperature range of water for bathing the client in bed should be 110-115
2. Meals on Wheels is a community service that provides hot, well-balanced meals to homebound people for a nominal fee.
3. The usual treatment for pediculosis is Lindane.

MULTIPLE-ANSWER MULTIPLE CHOICE

Circle the letter(s) corresponding to the appropriate answer(s). Circle all that apply.

1. When selecting the bathing method for the client, what should the nurse take into consideration?
    a. Nurse's energy level
    b. Method that allows the client the most independence in self-care
    c. Client's gender
    d. Nurse's ability to perform the bathing method without assistance
    e. Client's condition and abilities
    f. Client's preference

ORDERING

Items A through T are key steps to follow when making an occupied bed. Read the list carefully. Place each step in the correct sequence by numbering the items.

a. 1 Assemble equipment.
b. 20 Complete top covers in the same manner as for the unoccupied bed.
c. 8 Fanfold and tuck the dirty draw sheet and bottom sheet under the client's buttocks.
d. 15 Grasp the edge of the fanfold bottom sheet and secure it over the mattress.
e. 7 Help the client roll onto his or her side facing away from you.
f. 17 Help the client to the center of the bed.
g. 13 Help the client to roll over the folds of linen onto the opposite side.
h. 11 Lock the side rail on your side.
i. 2 Lock the side rail on the side of the bed opposite from where the clean linen is stacked.
j. 4 Loosen all top linen and remove the bedspread and blanket separately.
k. 5 Loosen the bottom sheet on your side.
l. 6 Lower the head of the bed to the flat position.
m. 12 Move to the opposite side and lower the side rail.
n. 9 Place the clean bottom sheet on the bed.
o. 10 Place the clean draw sheet on the bed.
p. 18 Place the top sheet over the client.
q. 3 Raise the bed to a comfortable working position.
r. 14 Remove the soiled linen.
s. 19 Remove the soiled top linen or bath blanket.
t. 16 Unfold the draw sheet by grasping at the center, then tuck the excess under the mattress.

CHAPTER 35

Mobility and Body Mechanics

CHAPTER OVERVIEW

In Chapter 35, the importance of mobility and proper body mechanics is discussed. The normal function of the musculoskeletal system is reviewed. Systemic effects of immobility and related nursing interventions are discussed.

LEARNING OBJECTIVES

After mastering the content in this chapter, you should be able to do the following:

1. Explain normal functions of the musculoskeletal system and characteristics of normal movement.
2. Identify factors, including lifespan considerations, that can affect or alter mobility.
3. Describe the impact of immobility on physiologic and psychological functioning.
4. Discuss appropriate subjective and objective data to collect to assess mobility status.
5. Demonstrate nursing interventions such as positioning, ambulating, providing range of motion, and using assistive devices.
6. Plan strategies to avoid musculoskeletal injury to the nurse and client during client care.
7. Develop appropriate community-based nursing interventions for preventing and managing mobility problems.

■ Mastering the Information

MATCHING

Match the terms in Column I with a definition, example, or related statement from Column II. Place the letter corresponding to the answer in the space provided.

COLUMN I

1. d Anaerobic exercise
2. h Ataxia
3. j Athetosis
4. i Chorea
5. c Contracture
6. b Festinating
7. f Isotonic exercises
8. g Range of motion
9. e School-age years
10. a Toddler and preschool years

COLUMN II

a. Marked by refinement of both gross- and fine-motor skills and by seeming boundless energy
b. Typified by walking on the toes as if being pushed
c. Progressive shortening of a muscle and loss of joint mobility due to fibrotic changes in tissue around the joints
d. Occurs when the muscle cannot extract enough oxygen from the blood
e. Physical growth slows, and refinement of gross- and fine-motor skills is often supported by group activity
f. A dynamic form of exercise in which there is constant muscle tension, muscle contraction, and active movement
g. The ability to move all joints through the full extent of intended function
h. A general term used to describe defective muscle coordination in which the gait is staggering and unsteady
i. Spontaneous, brief, involuntary muscle twitching of the limbs or facial muscles
j. Movement characterized by slow, irregular, twisting motions
k. Stiff walking and toes catching and dragging
l. A rhythmic, repetitive movement that can occur at rest or when movement is initiated

TRUE–FALSE

Indicate if the following statements are true or false.

T 1. Anything that interrupts full ROM of the joints, bone resiliency and strength, and muscle strength can impair mobility.

F 2. Diseases that impair the ability of the nervous system to control muscular movement and coordination actually have little effect on functional mobility.

F 3. Chronic health conditions primarily affect mobility by causing an emotional strain on the client.

F 4. Paraplegia is a term used to describe paralysis of the arms and legs.

F 5. Affective disorders result in limited mobility because of an associated physical impairment.

T 6. Short periods of immobility can impair activity tolerance.

T 7. Muscle strength and size decrease with immobility.

F 8. The formation of new connective tissue around joints and muscles is promoted by extended bed rest.

F 9. Extension contractures are the most common type of contractures in the immobilized client.

T 10. Orthostatic hypotension is a significant drop in systemic blood pressure when changing from a supine to an upright position.

FILL IN THE BLANK

Supply the missing term or the information requested.

1. The normal functions of the musculoskeletal system are proper posture, balance, body alignment, and coordinated movement

2. Performing activities such as bending, lifting, and moving in a safe and efficient manner is accomplished through proper body mechanics

3. Normal walking gait consists of the stance phase and the swing phase.

4. List five of the six factors needed for normal mobility.
   a. Intact musculoskeletal sy
   b. Regular exercise
   c. Optimal nutrition
   d. Circulation + oxygenat
   e. Nervous system contro

5. Four of the six basic symptoms of altered mobility are: Lack of coordination, pain, altered gait, and Falls.

6. Two North American Nursing Diagnosis Association (NANDA) nursing diagnoses in the functional area of mobility are impaired physical mobility and activity intolerance

7. Client goals concerning mobility should focus on promoting optimum mobility, increasing endurance and tolerance to exercise, preventing complications from immobility, and adapting to mobility restrictions.

8. Paralysis occurs when the client cannot move his or her entire body or a specific body.

9. Teenagers typically appear gangly and awkward due to rapid growth and variation of growth rates.

10. Movements of the newborn are random and reflexive.

11. State the two primary purposes for using proper body mechanics.
    a. Prevent injury
    b. Maintain balance

12. To move heavy clients, the nurse should use friction reducer or additional personel.

13. List three of the four general concepts related to body mechanics.
    a. assess situation
    b. use large muscle groups
    c. get help

14. When discharging a client with mobility problems, the nurse should address transfer and ambulation techniques and the use of specific equipment in the client and family teaching plan.

■ Applying Your Knowledge

CASE STUDY

Ms. Jones is a 5-foot 5-inch, 230-pound woman who was admitted to the hospital with a diagnosis of head trauma secondary to a head-on car collision. She is unconscious, on ventilatory support, and requires care.

1. Describe how Ms. Jones's present status affects the functional health pattern of activity and rest.
2. Determine the area of activity and exercise you would consider the priority area of concern.
3. Summarize the assessment data you would collect as a basis for your response in question 2.
4. Justify the precautions you should take to prevent injury to your musculoskeletal system while caring for Ms. Jones.

CRITICAL INQUIRY EXERCISE

Design a plan to teach a family member of a stroke victim good body mechanics for use when moving the client from the bed to a chair.

CRITICAL EXPLORATION EXERCISE

Tie the hands and feet of a classmate (to simulate paralysis) and transfer the classmate from a bed to a wheelchair and from the bed to a stretcher using good body mechanics.

■ Practicing for NCLEX

MULTIPLE CHOICE QUESTIONS

Circle the letter that corresponds to the best answer for each question.

1. When transferring a client to a wheelchair, make sure which of the following is true?
    a. The client's feet are touching the ground to stabilize the chair.
    b. The nurse is fully supporting the client's weight using back, not thigh, muscles.
    c. No weight is placed on the client's legs during the procedure.
    d. All the wheels are locked to avoid chair movement and falls.

2. Mrs. Wilson has a cold and is taking a medication that may affect her equilibrium. It is most important that the nurse caution Mrs. Wilson to do which actions?
    a. Move quickly when getting out of bed to avoid falling down
    b. Ambulate carefully to the restroom with assistance as needed
    c. Eat extra servings of meat or other protein to stabilize her balance
    d. Take a multivitamin daily to build up her red blood cell levels

3. Proper use of body mechanics during client transfer involves
    a. instructing the client not to assist in the procedure to avoid a possible strain on the nurse.
    b. lifting and carrying, rather than sliding or pulling, the client whenever possible.
    c. the nurse placing both feet side by side on the floor with knees straight to increase the base of support.
    d. the nurse tightening the abdominal and gluteal muscles before lifting or moving a client.

4. To maintain the workload near the center of gravity to prevent muscle strain and fatigue, the nurse should do which of the following when moving a client or heavy object?
   a. Carry the object close to the body.
   b. Hyperextend the arms and neck whenever possible during the move.
   c. Maintain the bed in its lowest position with the side rails up.
   d. Stand as far away from the work area as possible.

5. Which of the following steps may be altered if two nurses, not one, are positioning a client in bed?
   a. Both nurses stand on one side of the client's bed with feet together.
   b. Both nurses relax their knees and hips during the procedure to avoid using excessive force.
   c. The nurses may use a draw sheet to pull and reposition the client.
   d. The nurses do not need to place the head of the client's bed flat.

6. The nurse would report that a client has decreased muscle strength if which of the following were observed?
   a. Bilateral hand grasps are firm.
   b. Leg force against the nurse's hand is very resisting.
   c. Extended arms begin to drift down after a few minutes.
   d. Leg muscles can support body weight.

7. The most effective and appropriate nursing intervention for an immobilized client who is prone to pressure sores would be to
   a. maintain the client in one position for as long as tolerated.
   b. place the client in a chair for 6 to 8 hours twice daily with pressure greatest at the ischial tuberosities.
   c. position the client with greatest weight at bony prominences.
   d. turn the client every 2 hours and position on side with pillows.

8. Adequate intake of ________ is most essential to maintain bone resiliency and an intact skeletal system.
   a. fresh citrus fruits
   b. yellow vegetables
   c. milk and milk products
   d. white or whole-grain breads

9. Which of the following is a common effect of immobility on functional health?
   a. Bronchial airway constriction
   b. Greater-than-normal lung expansion
   c. Increased appetite and weight gain
   d. Thrombus formation and embolism

10. Immobility would have which of the following effects on lung secretions?
    a. Secretions become thicker due to an increased loss of body fluids.
    b. Cough reflexes are stimulated, resulting in an excess loss of lung secretions.
    c. Lung expansion is increased, and secretions are distributed through the lungs and thinned.
    d. Secretions are retained and provide a medium for microorganism growth and infection.

11. Which of the following is most likely to occur as a result of immobility?
    a. Anorexia
    b. Diarrhea
    c. Increased protein synthesis
    d. Osteogenesis

12. Noted client inability to reach up with arms due to a contracture and limited range of motion of arms would best support which of the following nursing diagnoses?
    a. Activity intolerance
    b. High risk for injury
    c. Impaired physical mobility
    d. Urinary retention

13. Logrolling is accomplished through which of the following procedures?
    a. Instructing the client to keep the body as relaxed as possible during the move
    b. Moving the client's legs and feet before turning the chest and head to the side
    c. Turning the upper part of the client's body first
    d. Using a draw sheet to turn obese clients smoothly

14. Which of the following is true of ROM exercises?
    a. ROM exercises should be avoided until 5 days after surgery.
    b. Clients at high risk for joint mobility problems may require more frequent ROM than indicated with other clients.
    c. Passive ROM occurs when the client performs exercises slowly with no assistance from the nurse or physical therapist.
    d. No physician's order is required for ROM for clients with arthritis or joint dislocation.

FILL IN THE BLANK

Supply the missing term or the information requested.

1. The procedure for using proper body mechanics requires that the nurse always ______________ movement before doing it.
2. Identify the following descriptions of joint motion.
    a. __________ involves decreasing the angle between two bones.
    b. __________ involves moving a joint or extremity toward the midline of the body.
    c. __________ involves turning a joint or an extremity on its axis away from the body's midline.
    d. __________ involves turning the body or body part to face upward.
    e. __________ involves turning the feet outward so the toes are pointing away from the midline.
    f. __________ involves moving a body part in widening circles.
    g. __________ involves straightening a joint.

MULTIPLE-ANSWER MULTIPLE CHOICE

Circle the letter(s) corresponding to the appropriate answer(s). Circle all that apply.

1. Indicate the appropriate crutch-walking gait for the client and description provided below: four-point gait, three-point gait, two-point gait, or swing-through gait.
    a. The two-point gait allows the client to bear weight on only one foot, with both crutches, and the weaker leg moves forward first.
    b. The swing-through gait requires the client to bear partial weight on each foot, as each crutch moves at the same time as the opposing leg.
    c. The swing-through is often used by paraplegics, with both crutches moving forward and then the body brought beyond the crutches to propel the client forward.
    d. The four-point gait allows the client to bear partial weight on both feet, with the right crutch placed forward, followed by the left foot; the left crutch is then moved forward, followed by the right foot.
    e. The two-point gait has crutch and foot movement that is similar to arm and leg movement in normal walking.

2. Indicate which step(s) are appropriate when one nurse is positioning a client in bed.
    a. ______ Review the client's chart for conditions that influence the ability to move or to be positioned.
    b. ______ Explain the procedure and rationale to the client.
    c. ______ Raise the head of the bed to 45 degrees.
    d. ______ Place the bed in its lowest position.
    e. ______ Place your feet together side by side.
    f. ______ Flex your knees and thighs.
    g. ______ Place one arm under the client's shoulders and one arm under the thighs.
    h. ______ Rock back and forth on front and back leg to the count of three; on three, the client pushes with feet as you lift and pull the client up in bed.

3. Indicate if the following interventions would be appropriate when providing care for the client with altered mobility.
   a. _____ Setting short-term, achievable goals
   b. _____ Performing a full bath on all clients with altered mobility
   c. _____ Assessing the client's alignment and balance
   d. _____ Asking the client to button a shirt to determine fine-motor skills
   e. _____ Ambulation of a client with complaints of dizziness to promote cerebral circulation
   f. _____ Increasing the activity level of a client with low hematocrit values to improve activity tolerance
   g. _____ Suggesting the use of area rugs at home to facilitate ambulation with crutches
   h. _____ Planning to place clients with mobility problems on the second floor of a two-story house for a pleasant view to prevent depression
   i. _____ Installing smoke detectors throughout the home for early warning

CHAPTER 36

Oxygenation: Respiratory Function

CHAPTER OVERVIEW

Chapter 36 examines and summarizes the role of respiratory function in the process of oxygenation of body tissue. Application of the nursing process in the care of clients with alterations in respiratory function is emphasized. Specific therapies used in the care of clients with altered respiratory function also are presented.

LEARNING OBJECTIVES

After mastering the content in this chapter, you should be able to do the following:

1. Identify factors that can interfere with effective oxygenation of body tissues.
2. Describe common manifestations of altered respiratory function.
3. Discuss lifespan-related changes and problems in respiratory function.
4. Describe important elements in the respiratory assessment.
5. List three appropriate nursing diagnoses and outcomes for the client with altered respiratory function.
6. Describe nursing measures to ensure a patent airway.
7. Discuss safe administration of oxygen using different modes of delivery.
8. Describe the impact of respiratory dysfunction on activities of daily living.
9. Identify home care considerations for the respiratory client.

■ Mastering the Information

MATCHING

Match the terms in Column II with a definition, example, or related statement from Column I. Place the letter corresponding to the answer in the space provided. (Use each letter only once; some letters may not be used.)

COLUMN I

1. ______ Stiff lungs or alveoli collapse
2. ______ Air trapping in alveoli secondary to floppy bronchial walls
3. ______ Coughing up frankly red and bloody mucus
4. ______ Bluish discoloration of the skin caused by decreased blood oxygen saturation
5. ______ pH less than 7.35

COLUMN II

a. Acidosis
b. Atelectasis
c. Cyanosis
d. Emphysema
e. Hemoptysis

TRUE–FALSE

Indicate if the following statements are true or false.

______ 1. Effective treatment of dyspnea addresses both its physical and psychological components.

______ 2. In the newborn, frequent periods of apnea lasting up to 30 seconds are a normal finding.

______ 3. The elderly client may experience activity intolerance and an increased incidence of respiratory infections due to normal changes that occur in the respiratory system with aging.

______ 4. You would expect the rate and depth of respirations to decrease during strenuous exercise.

______ 5. Chest pain occurs only in instances of cardiac dysfunction.

T 6. Central cyanosis is a grave sign because it is an indicator of serious tissue oxygenation problems.

T 7. Home care of the tracheostomy may be performed under clean conditions, rather than sterile conditions.

T 8. Clients receiving oxygen therapy are instructed not to smoke because of the fire hazard that smoking would create.

FILL IN THE BLANK

Supply the missing term or the information requested.

1. Identify the three major functions of breathing.
   a. O2 avail to the blood
   b. CO2 to be removed "
   c. Maintain PH balance
2. Essential observations that should be included as a part of inspection when assessing a client's respiratory status include the rate and pattern of respirations.
3. Identify the characteristics of lung secretions for the following situations.
   a. Normal lung secretions Clear, white no odor
   b. Asthma Stringy thickened egg white
   c. Infection yellow w/ putrid/musty odor
4. Identify four of seven diagnostic tests and procedures that are used in assessing respiratory status.
   a. Chest X-Rays
   b. Bronchoscopy
   c. Sputum Culture
   d. Skin test
5. Provide the definition, defining characteristics, and related factors for each of the following nursing diagnoses.
   a. Ineffective breathing pattern
      Definition:
      Defining characteristics:
      Related factors:
   b. Impaired gas exchange
      Definition:
      Defining characteristics:
      Related factors:
6. General indicators of the success of oxygen therapy include the client's color, Breathing effort, alertness, and heart Rate
7. Describe the five levels of dyspnea.
   a. Level I: Can walk 1 mile b4 shortness of breath
   b. Level II: SOB after 100 yds.
   c. Level III: SOB while talking or ADLs
   d. Level IV: SOB during no activity
   e. Orthopnea: SOB while laying do
8. To ensure accurate measurement Nail polish and fake nails should be removed when monitoring oxygenation via pulse oximetry.

■ Applying Your Knowledge

CASE STUDY

Christopher is a 15-year-old boy with chronic asthma. His asthma was diagnosed when he was 5 years old. He has been hospitalized on numerous occasions for acute asthma attacks. His mother states that he almost died one time because of his asthma. Christopher continues to have acute asthma attacks (usually no more than twice a year) but has not required hospitalization since he was 10 years old. His main reason for seeking healthcare at this time is not related to any acute illness. He is being seen because he recently tried out for and made the basketball team.

His mother is not sure this is a good idea and wants the physician to evaluate the situation.

1. Discuss how you would respond if you were asked if Christopher should be encouraged to play basketball.
2. Describe the treatment modalities you would expect Christopher to be using in the home setting and give your rationale for each treatment modality.
3. Develop a teaching plan to address potential needs that Christopher may have in the area of infection control.
4. Discuss ways that the nurse can foster Christopher's self-esteem, taking into consideration his developmental level.

CRITICAL INQUIRY EXERCISE

1. Develop a list of community resources that may be used by a client who experiences altered respiratory function when discharged home.
2. Search the Internet for organizations or resources for clients receiving home oxygen therapy.

CRITICAL EXPLORATION EXERCISE

1. Visit the respiratory therapy department in your assigned clinical agency.
   a. Identify services provided in the department and the purpose of each identified service.
   b. Identify the role of the nurse in assisting with respiratory therapies for the client on the clinical unit with a respiratory therapist in the department.

■ Practicing for NCLEX

MULTIPLE CHOICE QUESTIONS

Circle the letter that corresponds to the best answer for each question.

1. Gas exchange occurs in which of the following regions?
   a. Alveoli
   b. Bronchioles
   c. Trachea
   d. Mouth

2. In the elderly client, you would expect the PaO_2 to
   a. be the same as that of other adults.
   b. increase.
   c. decrease.
   d. be equal to the PCO_2 level.

3. The atmospheric concentration of oxygen is
   a. 21%.
   b. 45%.
   c. 82%.
   d. 100%.

4. Which of the following is placed in the category of restrictive lung disease?
   a. Asthma
   b. Bronchitis
   c. Pneumonia
   d. Epiglottitis

5. A client presents in the emergency room with alcohol intoxication and profuse vomiting. The most immediate concern in this situation would be
   a. possible respiratory arrest secondary to depression of the central nervous system.
   b. anemia secondary to insufficient nutritional intake.
   c. choking secondary to aspiration of stomach contents.
   d. alcohol addiction.

6. Breath sounds that indicate the presence of fluid in the lungs are referred to as
   a. pneumonic.
   b. rales.
   c. rhonchi.
   d. wheezes.

7. Adequate hydration assists with maintaining respiratory function by
   a. maintaining electrolyte balance.
   b. maintaining pH balance.
   c. maintaining moist and easily coughed up secretions.
   d. maintaining adequate circulation.

8. ______ is the most common midrange O_2 device and delivers 40% to 60% O_2 when operated at 6 to 10 L/minute.
   a. Cannula
   b. Oxyhood
   c. Simple mask
   d. Venturi mask

9. ______ is the most comfortable and convenient O_2 device and delivers 22% to 40% O_2 when operated at 1 to 6 L/minute.
   a. Cannula
   b. Oxyhood
   c. Simple mask
   d. Venturi mask

10. ______ provides precise O_2 delivery for infants and delivers 22% to 90% O_2 and up.
   a. Cannula
   b. Oxyhood
   c. Simple mask
   d. Venturi mask

11. Oxygen therapy may cause respiratory arrest in a client with which of the following conditions?
   a. Croup
   b. COPD
   c. Pneumonia
   d. Dyspnea

12. A 65-year-old man is admitted with a diagnosis of COPD. Which of the following would be the most appropriate action for the client with regard to morning care?
   a. Encourage him to complete hygiene care, eating, and dressing within the first hour after arising in the morning.
   b. Encourage him to dress daily when this is physically possible because dressing helps to prevent the client from thinking of himself as an invalid.
   c. Have the client take a tub bath, instead of a shower, because this conserves energy.
   d. Prepare a large breakfast for the client and tell him he should eat it all to build his strength.

FILL IN THE BLANK

Supply the missing term or the information requested.

1. What plays the primary role in determining the frequency and depth of ventilation? ______________
2. What is the single most important factor affecting pulmonary health? ______________
3. A substance that triggers the release of chemical mediators because of its perceived harm to the body is referred to as a(n) ______________.
4. The breathing technique used by clients with chronic obstructive pulmonary disease (COPD) and those with asthma for the purpose of removing trapped air from obstructed airways is referred to as ______________.

MULTIPLE-ANSWER MULTIPLE CHOICE

Circle the letter(s) corresponding to the appropriate answer(s). Circle all that apply.

1. When performing nasotracheal suction in the adult, the nurse should
   a. apply suctioning for a maximum of 10 seconds.
   b. apply suctioning for a maximum of 5 seconds.
   c. insert catheter during expiration.
   d. insert catheter during inspiration.
   e. retract catheter1 cm before applying suction.
   f. retract catheter 5 cm before applying suction.

2. When providing care to a patient with a chest tube, the nurse should notify the physician if
   a. there is bubbling in the water seal chamber when the patient coughs.
   b. the chest tube becomes dislodged.
   c. there is significant unexpected drainage from the chest tube.
   d. the client experiences dyspnea.

3. The appropriate catheter size for an adult requiring nasopharyngeal suctioning is
   a. 8 Fr.
   b. 10 Fr.
   c. 12 Fr.
   d. 14 Fr.
   e. 16 Fr.
   f. 18 Fr.
   g. 20 Fr.

4. The upper airway consists of which of the following structures?
   a. Mouth
   b. Nose
   c. Pharynx
   d. Trachea

ORDERING

Items A through N are key steps to follow when suctioning secretions from airways. Read the list carefully. Place each step in the correct sequence by numbering the items.

a. ______ Advance catheter until resistance is felt.
b. ______ Apply suctioning while withdrawing catheter.
c. ______ Attach catheter to connecting tubing, and test equipment function.
d. ______ Document procedure and observations.
e. ______ Don sterile gloves.
f. ______ Insert catheter into trachea during inspiration.
g. ______ Offer assistance with oral/nasal hygiene.
h. ______ Position client for ease of catheter insertion.
i. ______ Preoxygenate client with 100% O_2.
j. ______ Prepare sterile suction catheter kit.
k. ______ Remove gloves and discard them.
l. ______ Rinse catheter and suction oropharynx.
m. ______ Turn off suction.
n. ______ Turn on suction device.

HOT SPOT QUESTIONS

Place an "X" on the respiratory structure that prevents food from entering the airway.

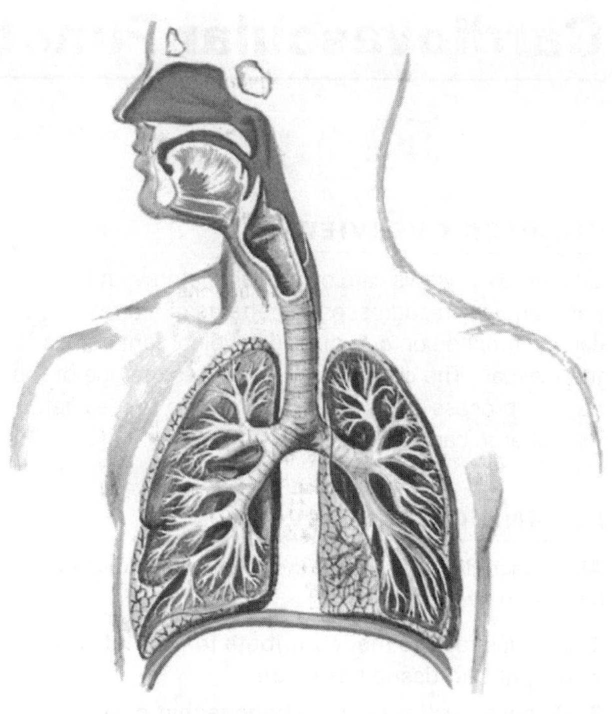

CHAPTER 37

Oxygenation: Cardiovascular Function

CHAPTER OVERVIEW

Chapter 37 reviews cardiovascular anatomy and physiology, and addresses the effects of altered cardiac function on growth and development across the lifespan. The chapter also discusses the use of the nursing process to plan and provide care to the client with altered cardiac function.

LEARNING OBJECTIVES

After mastering the content in this chapter, you should be able to do the following:

1. Discuss factors that contribute to normal cardiac output and tissue perfusion.
2. Discuss cardiovascular changes that occur across the lifespan.
3. Describe the causes of altered cardiovascular function.
4. Describe how altered cardiovascular function can have an impact on normal activities.
5. Perform a basic nursing assessment of cardiovascular function.
6. Identify common procedures and diagnostic tests used in the evaluation of the cardiovascular client.
7. State relevant nursing diagnoses for the client with cardiovascular dysfunction.
8. Discuss nursing measures directed at promoting and restoring cardiovascular function.

■ Mastering the Information

MATCHING

Match the terms in Column II with a definition, example, or related statement from Column I. Place the letter corresponding to the answer in the space provided. (Use each letter only once; some letters may not be used.)

COLUMN I

1. ______ The period between contractions of the ventricles when the heart muscle relaxes and chambers fill
2. ______ Outlines blood flow through vessels to identify blockages
3. ______ Capability of the heart to generate its own electrical impulse
4. ______ Limb pain caused by poor blood flow
5. ______ The natural strength of the heart muscle
6. ______ Vein inflammation
7. ______ Results in increased blood viscosity
8. ______ The flow of blood through the tissues of the body
9. ______ An inappropriate clot formation; usually occurs in deep leg veins
10. ______ Inadequate perfusion resulting in tissue hypoxia and starvation and pain

COLUMN II

a. Perfusion
b. Arteriosclerosis
c. Ischemia
d. Thrombus
e. Contractility
f. Aneurysm
g. Diastole
h. Automaticity
i. Intermittent claudication
j. Phlebitis
k. Polycythemia
l. Angiography

TRUE–FALSE

Indicate if the following statements are true or false.

______ 1. Positioning extremities higher than the level of the heart would result in increased venous return.

______ 2. A client with cardiac dysrhythmias may experience decreased tissue perfusion due to decreased pumping ability of the heart.

______ 3. Plaque formation on the arterial vessel wall is a common cause of low blood pressure.

______ 4. Capillary dysfunction may result from venous congestion and may cause tissue edema.

______ 5. Venous pooling decreases myocardial work by increasing stroke volume and cardiac output.

FILL IN THE BLANK

Supply the missing term or the information requested.

1. Good cardiovascular function depends on a ________________ to pump blood, an adequate ________________, and healthy ________________ to distribute blood to tissues.
2. To guarantee a near-constant level of perfusion, the brain relies on neural receptors located in the ________________, which supply blood to the brain.
3. Two of the three primary NANDA nursing diagnoses for the client with cardiovascular dysfunction include ________________ and ________________.
4. State one important role of the nurse in promoting optimum cardiovascular health.

   ____

   ____
5. What impact might cardiovascular dysfunction have on an individual?

   ____

   ____
6. List five manifestations of altered cardiovascular function.

   a.

   b.

   c.

   d.

   e.
7. Give one example of a condition in which altered cardiovascular function can occur in each of the following categories.

   a. The heart being less effective as a pump:

   ____

   b. The blood vessels being unable to deliver blood adequately to the tissues: ________________

   c. Abnormalities occurring within the blood:

   ________________ .
8. ________________ is a medical emergency for which cardiopulmonary resuscitation must be quickly and effectively performed to prevent ________________ and ________________.

■ Applying Your Knowledge

CASE STUDY

Mr. Presley, 59 years old, has come to the doctor today because he is concerned that he may be "getting sick." Mr. Presley states that he is experiencing intermittent periods of confusion that he initially attributed to getting old. He became more concerned because his speech is slurred sometimes, and he has begun to experience occasional numbness in his right hand and leg.

1. Identify the medical condition of which the above clinical picture is strongly suggestive and outline the changes in the normal cardiovascular function that would lead to the identified condition.
2. Develop a list of questions that you would ask Mr. Presley in order to identify factors that contribute to the manifestations he has described.

3. Identify nursing interventions that will be incorporated into Mr. Presley's plan of care. Provide a rationale for each intervention.

CRITICAL INQUIRY EXERCISE

1. Assess the risk factors for cardiovascular problems for yourself and those of an older relative—mother, father, aunt, or uncle.
2. Prepare a discharge teaching plan for a client admitted with chest pain without evident myocardial damage and for the client's significant others. Include activity precautions, medication administration, and emergency measures.

CRITICAL EXPLORATION EXERCISE

Spend a day in the cardiac care unit. Monitor the care provided to the client who has experienced acute myocardial infarction. Note the laboratory work ordered and results that confirmed the infarct. Contrast the laboratory results and nursing care provided this client with those of a client admitted with chest pain without cardiac damage.

■ Practicing for NCLEX

MULTIPLE CHOICE QUESTIONS

Circle the letter that corresponds to the best answer for each question.

1. Mrs. Wilson presents in the physician's office with symptoms of a transient ischemic attack (TIA). The nurse knows to observe Mrs. Wilson for which of the following characteristic disturbances?
   a. Cold skin
   b. Confusion
   c. Congestion
   d. Constipation

2. The nurse knows that TIAs are warning signs of possibly impending
   a. cerebrovascular accident.
   b. intermittent claudication.
   c. myocardial infarction.
   d. pulmonary embolism.

3. Increased blood flow to the skin, such as that which occurs with fever, would result in which of the following colorings?
   a. Ashen
   b. Cyanosis
   c. Pallor
   d. Rubor

4. Persons having problems with high blood pressure should be taught the importance of avoiding
   a. cigarette smoking.
   b. decaffeinated beverages.
   c. light alcohol intake.
   d. prescription vasodilators.

5. A client who stands for long periods of time while working or who has had trauma to his veins with resulting phlebitis could experience venous valve incompetency and
   a. arterial vessel occlusion.
   b. decreased capillary refill.
   c. decreased stroke volume.
   d. poor vascular resistance.

6. The nurse would be concerned if which of the following changes in vital signs were noted in one of the following clients?
   a. Amy, 5 years old, whose blood pressure is 10 mm Hg higher than noted 2 years previously
   b. Bryan, 2 months old, whose systolic blood pressure is 30 mm Hg higher than noted when he was a newborn
   c. Cynthia, 17 years old, whose resting pulse rate is 20 beats faster than noted during her preschool years
   d. Derrick, 28 years old, whose pulse rate is the same as noted when he was a teenager

7. To promote activity tolerance for the client with cardiovascular dysfunction, the nurse should teach the client to
   a. limit activity for 10 minutes after ingesting meals.
   b. monitor blood pressure during and after activity.
   c. take prescribed nitroglycerin after activity when pain is noted while performing an activity.
   d. plan heavy activity to alternate with 1- to 2-hour rest periods.

8. A client with edema should be instructed to
   a. avoid foods with high sodium content and excessive fluid intake.
   b. lower edematous areas to increase blood flow and tissue perfusion.
   c. maintain a dependent position to facilitate drainage of blood from extremities.
   d. wear constrictive clothing to limit the formation of edema in the extremities.

9. Mr. Wilson has a history of chest pain due to inadequate oxygen supply to the heart. He was discharged with instructions to use nitroglycerin as needed. He was washing his car and began to have dull pain in his left chest. Initially, Mr. Wilson should
   a. sit comfortably with head elevated and rest quietly.
   b. slow his pace and breathe deeply as he finishes washing his car.
   c. take three nitroglycerin tablets orally and continue his activity.
   d. call 911 and ask that an ambulance be sent to his home immediately.

10. Successful rehabilitation of the client with cardiovascular problems should include
    a. emphasizing the need for the client to lead a sedentary lifestyle to avoid stress on the heart.
    b. promoting activity tolerance after the client's medical problem has been identified and treated.
    c. explaining to most clients that they will be unable to enjoy a normal lifestyle.
    d. instructing the client to perform the Valsalva maneuver to treat chest pain.

FILL IN THE BLANK

Supply the missing term or the information requested.

1. The purpose of tissue perfusion is to supply oxygen to body tissues and to remove ________________.

2. A medical emergency for which CPR must be quickly and effectively performed to prevent morbidity and mortality is ________________.

MULTIPLE-ANSWER MULTIPLE CHOICE

Circle the letter(s) corresponding to the appropriate answer(s). Circle all that apply

1. When applying antiembolic stockings, the nurse should
   a. apply powder or light talc over the foot and leg first.
   b. measure the length from heel to knee for thigh-high stockings.
   c. order the size of stocking that will provide a firm constriction around the top of the calf or thigh.
   d. position the client with the legs dependent one-half hour before application.

2. Which of the following are appropriate initial questions to ask of the client experiencing chest pain?
   a. What does it feel like?
   b. Does the pain go anywhere?
   c. Does the pain increase with deep breathing or movement?
   d. When did the pain start?
   e. What were you doing when it began?

3. Which of the following nursing interventions are appropriate?
   a. Applying an ice compress to the extremities of a client with peripheral ischemic pain
   b. Placing a pillow case over a heating pad used on the extremities of a client with peripheral ischemic pain
   c. Assessing the cardiovascular client's physical, mental, and emotional readiness for rehabilitative measures before implementation of any measures
   d. Teaching the client with cardiovascular conditions to perform warm-up exercises before routine exercising
   e. Instructing the client with cardiovascular disease that exercise is the best cure for the condition

4. Which of the following are controllable cardiovascular risk factors?
   a. Age
   b. Being male or female after menopause
   c. Cigarette/tobacco use
   d. Diabetes mellitus
   e. High blood cholesterol
   f. High blood pressure
   g. Physical inactivity

5. Which of the following interventions would be most appropriate for the client who is in day 2 of treatment for congestive heart failure?
   a. Pulmonologist consultation
   b. Assess need for home healthcare social service referral
   c. Vital signs every 4 hours
   d. Daily weights
   e. O_2 saturation monitoring
   f. Clear liquids as tolerated
   g. IV diuretics

ORDERING

Indicate the appropriate order for the following steps in adult cardiopulmonary resuscitation by numbering the items.

a. ______ Ventilate two full breaths.

b. ______ Open airway using a head tilt—chin lift.

c. ______ Listen, look, and feel for breathing.

d. ______ Shake to determine responsiveness.

e. ______ Perform 15 cardiac compressions.

f. ______ Assess for carotid pulse for 5 seconds.

g. ______ Find correct hand placement for cardiac compressions.

h. ______ Pinch nostrils with thumb and index finger of your hand.

UNIT IX

Nutrition and Metabolism

CHAPTER 38

Fluid, Electrolyte, and Acid–Base Balance

CHAPTER OVERVIEW

Chapter 38 examines and summarizes the basic concepts of fluid, electrolyte, and acid–base balance. Application of the nursing process in the care of clients with alterations in fluid, electrolyte, and acid–base balance and interventions used to facilitate fluid, electrolyte, and acid–base balance are also emphasized.

LEARNING OBJECTIVES

After mastering the content in this chapter, you should be able to do the following:

1. Describe physiologic factors that affect fluid, electrolyte, and acid–base homeostasis.
2. Explain the impact of age on fluid and electrolyte status.
3. Discuss common alterations in fluid, electrolyte, and acid–base balance.
4. Describe assessment parameters for clients with potential or actual fluid, electrolyte, or acid–base imbalances.
5. Identify appropriate nursing diagnoses for clients with fluid, electrolyte, or acid–base imbalances.
6. Implement appropriate client teaching to prevent or manage fluid and electrolyte imbalance.

■ Mastering the Information

MATCHING

Match the terms in Column II with a definition, example, or related statement from Column I. Place the letter corresponding to the answer in the space provided. (Use each letter only once; some letters may not be used.)

COLUMN I

1. ______ Fluid that is dispersed between cells
2. ______ Proportion of dissolved particles in a fluid
3. ______ Any area where fluid accumulates and is physiologically unavailable
4. ______ Helps to maintain fluid and electrolyte balance by regulating sodium levels
5. ______ Used to evaluate acid–base balance

COLUMN II

a. Third spacing
b. Osmolarity
c. Aldosterone
d. Arterial blood gases
e. Interstitial fluid

TRUE–FALSE

Indicate if the following statements are true or false.

______ 1. A client history of altered mental status and stress would have no relevance in the evaluation of fluid and electrolyte balance.

______ 2. Edema is an early symptom indicative of fluid volume excess.

______ 3. Moment-to-moment maintenance of acid–base status is handled by the kidneys.

______ 4. Cations are positively charged electrolytes.

______ 5. A person is alkalotic when the pH is greater than 7.43.

______ 6. Medications such as insulin and antacids can contribute to fluid and electrolyte disturbances.

______ 7. With ECF volume excess, the pulse may be weak and thready.

______ 8. Water loss through the skin, respiration, urine, and stool is proportionally less for the young child than for the adult.

FILL IN THE BLANK

Supply the missing term or the information requested.

1. Identify three of the four routes through which water can be lost from the body.
   a.
   b.
   c.
2. The percentage of total body water for an individual varies depending on the individual's ________________, ________________, and ________________.
3. Identify three related nursing diagnoses that can occur when clients are experiencing fluid and electrolyte imbalances.
   a.
   b.
   c.
4. State two reasons for initiating intravenous (IV) therapy.
   a.
   b.

■ Applying Your Knowledge

CASE STUDY

Charity, age 4½ months, is admitted to the hospital with a diagnosis of dehydration. Her father states that she has been vomiting everything that she has been given for the past 24 hours. She is lethargic, her skin turgor is poor, and her mucous membranes are dry. Her pH is 7.31; Na, 130; Cl, 93; and K, 3.3. Her father states that she has had only two wet diapers in the last 24 hours.

1. Identify what type of fluid deficit the client is experiencing, and provide your rationale.
2. Based on the information in the situation, determine if the client is experiencing acidosis or alkalosis and if the imbalance is metabolic or respiratory. Explain your answers.
3. Identify the normal characteristics of the client that increase her risk for alterations in fluid and electrolyte balance.
4. Develop a plan of care to meet the fluid needs of the client.
5. Contrast the clinical picture and treatment for a client with diarrhea with those of a client with vomiting.

CRITICAL INQUIRY EXERCISE

Record your own intake and output for a 24-hour period. Compare intake to output. Is there a balance between the two? If not, give reasons that may account for the difference.

CRITICAL EXPLORATION EXERCISE

Review a client's electrolyte laboratory values. Are there any imbalances? If so, can any of the imbalances be associated with treatment? Provide a rationale for your response.

■ Practicing for NCLEX

MULTIPLE CHOICE QUESTIONS

Circle the letter that corresponds to the best answer for each question.

1. Which of the following is/are sign(s) of fluid volume excess?
   a. Warm, moist skin
   b. Distended neck veins
   c. Dyspnea on exertion
   d. Blue extremities

2. Mrs. Lewis presents in the doctor's office complaining of difficulty breathing. She has a history of asthma. Her respiratory rate is 28. The physician draws blood gases. The pH is 7.2, and the $PaCO_2$ is 65. Based on the assessment data, Mrs. Lewis is probably experiencing
   a. respiratory acidosis.
   b. respiratory alkalosis.
   c. metabolic acidosis.
   d. metabolic alkalosis.

3. The client presenting with vomiting is most likely to experience
   a. respiratory acidosis.
   b. respiratory alkalosis.
   c. metabolic acidosis.
   d. metabolic alkalosis.

4. The average daily amount of fluid intake that is necessary for the healthy adult to maintain fluid homeostasis is
   a. 300 mL.
   b. 600 mL.
   c. 1000 mL.
   d. 1300 mL.

5. Which of the following initial responses by the body would you expect with metabolic acidosis?
   a. Decreased heart rate
   b. Increased urinary output
   c. Increased rate and depth of respirations
   d. Increased blood pressure

6. Mrs. Brown, 72 years old, is seen in the emergency room with a diagnosis of possible fluid volume deficit. Which of the following signs and symptoms would reliably indicate a fluid volume deficit?
   a. Elastic skin turgor
   b. Rapid filling of peripheral veins
   c. Decreased urine output for the past 2 days
   d. Brown skin tone on a client of color

7. A client presents with dyspnea, rales, and orthopnea. These symptoms are often present in the client who has
   a. extracellular fluid deficit.
   b. extracellular fluid excess.
   c. water deficit.
   d. water excess.

8. Which of the following dietary sources is appropriately matched to the electrolyte it will replenish?
   a. Magnesium/tea
   b. Calcium/squash
   c. Potassium/bananas
   d. Protein/peaches

9. When evaluating intake and output, the nurse should
   a. check the output record for the best indication of intake volume.
   b. evaluate the trend of intake and output for at least 48 hours.
   c. suspect a fluid balance problem when urinary output is less than 300 mL/hour.
   d. encourage the client to drink enough fluid to keep urine dark yellow.

10. To minimize thirst for clients on fluid restrictions, the nurse should include all of the following except
    a. allowing the client to rinse the mouth frequently.
    b. encouraging the use of sugar-free gum and hard candy.
    c. encouraging the client to view television as a diversional activity.
    d. providing frequent oral care.

FILL IN THE BLANK

Supply the missing term or the information requested.

1. Pitting edema indicates that a client has experienced at least what percentage of increase in body weight? ____________________
2. The total milliliter fluid intake for a client consuming 8 oz of gelatin dessert, 4 oz of pureed peas, 8 oz of ice chips, and 4 oz of chicken broth is ____________________.

MULTIPLE-ANSWER MULTIPLE CHOICE

Circle the letter(s) corresponding to the appropriate answer(s). Circle all that apply.

1. Ms. Carpenter is placed on diuretic therapy as part of her treatment regimen for fluid volume excess. Ms. Carpenter may experience a depletion of which electrolyte secondary to diuretic therapy?
   a. Calcium
   b. Chloride
   c. Potassium
   d. Sodium
   e. Magnesium
2. When administering intravenous calcium, the nurse should
   a. administer the infusion slowly.
   b. implement seizure precautions as needed.
   c. monitor for cardiac dysrhythmias.
   d. prepare client for the possibility of needing peritoneal dialysis.
   e. restrict phosphate intake.
3. Which of the following factors can alter the surgical client's fluid and electrolyte status?
   a. Cellular trauma
   b. Emotional stress
   c. Increased insensible water loss
   d. Nausea and vomiting
   e. NPO status
   f. Pain
   g. Presence of nasogastric tubes and drains
4. Which of the following combination of findings best indicate that the client has experienced a decrease in vascular volume?
   a. Decreased urine output
   b. Dry mucous membranes
   c. Orthostatic decrease in blood pressure
   d. Poor skin turgor
   e. Weak pulse

CHAPTER 39

Nutrition

CHAPTER OVERVIEW

Chapter 39 discusses the function of the digestive system, nutrients essential for health, factors that affect nutrition, nutritional-assessment modalities, and manifestations of altered nutrition. Nursing interventions to promote optimal nutrition and techniques for evaluating client responses are also discussed.

LEARNING OBJECTIVES

After mastering the content in this chapter, you should be able to do the following:

1. Identify essential nutrients and examples of good dietary sources of each.
2. Describe normal digestion, absorption, and metabolism of carbohydrates, fats, and proteins.
3. Discuss nutritional considerations across the lifespan.
4. List factors that can affect dietary patterns.
5. Describe manifestations of altered nutrition.
6. Explain nursing interventions to promote optimal nutrition and health.
7. Discuss nursing responsibilities for interventions used to treat altered nutritional states.

■ Mastering the Information

MATCHING

Match the terms in Column II with a definition, example, or related statement from Column I. Place the letter corresponding to the answer in the space provided. (Use each letter only once; some letters may not be used.)

COLUMN I

1. ______ The actions related to tissue repair, converting simple substances into complex substances
2. ______ Polysaccharides that are not digested in the gastrointestinal tract
3. ______ Measures the energy obtained from food sources
4. ______ The act of breaking down complex substances into simpler substances
5. ______ The chemical process in the cells that allows for energy use and cellular growth and repair
6. ______ An opening into the stomach
7. ______ A condition in which the blood glucose level is higher than normal due to inadequate production or use of insulin
8. ______ A condition in which the BMI is 30 kg/m^2 or more
9. ______ A condition in which the blood glucose level is lower than normal
10. ______ A condition that exists when the amount of nitrogen excreted exceeds the intake
11. ______ A nutrient that contains sufficient amounts of amino acids to maintain body tissue and promote growth

COLUMN II

a. Metabolism
b. Hypoglycemia
c. Complete protein
d. Negative nitrogen balance
e. Obesity
f. Anabolic processes
g. Catabolic processes
h. Hyperglycemi
i. Kilocalorie
j. Fiber
k. Gastrostomy

TRUE–FALSE

Indicate if the following statements are true or false.

_____ 1. A nutritionally adequate diet is vital for promoting normal growth and development and preventing deficiency states.

_____ 2. Total parenteral nutrition is the only useful therapy for clients with impaired nutritional status.

_____ 3. The body uses nutrients for three major functions: building and maintaining body tissue, furnishing energy, and regulating body processes.

_____ 4. Fresh foods are usually the best source of vitamins.

_____ 5. Adequate nutritional intake is important to maintain body functions, promote healing, maintain healthy tissues, maintain body temperature, and build resistance to infection.

_____ 6. Therapeutic diets are prescribed only for the management of disease processes.

_____ 7. Nursing interventions to promote optimum nutrition include client teaching to help increase the individual's understanding/valuing of the importance of a healthy diet and creating an atmosphere that encourages healthy eating.

_____ 8. Anthropometric measurements, such as height and weight and arm circumference, along with calorie counts and swallowing ability, can provide objective data regarding an individual's nutritional status.

_____ 9. In addition to providing a substantial part of the daily nutritional needs of children, the school lunch program should make a valuable contribution in terms of nutrition education and developing good nutrition habits.

_____10. A nutritional assessment should include information about normal eating patterns, risk factors for nutritional deficits, and altered nutrition.

FILL IN THE BLANK

Supply the missing term or the information requested.

1. Essential nutrients include _______________, _______________, _______________, _______________, _______________, and _______________.

2. Foods that are good sources of iron are _______________, _______________, _______________, and _______________.

3. Problems of altered nutrition are often related to various factors. Four of these 10 factors are _______________, _______________, _______________, and _______________.

4. Calcium is essential for regulation of materials in and out of cells. It may be acquired from such foods as the following: _______________, _______________, _______________, _______________, _______________, and _______________.

5. Foods that have high sodium content include _______________, _______________, _______________, _______________, _______________, _______________, and _______________.

6. Foods that have high potassium content include _______________, _______________, _______________, _______________, and _______________.

7. Normal physiologic functions of the digestive system include _______________, _______________, _______________, and _______________.

8. Four indications of normal nutrition are:
   a.
   b.
   c.
   d.

9. List seven factors that affect the intake of nutrients.
   a. ______
   b. ______
   c. ______
   d. ______
   e. ______
   f. ______
   g. ______
10. Manifestations of altered nutrition include:
   a. ______
   b. ______
   c. ______
   d. ______
   e. ______

■ Applying Your Knowledge

CASE STUDY

Ms. Griggs, 75 years old, is being admitted to the hospital with a diagnosis of malnutrition and dehydration. She is 5 ft 6 in tall and weighs 90 lb on admission. Her skin and mucous membranes are dry, her skin turgor is poor, and her hair is dry and brittle. She reports nausea but is not vomiting currently. She also reports abdominal pain. Her abdomen is slightly distended, and her bowel sounds are hypoactive. Her son is with her. He states that his mother lives alone and that she has severe arthritis. He does not live in town but calls his mom frequently to check on her. He decided to go check on her after he spoke to her last because "she just didn't sound right, even though she told me she was fine." He states that when he arrived at her home, "she looked like she was about to pass out," but even at this point, she insisted that she was okay. He decided she needed to come to the hospital.

1. Discuss the priority nursing diagnosis you would address for Ms. Griggs, and provide your rationale for this choice.
2. Outline the initial nursing interventions that would be appropriate for this client.
3. Develop a discharge plan for Ms. Griggs addressing ways to prevent this from happening again.
4. Discuss some of the feelings Ms. Griggs' son may have regarding his mother's situation and how you would address these feelings.

CRITICAL INQUIRY EXERCISE

1. Use a telephone directory to identify and list the community-based programs for nutritional support of individuals of different ages in your community.
2. Observe the preparation of therapeutic or special diets in a hospital dietary department.
3. Observe during mealtime in one of the following settings: nursing home, newborn nursery, school lunch room, or cancer unit. Write a brief report of the methods used to promote health or correct nutritional deficits.

CRITICAL EXPLORATION EXERCISE

Perform a comprehensive nutritional assessment of a homebound client.

■ Practicing for NCLEX

MULTIPLE CHOICE QUESTIONS

Circle the letter that corresponds to the best answer for each question.

1. Ms. Petty has an extremely high serum cholesterol level. She should be instructed that dietary modifications will
   a. not lower fat and cholesterol intake that is not related to obesity, coronary artery disease, or several forms of cancer.
   b. lower fat and cholesterol intake, which is vital to preventing obesity, coronary artery disease, and several forms of cancer.
   c. not affect serum cholesterol levels but will reduce the risk of obesity, coronary artery disease, hypertension, diabetes, and stomach cancer.
   d. significantly lower serum cholesterol levels for all clients but do not have any relationship to hypertension, coronary artery disease, or various forms of cancer.

2. Melvin's record shows a 2-year history of inflammatory bowel disease. A likely nursing diagnosis is imbalanced nutrition
   a. less than body requirements related to inability to use ingested nutrients.
   b. less than body requirements related to inadequate intake of nutrients.
   c. less than body requirements related to eating habits, lifestyle, and ability to masticate foods.
   d. more than body requirements related to excessive absorption and digestion of nutrients.

3. Sara Jones has small bowel obstruction. Such a condition usually necessitates withholding
   a. all high-fiber and spicy foods until the problem is resolved or has been surgically corrected.
   b. all high-fiber foods and water until the problem is resolved or has been surgically corrected.
   c. all spicy and high-calorie foods until the problem is resolved.
   d. all oral intake until the obstruction is resolved or has been surgically corrected.

4. A low-sodium diet has been prescribed for Mr. Johnson, who has hypertension. Which of the following questions should the nurse ask to ascertain information about his values and knowledge?
   a. "Will you follow the prescribed diet?"
   b. "Do you know which foods to avoid and how to prepare your food?"
   c. "What changes in your diet do you think are necessary to promote health?"
   d. "Do you use prepackaged foods or do you have someone to prepare food for you?"

5. Mr. Sipps has a nasogastric tube in place for intermittent feedings. During feedings he should be placed in which position, unless contraindicated?
   a. Flat with head to one side
   b. Flat and supine
   c. High Fowler's
   d. Right lateral

6. The physician states that a postoperative client is in a state of negative nitrogen balance. The nurse should understand that this is
   a. a desirable state that promotes healing and rapid recovery; therefore, no nursing intervention relating to diet is necessary.
   b. an indication for vigorous regulation of caloric intake and reduction of fluid intake until there is complete wound healing.
   c. an undesirable condition that exists when a disease state is causing excessive tissue breakdown or when the diet is inadequate in protein, calories, or both.
   d. an undesirable condition related to excessive intake of sodium, potassium, iron, and water, resulting in tissue breakdown and slowed metabolism.

7. Ms. Shaw is 2 months pregnant. Which statement is proper in response to her question about her dietary intake?
   a. A pregnant woman does not have to make substantial changes in her dietary habits.
   b. Minor deficiencies in the pregnant woman's diet are more likely to influence the baby's development than the mother's health.
   c. Individual food preferences, lifestyle, and economic, religious, and cultural factors should determine what the pregnant woman eats.
   d. The pregnant woman's dietary intake may include a substantial increase in calories, protein, calcium, folic acid, and iron.

8. Ms. Asp is a frail 70-year-old woman who has difficulty swallowing after experiencing a stroke. A stated nursing diagnosis is impaired swallowing related to weakness of muscles required for mastication and swallowing. Which of the following goals is specifically related to the nursing diagnosis?
   a. Client will avoid food that cannot be swallowed.
   b. Client will accept nutritional supplements.
   c. Client will maintain oral intake adequate to meet caloric demands.
   d. Client will maintain dietary intake adequate to meet expenditures of the body.

9. A client is known to have vitamin K deficiency. The nurse should be alert for signs of
   a. bleeding.
   b. swelling.
   c. vomiting.
   d. choking.

10. The newborn needs more calories per pound of body weight because the basal metabolic rate is
    a. low.
    b. moderate.
    c. high.
    d. unstable.

FILL IN THE BLANK

Supply the missing term or the information requested.

1. The upper limit for a normal fasting blood glucose is _____________.
2. The recommended daily allowance (RDA) of calcium for adults is ____________.
3. Two survey methods that may be used when accurate information about dietary patterns is needed are the 24-hour recall and the _______________.

MULTIPLE-ANSWER MULTIPLE CHOICE

Circle the letter(s) corresponding to the appropriate answer(s). Circle all that apply.

1. Nursing responsibilities for a client receiving nasogastric tube feedings include
   a. preventing and assessing potential complications, such as nausea, vomiting, aspiration, and fluid or electrolyte imbalance.
   b. keeping the client flat in bed to promote gravity flow of the formula and to provide for rest.
   c. checking residuals and decreasing or stopping the flow rate if the residual is greater than 100 mL.
   d. flushing the tube after each feeding and recording responses to various types of formula.

2. Values and attitudes concerning eating develop during which period?
   a. Newborn
   b. Infancy
   c. Toddler
   d. Preschooler
   e. Adolescence
   f. Young adulthood

3. The most common laboratory data used to specify nutritional deficiencies are
   a. hematocrit and hemoglobin.
   b. serum albumin.
   c. serum transferring.
   d. total lymphocyte count.

4. In the older adult, metabolic rate declines. The need for calories decreases, but the need for which nutrients remains high?
   a. Fats
   b. Iron
   c. Minerals
   d. Proteins
   e. Vitamins

5. Objective data about the nutritional status of a client are best obtained by
   a. observing the client.
   b. anthropometric measurements.
   c. calorie counts.
   d. evaluation of swallowing ability.
   e. reviewing laboratory and diagnostic test reports.

CHAPTER 40

Skin Integrity and Wound Healing

CHAPTER OVERVIEW

Chapter 40 examines the structure, function, and characteristics of normal skin, as well as manifestations of altered skin integrity. It presents interventions to prevent altered integumentary function and to promote wound healing.

LEARNING OBJECTIVES

After mastering the content in this chapter, you should be able to do the following:

1. Discuss factors that affect integumentary function.
2. Identify manifestations of impaired integumentary function.
3. Describe normal wound healing and factors that affect it.
4. Discuss nursing assessment of skin integrity and wound healing.
5. List categories of support surfaces used to prevent pressure ulcers.
6. Discuss nursing interventions to promote skin integrity.
7. Explain scientific principles in the application of heat and cold to injured areas.
8. Describe categories of wound dressings and their indications.

■ Mastering the Information

MATCHING

Match the terms in Column II with a definition, example, or related statement from Column I. Place the letter corresponding to the answer in the space provided. (Use each letter only once; some letters may not be used.)

COLUMN I

1. _b_ A break in skin integrity
2. _e_ The outer layer of the skin
3. _d_ Regeneration of tissue, a complex restorative process following any injury
4. _g_ The external covering of the body; its largest organ
5. _a_ The removal of foreign material or dead tissue from a wound
6. _h_ Skin continually exposed to moisture that has become more easily damaged
7. _f_ Full-thickness wound healing
8. _c_ A dark black crust that develops on pressure ulcers or other wounds

COLUMN II

a. Débridement
b. Wound
c. Eschar
d. Wound healing
e. Epidermis
f. Proliferation
g. Integument
h. Macerated

COLUMN I

1. _e_ Protective cover for areas exposed to friction
2. _d_ Minor burns
3. _b_ Packing of deep wounds
4. _a_ Deep, draining wounds
5. _c_ Venous leg ulcers

COLUMN II

a. Alginate
b. Gauzes
c. Hydrocolloid wafer
d. Hydrogels
e. Transparent adhesive

TRUE–FALSE

Indicate if the following statements are true or false.

T 1. The very young and the very old are most susceptible to skin disruption.

F 2. The presence of skin odor is always indicative of impaired skin function.

F 3. Healing by first intention occurs when a wound is closed after the wound surface has started to granulate.

T 4. Wounds that fill with soft, pinkish-red buds that easily bleed and finally grow epithelial cells are said to heal by second intention.

F 5. Most hospitalized or homebound clients do not require planned nursing intervention to prevent development of pressure sores or trauma to the skin.

T 6. Wound support can be provided by sutures, staples, clips, steristrips, bandages, and binders.

T 7. Effective management of drain systems may include ensuring that drainage systems function properly and dressings are intact to promote optimal wound healing.

T 8. Family members' acceptance of the skin impairment and their willingness to assist with care can boost the client's self-esteem.

T 9. Regeneration follows the inflammatory phase in healing of partial-thickness wounds.

FILL IN THE BLANK

Supply the missing term or the information requested.

1. The health of skin depends on adequate blood flow, sufficient nutrition, intact epidermis, and proper hygene.
2. List five physiologic functions of normal skin.
   a. protection
   b. thermoregulation
   c. sensation
   d. metabolism
   e. communication
3. Altered skin integrity may be manifested by pruritus, rashes, lesions, pain, and inadequate wound healing
4. Understanding the types of wound healing (primary, secondary, and tertiary) is vital for proper wound assessment and management
5. Five major factors that affect integumentary function are:
   a. allergies
   b. infection
   c. trauma
   d. circulation
   e. nutrition
6. List five principles that relate to skin care.
   a. skin nourishment
   b. hygeine
   c. sensitivity
   d. intact skin
   e. prevention of breakdown
7. Subjective data about a client's skin should include information about the following:
   a. normal status
   b. risk for impairment
   c. past history
8. Local application of heat causes vasodilation and promotes removal of metabolic waste.

■ Applying Your Knowledge

CASE STUDY

Jennifer is an 11-year-old girl with chickenpox. The lesions are more numerous on her face and head. Her mother states that she constantly has to remind Jennifer not to scratch the lesions. She also states that she is very concerned because Jennifer stares at her face in the mirror saying that she never wants to leave her room again.

1. Identify two physiologic diagnoses and one psychosocial diagnosis appropriate for this client situation.
2. State your rationale for each of the above nursing diagnoses.
3. Identify nursing interventions that should be included in the plan of care for this client situation.
4. How would you address Jennifer's mother's concern about Jennifer staring in the mirror and saying she never wants to leave her room?

CRITICAL INQUIRY EXERCISE

1. Practice applying bandages, binders, slings, dressings, Montgomery straps, and ties in a skills laboratory or at home.
2. Design a discharge teaching plan for a client going home with a pressure sore.

CRITICAL EXPLORATION EXERCISE

1. Tour a hospital emergency room or first aid station. Write a short observation report regarding the following:
   a. Types of wounds noted
   b. Types of wound support devices used
   c. Follow-up instructions given
2. During a clinical experience, note the medical diagnoses of clients at risk of integumentary malfunction.

■ Practicing for NCLEX

MULTIPLE CHOICE QUESTIONS

Circle the letter that corresponds to the best answer for each question.

1. A client who sustained a small laceration on her finger while peeling potatoes should be instructed to
   a. cleanse it well and apply heat immediately to promote healing.
   b. cleanse it well and apply ice to promote blood clotting.
   c. cleanse it well with water and mild soap.
   d. cleanse it well with alcohol and apply a Band-Aid.

2. When bathing a client, a complete skin assessment is possible. The recorded assessment data should include which of the following information about the skin?
   a. Color, texture, and moisture
   b. Temperature, drainage, and odor
   c. Odor, turgor, and hair color
   d. Suspected illness, odor, and temperature

3. A 68-year-old obese woman is confined to the bed or a wheelchair. A likely nursing diagnosis is
   a. impaired skin integrity related to decreased nutritional status.
   b. risk for impaired skin integrity related to limited mobility and exercise.
   c. altered integumentary function related to decreased perception.
   d. potential for tissue wasting related to poor circulation.

4. To prevent development of pressure sores in a bedridden client, the nurse should
   a. change the client's position at least once during the 8-hour shift.
   b. limit food intake to minimize the risk of skin breakdown secondary to obesity.
   c. provide fluids for adequate hydration.
   d. keep bony prominences moist.

5. Two common skin disorders of infants are
   a. overgrowth of the epidermis and pruritus.
   b. diaper rash and eczema.
   c. overgrowth and hematomas.
   d. hematomas and pruritus.

6. In addition to physiologic functions, the skin plays an important role in self-concept development by
   a. providing the basis for personal appearance and a means of communication between people.
   b. reacting to touch by loved ones and changing complexion.
   c. responding to temperature changes and serving as a gauge for proper dress.
   d. collecting bacterial contaminants, which might invade the body and cause illness.

7. Special care is needed to maintain skin integrity in neonates because the skin is
   a. thicker and coarser than that of older infants or adults.
   b. thicker and more moist than that of older infants or adults.
   c. thinner and more sensitive than that of older infants or adults.
   d. thinner and less sensitive than that of older infants or adults.

8. Client teaching regarding the maintenance of skin integrity should include
   a. keeping infants clean and dry and avoiding overexposure to sun rays.
   b. pruritus relief measures, wound-healing techniques, and application of moisturizing skin cream to skin folds.
   c. daily bathing with a deodorant soap and limiting dietary intake of protein.
   d. periodic sun bathing, using moisturizers, and limiting fluid intake.

FILL IN THE BLANK

Supply the missing term or the information requested.

1. The wound cleansing solution of choice for chronic wounds is Saline.

2. How many days after surgery are sutures usually removed from well-approximated incisions? 7-10

3. Two commonly used closed systems for wound drainage are the Penrose drain and the Hemovac.

4. Prevention of communicable diseases, impetigo, and lice infestation are the goals of prevention for which population of children? School-age

MULTIPLE-ANSWER MULTIPLE CHOICE

Circle the letter(s) corresponding to the appropriate answer(s). Circle all that apply.

1. Which of the following measures is appropriate to use for an electrical burn?
   a. Remove from source
   b. Stop, drop, and roll
   c. Remove clothing
   d. If smothering, douse with water

2. Which of the following would be considered primary lesions?
   a. Fissure
   b. Macule
   c. Nodule
   d. Scale
   e. Tumor

3. Which of the following are considered to be systemic factors that affect wound healing?
   a. Circulation
   b. Drug therapy
   c. Nature & location of injury
   d. Obesity
   e. Presence of infection

4. Which of the following is/are complication(s) of wound healing?
   a. Dehiscence
   b. Evisceration
   c. Fistula formation
   d. Hematoma
   e. Hemorrhage
   f. Interstitial fluid loss

ORDERING

Items A through I are key steps to follow when changing a dry sterile dressing. Indicate the correct sequence by numbering the steps.

a. 9 Apply sterile dressing.
b. 6 Clean drainage from wound.
c. 7 Dry surrounding skin.
d. 8 Inspect incision.
e. 1 Put on clean gloves.
f. 5 Put on sterile gloves.
g. 3 Dispose of clean gloves.
h. 2 Remove dressing from wound and discard.
i. 4 Set up sterile supplies.

HOT SPOT QUESTIONS

Place an "X" on the sweat glands.

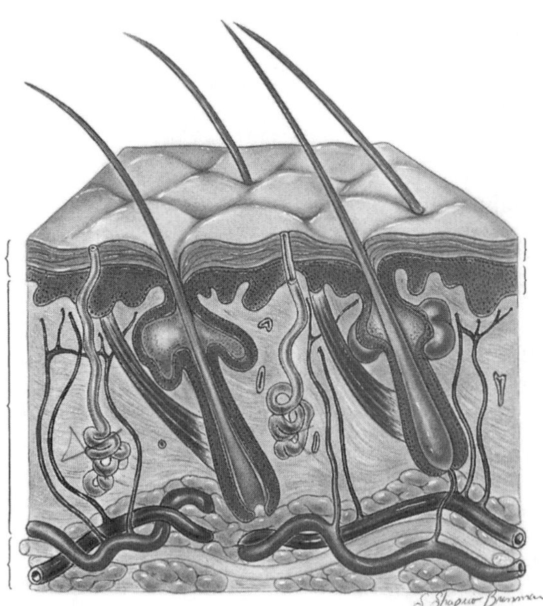

CHAPTER 41

The Body's Defense Against Infection

CHAPTER OVERVIEW

Chapter 41 examines and summarizes the basic concepts of the immune system, infection, and the infectious processes; the application of the nursing process in the care of clients with infections; and measures used to increase clients' defense mechanisms against infection.

LEARNING OBJECTIVES

After mastering the content in this chapter, you should be able to do the following:

1. Name the major components of the body's normal resistance to infection and the role of each.
2. Differentiate between cellular and humoral immunity and between active and passive immunity.
3. Identify possible risk factors for infection or infectious disease.
4. Name four common nosocomial infections.
5. Recognize common manifestations of infections.
6. Identify common laboratory and diagnostic tests used to identify or confirm an infectious process.
7. Describe major consequences of an infectious process.
8. Describe nursing measures that strengthen defense mechanisms against infection.

■ Mastering the Information

MATCHING

Match the terms in Column II with a definition, example, or related statement from Column I. Place the letter corresponding to the answer in the space provided. (Use each letter only once; some letters may not be used.)

COLUMN I

1. ____ A nonspecific chemical inhibitor the body cells secrete in response to viral invasion
2. ____ Microorganisms normally not considered pathogens that cause diseases when the immune system is compromised
3. ____ Drainage containing pus
4. ____ An infection acquired while receiving healthcare
5. ____ Microorganisms that live on the skin, in the nasopharynx, in the gastrointestinal tract, and on other body surfaces
6. ____ Foreign particles that invade the host, usually microbes but may be the person's own cells
7. ____ An increase in the circulation of white blood cells (WBCs), about 10,000 cells/mL
8. ____ Sample specimens of blood, sputum, and stool used to identify microorganisms and tested for antibiotic sensitivity or resistance

COLUMN II

a. Purulent
b. Leukocytosis
c. Normal flora
d. Culture and sensitivity
e. Interferon
f. Opportunistic
g. Nosocomial infection
h. Antigen

COLUMN I

1. b Immunity takes place in the bloodstream.
2. d Temporary immunity is provided in the form of immune globulins or antitoxins.
3. a The immune system is stimulated by infection or vaccination to produce antibodies.
4. c Composed of T-lymphocytes, it is stimulated by fungi, protozoa, some viruses, and bacteria.

COLUMN II

a. Active immunity
b. Humoral immunity
c. Cellular immunity
d. Passive immunity

TRUE–FALSE

Indicate if the following statements are true or false.

F 1. The most important barriers to infection are the phagocytes and inflammatory response.

T 2. Nutrition and stress are two factors affecting normal resistance to infection.

T 3. The immune system does not become fully operational until about 6 months of age.

F 4. Antibiotics are given to cure clients of infections.

T 5. Elderly clients and newborns have improperly functioning immune systems.

T 6. Bacteremia and septicemia are terms used to describe systemic infections.

FILL IN THE BLANK

Supply the missing term or the information requested.

1. The hospitalized client is predisposed to many nosocomial infections, most involve the following: UTI, wound infection, respiratory tract infection, and bacteremias.

2. Five nonspecific natural defense barriers are chem/anatomic, WBC, mechanical fever, inflam response, and culture.

3. Five factors affecting normal resistance to infection resulting in a compromised host are breaks in skin, invasive devices, stasis of fluid, poor nutrition, and stress.

4. The four signs of inflammatory response are redness, warmth, swelling, and pain.

5. The four stages in the progress of an infection are incubation, prodromal, accute, and convalescent.

■ Applying Your Knowledge

CASE STUDY

Mr. Lawrence, age 47 years, had an exploratory laparotomy. On the second postoperative day, he becomes febrile; his WBC count is 15,000 cells/mL, and he reports increased incisional pain. The physician states that Mr. Lawrence is experiencing a wound infection and orders a culture and sensitivity test. After the specimen for the culture and sensitivity test is obtained, Mr. Lawrence begins antibiotic therapy.

1. Discuss ways in which the nurse can intervene to prevent or minimize the occurrence of nosocomial wound infections.
2. Discuss how Mr. Lawrence's risk for infection would differ if he were 87 years old, instead of 47 years old.
3. Describe the nursing interventions that would be required when collecting the specimen for the culture and sensitivity test.
4. Explain when you would expect to collect the specimens for the peak and trough levels ordered by the physician.

CRITICAL INQUIRY EXERCISE

Many diagnostic tests are used to determine if clients are experiencing an inflammatory response. Listed below are the various diagnostic tests discussed in this chapter. For each test, write the specific values that would indicate an infectious process.

a. WBC
b. Urinalysis
c. Erythrocyte sedimentation rate
d. Culture and sensitivity

CRITICAL EXPLORATION EXERCISE

Visit the areas listed below. Collect information on common infections or diseases, treatment and control, percentages of clients actually contracting diseases or infections, evaluation of effectiveness of treatment, and when diseases or infections present a risk for others in the community or on a particular hospital unit.

a. Public health department: collect information on immunization and community-acquired infections.
b. Clinical agencies: collect information on nosocomial infections and commonly treated diseases.

■ Practicing for NCLEX

MULTIPLE CHOICE QUESTIONS

Circle the letter that corresponds to the best answer for each question.

1. Nonspecific symptoms of infection include
   a. fever.
   b. increased pulse and respiratory rate.
   c. inflammatory symptoms.
   d. tachypnea.

2. John Steven, 4 years old, is admitted with a diagnosis of diarrhea. Which statement is correct in regard to stool culture or specimens?
   a. Stools for leukocytes are collected daily for 3 days.
   b. Clean-catch technique is used to collect stool specimens.
   c. Stool specimens can be affected by antibiotics and antacids.
   d. Moving organisms can be easily detected in 1-day-old specimens.

3. The most common type of infection during early childhood is
   a. roundworm infestation and lice.
   b. respiratory tract infection.
   c. impetigo.
   d. streptococcal infections.

4. Ms. Roberts is being seen in the emergency room and reports chills and fever for 3 days; a dry, hacking cough; and chest pain when breathing. What additional related information should the nurse elicit during the assessment of the client?
   a. Diet preferences
   b. Client's general health
   c. Bowel pattern
   d. Ethnic background

5. Which of the following clients is most likely to experience a secondary superimposed infection?
   a. The client who has leukemia and is receiving antibiotics for a respiratory tract infection
   b. The client who is receiving 200,000 units of penicillin G intramuscularly as a single dose
   c. The client who is receiving routine immunizations
   d. The client who is applying topical antibiotics to a knee abrasion for 2 to 3 days

6. Which of the following diagnostic imaging tests is useful in differentiating the density among organs and locating abscesses?
   a. X-rays
   b. MRIs
   c. CT scans
   d. Endoscopic procedures

7. Which of the following diagnostic tests will confirm the presence of an inflammatory disease process?
   a. Culture and sensitivity
   b. ESR
   c. Serology
   d. WBC

8. During the assessment of a febrile client, the nurse would expect the to find what alteration in the vital signs?
   a. Decreased pulse
   b. Increased respiratory rate
   c. Shallow respirations
   d. Thready pulse

9. A peak drug level specimen should be collected
   a. just after the medication is given.
   b. midway through the administration of the medication.
   c. just before the next dose of the medication.
   d. just after the final dose of the medication.

10. When teaching the client how to manage a fever during the chill phase, it would be correct to tell the client to
    a. remove heavy covers.
    b. increase activity.
    c. decrease fluid intake.
    d. avoid tepid sponging.

FILL IN THE BLANK

Supply the missing term or the information requested.

1. Which temperature control measure is contraindicated for children who are exhibiting flu-like symptoms? ____________________
2. When giving a tepid bath for a temperature elevation, the caregiver should check the temperature how many minutes after starting the bath? ________________
3. Sputum specimens should be collected at what time of the day? _______________

MULTIPLE-ANSWER MULTIPLE CHOICE

Circle the letter(s) corresponding to the appropriate answer(s). Circle all that apply.

1. Which of the following nursing interventions is appropriate for the collection of blood cultures?
   a. Use a needle for collection
   b. Wear gloves while aspirating blood
   c. Remove gloves after injecting specimen into vacuum bottles
   d. Draw the specimen before or after a rise in temperature
   e. Use a central venous line to draw the specimen

2. Which of the following factors predispose a person to the development of a urinary tract infection?
   a. Age
   b. Catheterization
   c. Decreased diaphragmatic movement
   d. Fecal incontinence
   e. Inadequate fluid intake
   f. Malnutrition
   g. Sexual intercourse

3. Neutropenia precautions require that the client
   a. avoid fresh fruits and undercooked meats.
   b. avoid flossing.
   c. be placed in a private room.
   d. use a mask if he/she must leave the room.
   e. limit visitors, especially children.

4. Which of the following measures are appropriate for the prevention of measles?
   a. Administer the measles vaccination
   b. Give immune globulin
   c. Isolate the person with measles until lesions have crusted over
   d. Wear a mask if contact with infected person is necessary

5. Karen, age 4 months, is in the physician's office today for a well-baby check-up. The nurse would expect that Karen will receive the HB-2, if she has not already received it, along with which of the following vaccines?
   a. DTaP
   b. Hib
   c. IPV
   d. MMR
   e. PCV

UNIT X

ELIMINATION

CHAPTER 42

Urinary Elimination

CHAPTER OVERVIEW

Chapter 42 examines and summarizes the basic concepts of urinary elimination. The application of the nursing process in the care of clients with alterations in urinary elimination is discussed, and measures used to facilitate adequate urinary function are reviewed.

LEARNING OBJECTIVES

After mastering the content in this chapter, you should be able to do the following:

1. Describe the structure and function of the urinary system.
2. Outline the process of micturition.
3. Describe alterations in normal voiding patterns.
4. Recognize age-related differences in urinary elimination.
5. Describe factors that can alter urinary function.
6. Identify nursing diagnoses related to urinary elimination.
7. Describe measures for facilitating adequate elimination.
8. Discuss interventions for altered urinary function.
9. Develop appropriate collaborative and community-based nursing interventions to manage problems with voiding.

▪ Mastering the Information

MATCHING

Match the terms in Column II with a definition, example, or related statement from Column I. Place the letter corresponding to the answer in the space provided. (Use each letter only once; some letters may not be used.)

COLUMN I

1. __c__ Formation and excretion of less than 500 mL of urine in 24 hours
2. __e__ Subjective feeling of being unable to delay voluntarily the desire to void
3. __b__ Voiding during normal sleeping hours
4. __a__ Involuntary voiding with no underlying pathophysiologic origin

COLUMN II

a. Enuresis
b. Nocturia
c. Oliguria
d. Pyuria
e. Urgency

COLUMN I

1. __h__ Clean specimen of urine collected in a urinal, bedpan, or hat
2. __j__ First voided specimen discarded
3. __f__ Sterile specimen obtained directly from the bladder
4. __b__ Most appropriate for infants and small children
5. __a__ The more concentrated the urine, the higher the value
6. __g__ Used by the nurse to determine the amount of substances (e.g., protein or glucose) in the urine

7. d Can identify organisms present and an effective antibiotic
8. e Indicates a buildup of nitrogenous waste due to increased intake or low renal output
9. i A reliable indicator of impaired renal function
10. c Includes a blood test and a urine test to determine adequacy of renal function

COLUMN II

a. Specific gravity
b. Plastic collection bag
c. Creatinine clearance
d. Culture and sensitivity
e. Elevated blood urea nitrogen level
f. Catheterized specimen
g. Reagent strips
h. Random specimen
i. High serum creatinine level
j. 24-hour specimen

TRUE–FALSE

Indicate if the following statements are true or false.

F 1. Clients find it easier to describe their normal elimination pattern than to describe alterations in urinary elimination.

T 2. The nurse should ask how often the client voids, the time of day voiding occurs, and the usual amount of each voiding.

F 3. The nurse should not use words such as "potty" or "peeing" because this is unprofessional.

F 4. A client history of heart disease, spinal injury, or previous urinary tract problems would have no relevance in a urinary system evaluation.

T 5. Both urinary retention and nocturia are common complaints of the elderly and occur because of age-related changes in the urinary tract.

T 6. Clients who have experienced problems with urinary retention, incontinence, and flow over long periods of time may not report these conditions unless specifically asked.

F 7. When recording intake and output, the nurse focuses on the amount of intake and the amount of each voiding. The time of fluid intake or time of voiding is not important.

F 8. If no urine output has been noted during an 8-hour period, or if small, frequent voiding is noted, the nurse should avoid touching the client's lower abdominal area.

F 9. Inspection of the lower abdomen is the most reliable method for determining the degree of bladder distention.

T 10. In percussing the lower abdomen, a distended bladder produces a dull sound; a nearly empty bladder produces a hollow sound.

FILL IN THE BLANK

Supply the missing term or the information requested.

1. The two major functions of the kidney are to regulate volume and the composition of extracellular fluid
2. Urine formation occurs in the nephron, which is the functional unit of the kidney, through the processes of filtration, reabsorption, and secretion.
3. An important assessment, which might help to prevent an anaphylactic reaction, that should be made before a client has an intravenous pyelogram would be allergy to iodine.
4. During the period after a client has had a cystoscopy with biopsy, the nurse should monitor for Hematuria as a sign of hemmorage, signs of infection, bladder spasms, and urinary retention
5. State one of the three general client goals that would be most appropriate for the client with a history of urinary dysfunction. Reestablish control of voiding

■ Applying Your Knowledge

CASE STUDY

Jeanine Wiseman, 72 years old, is being discharged in 2 days. Her problem on admission was urinary retention. She was evaluated and has had an indwelling catheter in for the past 4 days. The physician ordered removal of the catheter after bladder training but states that if the urinary retention returns, Ms. Wiseman may have to go home with an indwelling catheter.

1. Design a plan for bladder training and criteria you would use to judge the effectiveness of that training.
2. Design a discharge teaching plan for Ms. Wiseman if she is going home with an indwelling catheter, with highlights on the following:
   a. Care and cleansing of the perineum and catheter
   b. Positioning of the drainage bag
   c. Signs and symptoms of infection

CRITICAL INQUIRY EXERCISE

1. Tour a dialysis unit or a floor on which peritoneal dialysis is performed. Write a short observation report, including information regarding the following:
   a. The effects of dialysis on a client's vital signs
   b. Changes noted in the client's weight and laboratory values from before dialysis to after dialysis
   c. A description of the apparatus used in the dialysis procedure, with an explanation of the purpose of the equipment

CRITICAL EXPLORATION EXERCISE

During a clinical experience, monitor the types of urine specimens collected from the clients throughout the shift. Note the medical diagnoses of the clients for which various types of specimens are collected (for example, a client with "fever" or "infection" may have a midstream urine for culture and sensitivity ordered). Look for a variety of types of clients and specimens.

■ Practicing for NCLEX

MULTIPLE CHOICE QUESTIONS

Circle the letter that corresponds to the best answer for each question.

1. Mrs. Wilson presents in the physician's office for a routine check-up. A urine specimen is obtained and is noted to be 250 mL of light yellow, cloudy, odorless urine. All of the specimen's characteristics are normal except
   a. amount.
   b. clarity.
   c. color.
   d. odor.

2. Which of the following factors influences urinary elimination?
   a. Ethnic background
   b. Upper body shape
   c. Intake of fresh fruits
   d. Carbon dioxide level

3. Mrs. Peters reports that she often urinates by accident when she laughs or sneezes. Mrs. Peters' complaint matches the definition for
   a. bladder retention.
   b. stress incontinence.
   c. urinary tract infection.
   d. urge incontinence.

4. Which of the following would be an appropriate nursing diagnosis for a client experiencing an involuntary loss of urine when a specific bladder volume is reached?
   a. Urge incontinence
   b. Functional retention
   c. Reflex incontinence
   d. Urinary retention

5. Which of the following measures might the nurse discuss with a client to help in the control of urinary incontinence?
   a. Avoiding the intake of sodium and cholesterol
   b. Increasing daily fluid intake to 10 to 12 glasses
   c. The importance of cleaning the perineum from back to front
   d. Weight loss methods if the client is obese

6. The nurse should always clear a client's room of environmental barriers to the bathroom to prevent
   a. functional incontinence.
   b. reflex incontinence.
   c. stress incontinence.
   d. total incontinence.
7. Which of the following related factors is appropriately matched to the condition to which it might lead?
   a. Consumption of a large amount of fluid, particularly fluids containing alcohol or caffeine, often causes reflex incontinence.
   b. Pregnancy or excessive body weight commonly result in problems with urge incontinence.
   c. Spinal cord lesion above T12 involving both motor and sensory tracts is a frequent cause of stress incontinence.
   d. Visual deficits or cognitive deficits, such as lethargy, dementia, or confusion, may result in functional incontinence.
8. The elderly often experience a loss of muscle tone, which could predispose them to
   a. bladder spasm.
   b. fluid overload.
   c. oliguria.
   d. urinary retention.
9. The nurse should instruct adult clients regarding the need to drink 1500 to 2000 mL of fluid daily because this fluid will help to
   a. flush microorganisms out of the urinary system.
   b. produce more concentrated, hyperosmolar urine.
   c. relax the tone of the bladder and prevent influx.
   d. stimulate the atrophy of the detrusor muscle.
10. Measures to help prevent urinary tract infection include
    a. abstaining from washing the perineal area during menstruation.
    b. cleansing the perineum from front to back after elimination.
    c. not voiding for at least 1 hour after sexual intercourse.
    d. taking a warm bubble bath at least three times a week.
11. Kegel exercises should be taught to the incontinent client to facilitate urinary control and prevent incontinence by
    a. strengthening the bladder wall.
    b. strengthening the renal pyramids.
    c. tightening the distal ureters.
    d. tightening the perineal muscles.
12. To facilitate urinary elimination in the client who is bedridden or has limited mobility, the nurse might
    a. ask the doctor to allow the client bathroom privileges.
    b. offer the client the bedpan, urinal, or bedside commode.
    c. position the client prone in the bed for each voiding.
    d. use a hat in the toilet to catch urine output.

FILL IN THE BLANK

Supply the missing term or the information requested.

1. The body of the bladder is composed of three layers of smooth muscle. Collectively, these three layers are called the ____________.
2. A noninvasive procedure useful in determining the need for catheterization to relieve urinary retention is ____________.

MULTIPLE-ANSWER MULTIPLE CHOICE

Circle the letter(s) corresponding to the appropriate answer(s). Circle all that apply.

1. When inserting a urethral catheter, the nurse should
   a. instruct the client that the procedure will cause no pain or discomfort.
   b. determine whether or not the client is allergic to iodine solutions.
   c. insert the catheter an additional 2.5 inches after the flow of urine begins.
   d. inflate balloon with prefilled syringe to check for defective balloon, if continuous drainage is ordered.

2. Teaching regarding home care of modifications for the client discharged with an indwelling catheter should include
   a. explanation regarding the need to place the catheter bag on the side rail of the bed.
   b. instructions on methods of kinking the catheter tubing to relieve intermittent bladder spasms.
   c. information on signs and symptoms of urinary tract infection with directions about who to contact.
   d. the need to limit fluid intake to concentrate urine and promote urinary function.

3. Which of the following is true regarding the irrigation of a urinary catheter?
   a. It involves separating the drainage tubing from the catheter or the sterile insertion of a syringe into the catheter.
   b. It is always performed before removal of the catheter to prevent postcatheterization urinary retention.
   c. It requires the use of an indwelling triple lumen catheter.
   d. If the catheter becomes encrusted or obstructed, the entire system, including the catheter, should be changed.
   e. The catheter lumen used for removal of urine can be left open to allow outflow of urine throughout the procedure.
   f. The specified type and amount of irrigating solution is prescribed by the physician or by written protocol.

4. Which of the following areas of the catheter must be kept sterile during a catheter insertion?
   a. Tip
   b. Shaft
   c. Balloon port
   d. Drainage tubing

5. Which of the following statements is true about bladder training?
   a. It begins with scheduled voidings.
   b. It can be facilitated by the intake of caffeine.
   c. A fluid intake of at least 2000 mL daily is recommended.
   d. It works best with female clients.

6. Which of the following statement(s) is/are important for the nurse to consider when applying a condom catheter?
   a. Excess pubic hair should be trimmed from the base of the penis as needed.
   b. A thin film of skin protector should be applied before placement of the adhesive liner.
   c. Frequent inspection of the skin and skin care are necessary to prevent skin breakdown.
   d. When the penis is grasped in the older male client, it may retract and make application difficult.
   e. The adhesive strip should be wrapped in a spiral fashion around the shaft of the penis.

CHAPTER 43

Bowel Elimination

CHAPTER OVERVIEW

Chapter 43 examines and summarizes the basic concepts of bowel elimination, the application of the nursing process in the care of clients with alterations in bowel elimination, and measures used to facilitate adequate bowel function.

LEARNING OBJECTIVES

After mastering the content of this chapter, you should be able to do the following:

1. Describe the normal anatomy and physiology of bowel function.
2. Understand the process of defecation.
3. List several factors that influence bowel elimination.
4. List and describe the manifestations of altered bowel elimination.
5. List age-related differences in bowel elimination.
6. Describe measures for facilitating adequate elimination.
7. Use the nursing process to detect and address potential and actual problems in bowel elimination.

■ Mastering the Information

MATCHING

Match the terms in Column II with a definition, example, or related statement from Column I. Place the letter corresponding to the answer in the space provided. (Use each letter only once; some letters may not be used.)

COLUMN I

1. __d__ A medication prepared in a base and when inserted rectally melts and absorbs for systemic or local effects
2. __f__ A medication that acts directly on the intestine to slow bowel motility or absorb excess fluid in the bowel
3. __c__ A medication that is the treatment of choice to promote evacuation of hardened stool from the bowel
4. __b__ An agent given to relieve gas

COLUMN II

a. Antidiarrheal
b. Antiflatulent
c. Laxative
d. Suppository

COLUMN I

1. __e__ A nasogastric tube inserted to irrigate the stomach in case of accidental poisoning or drug overdose
2. __f__ A short piece of plastic tubing inserted about 4 inches into the rectum to relieve flatulence
3. __b__ A nasogastric tube that delivers food to the stomach for a client unable to obtain nutritional requirements orally
4. __d__ A thin, plastic tube inserted into a client's nose and threaded into the stomach
5. __a__ A nasogastric tube used to relieve the stomach and intestines of pressure caused by accumulation of air and fluid
6. __c__ A tube for intestinal decompression used for mechanical or nonmechanical bowel obstruction

COLUMN II

a. Gastric decompression
b. Gastric gavage
c. Nasointestinal tube
d. Nasogastric tube
e. Gastric lavage
f. Rectal tube

TRUE–FALSE

Indicate if the following statements are true or false.

T 1. The decreased dietary intake of fiber causes less frequent bowel movements.

F 2. Meconium is a dark, greenish-colored stool seen in the toddler.

T 3. The client's beliefs about "normal" bowel functions are important in determining if a bowel elimination dysfunction occurs.

F 4. Normal bacteria found in a stool for culture includes *Salmonella shigella*.

T 5. When percussing the left upper quadrant of the abdomen, it is normal to hear a high-pitched, hollow sound called tympany.

F 6. A bowel diversion surgery that brings a segment of the large colon out to the abdominal skin is called an ileostomy.

T 7. A client who has a nasogastric or nasointestinal tube for decompression will usually be NPO.

T 8. The bowel sounds of a client who has undergone abdominal surgery are hypoactive or absent for a period of 1 to 3 days after surgery.

T 9. Elderly clients erroneously report constipation because of normal age-related changes in the gastrointestinal tract.

F 10. The nurse should not make special attempts to separate stool and urine during a stool specimen collection.

FILL IN THE BLANK

Supply the missing term or the information requested.

1. Five of the 11 factors that have the potential to disrupt normal bowel function are nutrition, fluid intake, pregnancy, meds, and surgery.
2. The functions of the intestine include motility, absorption, and defication.
3. The manifestations of altered bowel elimination are constipation, fecal impaction, diahrhea, fecal inct, flatulence, and distention.
4. One of the three goals for clients with altered bowel elimination is acceptable pattern of bowel elimination.

■ Applying Your Knowledge

CASE STUDY

A 2-year-old is being seen today in the clinic. You are the nurse on duty, and you note that the child's mother expresses concern that the child seems to experience severe diarrhea when teething. She says, however, that the toddler has constipation when not teething.

1. Explain how you would assess if the child's symptoms were truly diarrhea and constipation.
2. Identify the data you would gather from the child's mother that might help you determine factors contributing to the occurrence of constipation and diarrhea.
3. Create a teaching plan that would prepare the toddler's mother to provide appropriate care at home if severe constipation or diarrhea occurs.

CRITICAL INQUIRY EXERCISE

1. Identify drugs used to address alterations in bowel elimination. Make notes related to the purpose of each drug, pharmacologic action, usual dosage, and various forms of the drug.
2. Keep a record of your bowel function for 2 weeks. Identify the following: characteristics of the stool, frequency, changes in the nature of the stools that occur with intake of various fluids or foods, and the effect that changes in the environment (e.g., different toilet facility and lack of privacy) have on bowel elimination.

CRITICAL EXPLORATION EXERCISE

1. Perform a thorough bowel assessment on a client in the clinical area. Identify bowel alterations and appropriate nursing interventions that may be used.
2. In a clinical setting, visit the radiology department and observe procedures involving the bowel. Collect information on the procedures invasive and noninvasive; purpose; process; and hospital policies related to the preprocedure, intraprocedure, and postprocedure care.

■ Practicing for NCLEX

MULTIPLE CHOICE QUESTIONS

Circle the letter that corresponds to the best answer for each question.

1. Which of the following factors influences bowel elimination?
   a. Dietary intake
   b. Body position
   c. Privacy
   d. All of the above
2. The nurse is about to perform a guaiac test on the client's stool. The client asks the nurse, "What are you looking for?" The most appropriate response by the nurse would be
   a. bacteria formation.
   b. hidden blood.
   c. bright red blood.
   d. mucus and fat deposits.
3. The most desired position for a client during a sigmoidoscopy procedure is
   a. Lithotomy.
   b. prone with head elevated 45 degrees.
   c. knee-chest position.
   d. Sims.
4. One of the most common signs of fecal impaction is
   a. painful burning of the anus.
   b. hyperactive bowel sounds.
   c. abdominal tenderness.
   d. passage of liquid or semiliquid stool.
5. Which of the following is the proper technique used to check for nasogastric tube placement?
   a. Insert the tube in a glass of water and observe for bubbles.
   b. Hold the tube close to the ear and listen for air exchange.
   c. Aspirate gastric contents.
   d. Insert 10 mL of air while listening over the right upper quadrant of the abdomen.
6. According to the Rome II Criteria, which of the following indicates constipation in the infant or child?
   a. Fewer than three bowel movements per week
   b. Firm stool more than two times per week for at least 2 weeks
   c. Straining during more than 25% of bowel movements
   d. Lumpy or hard stool in more than 25% of bowel movements

FILL IN THE BLANK

Supply the missing term or the information requested.

1. The color that indicates that a Hemoccult stool is positive for the presence of occult blood is ______________.
2. An important nursing intervention after a barium enema radiologic procedure is ______________.
3. The nurse who correctly performs a stoma assessment knows the color of a healthy stoma is ______________.

MULTIPLE-ANSWER MULTIPLE CHOICE

Circle the letter(s) corresponding to the appropriate answer(s). Circle all that apply.

1. Which of the following nursing interventions used by nurses when caring for clients with nasogastric tubes are appropriate?
   a. Irrigate the tube with an irrigating solution to maintain patency.
   b. Apply a water-soluble lubricant to the nares.
   c. Secure the nasogastric tube by pinning the tube to the client's pillow.
   d. Monitor intake and output, including amount, color, and type, of gastrointestinal drainage and record every 8 hours.
   e. Provide mouth care using lemon glycerin oral swabs.
   f. Allow the client with a nasogastric tube for decompression to have sips of water and small feedings for nutritional purposes.

2. Which of the following instructions/actions by the nurse promote(s) patient safety?
   a. Teach high-risk patients (i.e., cardiac patients) to inhale slowly during defecation.
   b. Administer no more than three large-volume, tap water enemas in succession.
   c. Use water soluble lubricant during nasogastric intubation.
   d. Avoid use of hooking motion during disimpaction.
   e. Use only tap water when administering enemas to infants and children.

3. Which of the following statements is true with regard to the normal bowel elimination pattern?
   a. A person's bowel elimination pattern is high individualized.
   b. The normal frequency of bowel elimination can be one to two bowel movements per day.
   c. The normal frequency of bowel elimination can be once every 2 to 3 days.
   d. Infants may pass stool with every feeding.

ORDERING

Items A through G are the steps for enema administration. Number these steps in the order that should be followed.

a. ______ Lubricate the tip of the tube with a water-soluble lubricant.

b. ______ Reclamp the tube and remove it; instruct the client to retain the solution as long as possible.

c. ______ Position the client in a Sim's position.

d. ______ Raise the container 18 inches above the anus; allow the solution to flow for 5 to 10 minutes.

e. ______ Provide privacy.

f. ______ Separate the buttocks and assess the anal area; insert the tube gently while instructing the client to take a deep breath.

g. ______ Open the clamp on the tubing to remove air and reclamp the tubing.

UNIT XI

SLEEP AND REST

CHAPTER 44

Sleep and Rest

CHAPTER OVERVIEW

Chapter 44 examines and summarizes the basic concepts of sleep and rest. Normal patterns of sleep and rest as well as common variations and disturbances are presented. Particular emphasis is placed on the use of the nursing process to address various sleep pattern disturbances.

LEARNING OBJECTIVES

After mastering the content in this chapter, you should be able to do the following:

1. Describe the five stages of sleep.
2. Describe normal patterns of sleep and rest throughout the lifespan.
3. Identify factors that affect sleep and rest.
4. Conduct an assessment interview regarding normal sleep patterns, risk for disturbance, and actual sleep problems.
5. Develop a daily schedule with a client, incorporating his or her unique needs and patterns for sleep and rest.
6. Discuss interventions to promote rest and sleep.
7. Develop a nursing plan of care for a client with sleep pattern disturbance.

▪ Mastering the Information

MATCHING

Match the terms in Column II with a definition, example, or related statement from Column I. Place the letter corresponding to the answer in the space provided. (Use each letter only once; some letters may not be used.)

COLUMN I

1. _____ A normally occurring altered state characterized by decreased awareness and responsiveness to stimuli; a total body phenomenon
2. _____ A state in which motor or cognitive response is decreased and awareness of environment is maintained
3. _____ A perceived difficulty in sleeping
4. _____ An urge of varying intensity to go to sleep
5. _____ A subjective state of weariness in which physical activity is accompanied by intense or rapid tiring

COLUMN II

a. Fatigue
b. Insomnia
c. Rest
d. Sleep
e. Sleepiness

TRUE–FALSE

Indicate if the following statements are true or false.

_____ 1. Infant sleep patterns differ from those of adults in that the sleep cycle is shorter.

_____ 2. The most frequently reported problem associated with sleep for toddlers and preschoolers is night terrors.

_____ 3. Older adults frequently express concern about taking longer to fall asleep and about awakening more frequently.

______ 4. Noises and extreme temperatures are the most frequent disturbers of sleep in institutional settings.

______ 5. Signs and symptoms associated with sleep deprivation are fatigue, headache, nausea, increased sensitivity to pain, decreased neuromuscular coordination, general irritability, and inability to concentrate.

______ 6. Manifestations of altered sleep function may include narcolepsy, sleep apnea, periodic limb movements, circadian-rhythm sleep disorders, and parasomnias.

______ 7. Exposure to bright light therapy, combined with good sleep habits, can effectively alter circadian rhythms.

______ 8. Health promotion includes environmental modifications, provision of intimacy and security, sleep rituals, and managing individuals' sleep needs.

FILL IN THE BLANK

Supply the missing term or the information requested.

1. Two basic research approaches that provide building blocks for developing concepts relating to mechanisms and functions of sleep are the ________________ approach and the ________________ approach.
2. Identify and briefly describe the stages of sleep.
   a.
   b.
   c.
   d.
   e.
3. The time period of 10 to 30 minutes required by most people to fall asleep is termed ____________.
4. Describe two changes in their activity and rest patterns that the elderly client may report that are a result of the normal process of aging.

■ Applying Your Knowledge

CASE STUDY

Mary Beth and her husband have three children: Mark, 5 years old; Kathy, 3 years old; and Iona, 5 weeks old. Realizing that sleep and rest are essential for normal growth and development, propose a plan to care for the family.

1. Identify additional data needed to determine actual or risk for sleep pattern disturbances, and describe how you will obtain the data.
2. Discuss goals that are appropriate for each family member relative to sleep/rest functions.
3. Describe areas in which counseling is likely needed.

CRITICAL INQUIRY EXERCISE

Write a list of sleeping problems you have experienced, identify strategies you used to promote rest and sleep, and discuss the effectiveness of each strategy.

CRITICAL EXPLORATION EXERCISE

Interview one of the following people about sleep pattern disturbance:

a. The parent of a newborn
b. Someone who has traveled across three or more time zones within the past 48 hours
c. A nurse who has rotated, 7-to-3 and 11-to-7 shifts during the past weeks

■ Practicing for NCLEX

MULTIPLE CHOICE QUESTIONS

Circle the letter that corresponds to the best answer for each question.

1. The most important indicator of the adequacy of an individual's sleep and rest patterns is
   a. presence or absence of circles under the eyes.
   b. concentration ability.
   c. the client's statement regarding sleep adequacy.
   d. number of hours of actual sleep time.

2. Which of the following are characteristic of an individual experiencing sleep apnea?
   a. Excessive daytime sleepiness
   b. Body position
   c. Ingestion of fresh fruits
   d. All of the above

3. ________ refers to an activity that is normal during waking hours but is abnormal during sleep.
   a. Insomnia
   b. Myoclonus
   c. Narcolepsy
   d. Parasomnia

4. A client has been admitted to the hospital for a diagnostic evaluation to rule out sleep apnea. The client reports difficulty sleeping in the hospital. The best way to promote sleep for the client would be to
   a. arrange for the client to have a roommate if the client is married.
   b. incorporate sleep rituals that are practiced at home as much as possible.
   c. give a sleeping pill (hypnotic) if the client is not asleep by midnight.
   d. assist client to bathroom before retiring to bed.

5. The average time required for an adult to fall asleep is
   a. 5 minutes.
   b. 10 to 30 minutes.
   c. 30 to 40 minutes.
   d. 40 to 60 minutes.

6. Which one of the following is most supportive of the nursing diagnosis Disturbed Sleep Pattern?
   a. Report of working rotating shifts
   b. Report of recently experiencing an acute illness
   c. Report of not feeling well-rested after sleep
   d. Report of awakening early each morning

FILL IN THE BLANK

Supply the missing term or the information requested.

1. ______________ are biologic rhythms that follow a cycle of about 24 hours.
2. ______________ is a subjective state of weariness in which intense or rapid tiring accompanies physical activity.

MULTIPLE-ANSWER MULTIPLE CHOICE

Circle the letter(s) corresponding to the appropriate answer(s). Circle all that apply.

1. Which of the following types of data should be elicited for the individual suspected of experiencing sleep pattern disturbance?
   a. Type of work
   b. Sleep pattern
   c. Frequency of sexual activity
   d. Intake of caffeine and alcohol

2. Which activity is influenced by circadian rhythm?
   a. Temperature regulation
   b. Sleep–wake cycle
   c. Eating pattern
   d. Hormone secretion

UNIT XII

COGNITION AND PERCEPTION

CHAPTER 45

Pain Perception and Management

CHAPTER OVERVIEW

Chapter 45 examines and summarizes concepts related to pain perception and comfort, the application of the nursing process for clients with pain dysfunction, and measures for reducing or inhibiting pain and promoting comfort. It describes alternate methods of pain relief based on individual needs.

LEARNING OBJECTIVES

After mastering the content in this chapter, you should be able to do the following:

1. Explain the transmission of pain sensation.
2. Outline how pain transmission is facilitated or inhibited.
3. Describe the four sensory pain components that must be included in the nursing database.
4. Examine nonpharmacologic methods of pain relief based on individual needs.
5. Describe the types, actions, and adverse effects of analgesics.
6. List nursing implications for various classes of drugs used for pain management.
7. Develop a nursing plan for a client experiencing pain.

■ Mastering the Information

MATCHING

Match the terms in Column II with a definition, example, or related statement from Column I. Place the letter corresponding to the answer in the space provided. (Use each letter only once; some letters may not be used.)

COLUMN I

1. _____ Stimulating the opposite area to relieve pain
2. _____ Occurs when the client learns voluntary control over autonomic functions, such as heart rate and muscle temperature
3. _____ Pain that occurs abruptly and persists until healing occurs
4. _____ Pain that persists beyond the normal healing period with a cause that is not amenable to treatment
5. _____ A pain sensation produced by an innocuous stimulus

COLUMN II

a. Acute pain
b. Allodynia
c. Biofeedback
d. Contralateral stimulation
e. Chronic pain

COLUMN I

1. _____ Pain that resists cure or relief
2. _____ An enhanced sensation to pain produced by a noxious stimulus
3. _____ Free nerve endings that respond to physiologic stimuli
4. _____ Nervous system adaptation after pain
5. _____ The highest intensity of pain that the person is willing to tolerate
6. _____ The amount of pain stimulation required before pain is felt

COLUMN II

a. Hyperalgesia
b. Malignant pain
c. Neural plasticity
d. Nociceptors
e. Pain threshold
f. Pain tolerance

TRUE–FALSE

Indicate if the following statements are true or false.

_____ 1. One of the most important areas of pain modulation is the spinal dorsal horn where complex processing of messages occurs.

_____ 2. Endogenous opioids (administered to the person) and exogenous opioids (produced by the body) are important to inhibition of pain perception.

_____ 3. The gate-control theory proposes that the dorsal horn acts as a gate that closes to prevent pain impulses from reaching the brain or opens to allow nociceptive impulses to be transmitted to the brain.

_____ 4. Suffering is associated with events that threaten the person's intactness, whereas pain is associated with events that threaten tissue.

_____ 5. A sense of not knowing and emotional responses to pain, such as fear and anxiety, increase muscle tension, thereby increasing pain perception and intensity.

_____ 6. Pain is a highly individualized experience existing whenever and wherever the person says it does.

_____ 7. Lack of pain expression (response) means lack of pain.

_____ 8. Neonates and toddlers do not experience pain.

_____ 9. If pain persists, a school-age child may regress to an earlier stage of development in an attempt to handle the situation.

_____ 10. Unrelieved pain can be harmful to recovery, lead to abnormal anatomic and genetic changes, and interfere with the quality of life.

FILL IN THE BLANK

Supply the missing term or the information requested.

1. Initially, pain serves a _______________ function, but unrelieved pain can be harmful.
2. Pain sensation is transmitted to the brain by _______________ pathways and _______________ pathways convey information from the brain to the spinal dorsal horn.
3. The sensation of pain may be altered by modulation at the _______________ nerve, the _______________, and several _______________ sites.
4. The gate-control theory emphasizes _______________, _______________, _______________, and _______________ dimensions of pain as playing a role in the modulation of the physiologic dimension.
5. Sensory characteristics of pain are described by its _______________, _______________, _______________, and _______________ pattern.

■ Applying Your Knowledge

CASE STUDY

A client is hospitalized for diagnostic tests because of urinary retention and dribbling. The client reports sudden onset of pain in the chest. The client says, "It feels as if someone is stabbing me in the chest." Apply what you have learned about characteristics of pain, pain function, factors affecting pain function, altered function resulting in pain, manifestation of pain, impact of pain on daily living, and pain management to this client.

1. Give your opinion of the client's thoughts and feelings after experiencing such pain.
2. Relate body language to the description of pain.
3. Describe the additional assessment data needed to develop a plan for managing this client's pain.

4. Explain the rationale, for or against, using positioning, heat or cold, anticipatory guidance, relaxation techniques, biofeedback, and analgesic medications as methods of pain relief for this client.
5. Describe at least two diagnostic tests or procedures that might be performed before the pain management plan is completed.

CRITICAL INQUIRY EXERCISE

1. Design a discharge teaching plan for a client going home with a non-narcotic analgesic with highlights on the following:
   a. Schedule for administration of the analgesic
   b. Lifestyle changes to avoid precipitation of pain and dysfunction

CRITICAL EXPLORATION EXERCISE

1. Spend a day on an oncology service or in an oncology clinic.
   a. Review the records of various clients.
   b. Outline the pain management plan of at least one client for the past 3 months, and list the outcomes.
   c. Observe the physician or the nurse during a pain assessment interview.
2. Visit the recovery room or surgical floor of a hospital.
   a. Review the records for instructions given before the painful procedure.
   b. List the narcotic and non-narcotic analgesic commonly used by reviewing the medication administration record.
   c. List noninvasive techniques being used for pain relief.

■ Practicing for NCLEX

MULTIPLE CHOICE QUESTIONS

Circle the letter that corresponds to the best answer for each question.

1. Pain assessment is best accomplished when
   a. the nurse validates, with the family, whether or not the client is experiencing pain.
   b. the nurse considers past experiences with clients who have reported similar pain.
   c. the client is calm and emotional during the assessment.
   d. the nurse acknowledges that pain is a subjective experience.
2. Comprehensive documentation of a client's pain requires that the nurse record
   a. the nurse's ideas about the level of pain.
   b. physician's orders and client diagnosis.
   c. verbal and nonverbal expressions of pain.
   d. all of the above.
3. Which one of the following precautions should be included for the client who is receiving amitriptyline?
   a. Administer the medication in the morning, instead of at night, to avoid sleep disturbances.
   b. Have an artificial airway and suction equipment readily available.
   c. Have the client rest in a sitting position before shifting from a reclining position to a standing position.
   d. Have the client take the medication with food to avoid gastrointestinal upset.
4. Which one of the following statements best describes the nurse's responsibility when giving an analgesic?
   a. Calculate and administer the amount of medication the client should receive.
   b. Evaluate and document the effectiveness of the medication.
   c. Give the medication as ordered by the physician.
   d. Change the dosage of the medication if there are adverse reactions.
5. A client who had an above-the-knee amputation of the right leg 5 hours ago is to receive Demerol 50 mg to 75 mg every 3 to 4 hours. To evaluate the effectiveness of the pain management regimen, the nurse must
   a. anticipate the client's level of pain.
   b. observe the client and ask questions.
   c. question family members about usual pain relief measures.
   d. offer the medication as scheduled.
6. The nurse would be correct to question the use of transcutaneous electrical stimulation (TENS) for pain management if the client
   a. has a pacemaker.
   b. is receiving an analgesic.
   c. is in active labor.
   d. reports a tingling sensation.

7. Which one of the following medications should be on hand when a client is receiving a narcotic analgesic?
   a. Acetylsalicylic acid
   b. Dexamethasone
   c. Indomethacin
   d. Naloxone

8. A client is recovering from anesthesia immediately after an appendectomy. To best minimize pain, the nurse should
   a. administer prescribed pain medication every 3 to 4 hours if the client verbalizes the presence of pain.
   b. validate the presence of pain with objective data before administering pain medication.
   c. collaborate with the physician to prescribe an opioid around the clock, instead of prn for the first 36 hours.
   d. Attempt to control pain with nonpharmacologic measures before using narcotic analgesics.

9. A client who has breast cancer with metastasis to the long bones has intractable pain. Which pain management regimen is most likely to provide a measure of comfort?
   a. Oral administration of large doses of analgesics and relaxation techniques
   b. Frequent intramuscular injections of small doses of an analgesic and distraction techniques
   c. Good hygiene, frequent backrubs, and massage of the long bones
   d. Alcohol injection via transnasal approach of the pituitary gland and good hygiene

10. Destruction or interruption of a nerve root or pain pathway is most likely to be used for which of the following conditions?
   a. Peptic or duodenal ulcers
   b. Menstrual cramps
   c. Tic douloureux (trigeminal neuralgia)
   d. Labor pains

FILL IN THE BLANK

Supply the missing term or the information requested.

1. The maximum amount of acetaminophen a person should receive in a 24-hour period is ____________________

2. Transdermal opioids, such as fentanyl have a duration of up to ___________.

3. A client is receiving 120 mg of morphine in a 24-hour period. Using the recommended guidelines for tapering the dose, determine the amount of medication the patient should receive per dose during the first 2 days. __________________

MULTIPLE-ANSWER MULTIPLE CHOICE

Circle the letter(s) corresponding to the appropriate answer(s). Circle all that apply.

1. Which of the following descriptions of pain provide information about the quality of the pain?
   a. Excruciating
   b. Gnawing
   c. Nagging
   d. Severe
   e. Shooting
   f. Terrifying

2. Which of the following are nonverbal indicators of pain?
   a. Bracing
   b. Eating
   c. Grimacing
   d. Reading
   e. Thrashing

3. Which of the following statements describes a behavioral coping strategy for pain?
   a. I do anything to get my mind off of it.
   b. I do something like house chores or crafts.
   c. I go out to the movies or shopping.
   d. I have faith that some day there will be a cure.
   e. I pray to God it won't last long.
   f. I pretend it is not there.
   g. I try to think of something special.

HOT SPOT QUESTIONS

Place an "X" on the areas associated with referred pain for both the ovaries and kidneys.

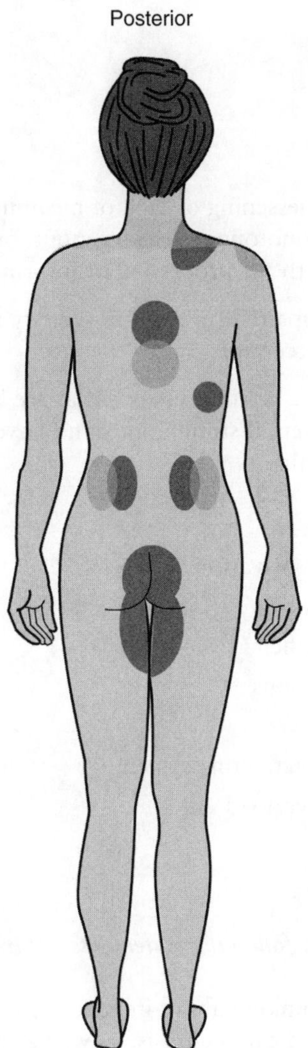

CHAPTER 46

Sensory Perception

CHAPTER OVERVIEW

Chapter 46 identifies factors and behavioral manifestations of sensory overload and sensory deprivation. Application of the nursing process in the care of people with altered sensory perception is emphasized. Nursing interventions that facilitate sensory function are presented.

LEARNING OBJECTIVES

After mastering the content in this chapter, you should be able to do the following:

1. Associate stress and sensoristasis with the sensory-perceptual process.
2. Describe the five senses and their roles in sensory perception.
3. Summarize factors affecting sensory perception.
4. Specify how sensory overload, deprivation, and deficit can occur, with interventions for each.
5. Relate manifestations of altered sensory function to their causes.
6. Identify clients at risk for altered sensory function in healthcare settings and in the home.
7. Discuss the relationship of safety to sensory dysfunction.

▪ Mastering the Information

MATCHING

Match the terms in Column II with a definition, example, or related statement from Column I. Place the letter corresponding to the answer in the space provided. (Use each letter only once; some letters may not be used.)

COLUMN I

1. ______ Controls arousal and awareness to stimuli
2. ______ Occurs when a person is unable to process or manage the intensity or quantity of incoming sensory stimuli
3. ______ A lessening or lack of meaningful stimuli, monotonous sensory input, or interference with the processing of information
4. ______ Impaired function in sensory reception or perception
5. ______ Sensory impressions that are based on internal stimulations and have no basis in reality

COLUMN II

a. Sensory deprivation
b. Sensoristasis
c. Sensory deficit
d. Hallucinations
e. Delusions
f. Reticular activating system
g. Sensory overload

TRUE–FALSE

Indicate if the following statements are true or false.

______ 1. Thinking about impending surgery or a medical diagnosis, as well as pain, lack of sleep, worry, medication, and brain injury, contribute to sensory overload.

______ 2. A sudden loss of sensory perception through a sensory deficit does not affect orientation.

______ 3. Marked decrements in sensory-perceptual behaviors begin as people approach 60 to 70 years of age, requiring more time for the processing of sensory input.

______ 4. Altered sensory perception frequently leads to anxiety, just as anxiety can further lead to additional altered sensory perception.

______ 5. Sensory perception dysfunction may have profound effects on activities of daily living.

______ 6. Assessment for sensory perception focuses only on cognitive behaviors, such as remembering, problem solving, and decision making.

______ 7. The nurse who occasionally plays the television or radio, encourages visitors, opens drapes, and places the bed or chair so that a client can hear or see activities in the area, is providing sensory stimulation.

______ 8. Nursing interventions to promote sensory health and function include teaching healthcare, objectively and specifically describing procedures, educating about why a procedure will be done, and individualizing frequent nurse-client interactions.

______ 9. Depression and withdrawal are two manifestations of altered sensory function that may result from sensory overload.

______ 10. All sensory aids are physical and include such items as hearing aids, eyeglasses, and canes.

FILL IN THE BLANK

Supply the missing term or the information requested.

1. Sensory perception depends on sensory receptors, the reticular activating system (RAS), and functioning nervous ________________ to the brain.
2. The senses receiving stimuli externally are ________________, ________________, ________________, ________________, and ________________.
3. Characteristics of normal vision include acuity near ________________, full ________________ of vision, and ________________ vision.
4. Two necessary time periods are crucial in helping a person deal with new stimuli. They are ________________ and ________________.
5. Seven factors that affect normal sensory perception are previous ________________, ________________, ________________, ________________, ________________, ________________, and ________________.
6. The newborn and infant receive most stimulation by ________________; they need to ________________ objects in the environment.
7. Lack of meaningful stimulation can lead to ________________ and motor delays in the toddler or preschooler.

■ Applying Your Knowledge

CASE STUDY

A 72-year-old client is scheduled for discharge from the hospital with the diagnosis of left-sided cardiovascular accident. The client lives alone in a senior citizens building. The client taught school for many years until experiencing significant visual impairment. You have been assigned to coordinate discharge planning.

1. Identify the additional information you would need to prepare a discharge plan.
2. Explain at least three factors that may contribute to the client's sensory dysfunction.
3. Outline the instructions that should be given to the client or significant others.
4. Identify the community agencies that may be helpful for the client after discharge.

CRITICAL INQUIRY EXERCISE

1. Divide into groups and experience sensory alteration by wearing gloves, smeared eyeglasses, and earplugs. Then perform basic activities of daily living, such as buttoning a shirt, ambulating, and communicating. For safety, have a partner assist. Then share your experiences with your classmates.

2. Divide into groups. Assign one student in your group to be a client with alteration in sensory function. Demonstrate appropriate nursing interventions for the client through role play.

CRITICAL EXPLORATION EXERCISE

1. Visit a rehabilitation unit or hospital.
   a. Observe the clients.
   b. Identify the contributing factors for sensory alteration.
2. Identify a client's clinical manifestations for altered sensory function.
3. Discuss nursing measures used by the staff to accomplish and maintain the goal of sensoristasis.

■ Practicing for NCLEX

MULTIPLE CHOICE QUESTIONS

Circle the letter that corresponds to the best answer for each question.

A 68-year-old client who was involved in an automobile accident is admitted to the hospital with a diagnosis of multiple bruises and facial lacerations. Both eyes are swollen, bandages have been applied, and the client is extremely restless. The client has been placed on bed rest and has no visitors.

1. During the assessment, the nurse should inquire about the client's typical day, lifestyle and habits, history of illness, and ability to see and hear, as well as the client's
   a. living and social situation.
   b. understanding of the seriousness of the diagnosis.
   c. financial status and usual income.
   d. insurance coverage and limits.

2. In addition to a client history, the nurse should initially collect data about the client's
   a. background.
   b. blood chemistry.
   c. education.
   d. prior hospitalizations.

3. The data given best support which one of the following diagnoses?
   a. Disturbed sensory perception related to altered sensory reception
   b. Disturbed sensory perception related to biochemical imbalances
   c. Disturbed sensory perception related to psychological stress
   d. Disturbed sensory perception related to excessive environmental stimuli

4. On the second day after admission, the nurse serves the client breakfast. The client refuses the meal after one bite and states, "This food has poison in it." Which manifestation of altered sensory function is evident?
   a. Hallucination
   b. Delusion
   c. Cognitive dysfunction
   d. Withdrawal

5. Which of the following are the most important nursing considerations in providing safety for the client?
   a. Age and habits
   b. Environment and medications
   c. Age and bed rest
   d. Food and habits

FILL IN THE BLANK

Supply the missing term or the information requested.

1. A conscious process of selecting, organizing and interpreting sensory stimuli is called ______________________.

2. A state of optimum arousal, not too much and not too little, is referred to as ____________________.

3. Selected products from this class of medications have been linked to the occurrence of hearing impairment. ____________________

MULTIPLE-ANSWER MULTIPLE CHOICE

Circle the letter(s) corresponding to the appropriate answer(s). Circle all that apply.

1. Which of the following nursing interventions would be appropriate for the client who is experiencing sensory deprivation or sensory deficit?
   a. Playing the television or radio
   b. Speaking slowly and unhurriedly
   c. Providing a thermometer to measure the temperature of bath water
   d. Enlisting help from significant others
   e. Limiting visitors

2. Which of the following internal factors can contribute to a person's vulnerability to sensory overload?
   a. Spinal cord injury
   b. Hypoxemia
   c. Brain damage
   d. Electrolyte disturbances

3. Which of the following assessment techniques would be appropriate to use in the assessment of somatic sensations?
   a. Use test tubes filled with warm and cold water
   b. Perform Weber and Rinne test
   c. Have client identify a common object by feeling the object
   d. Observe client's conversation with others

4. When assisting a visually impaired client with ambulation, the nurse should
   a. stand on the client's dominant side.
   b. have the client use the nondominant hand to feel around for landmarks.
   c. stand about one foot behind the client.
   d. ensure that the environment is uncluttered.

CHAPTER 47

Cognitive Processes

CHAPTER OVERVIEW

In Chapter 47, the cognitive process and function are reviewed. Changes occurring in cognition as a result of aging and varied disease processes are also reviewed. The use of the nursing process to address the needs of clients with altered thought processes is discussed.

LEARNING OBJECTIVES

After mastering the content in this chapter, you should be able to do the following:

1. Identify the components of cognitive and thought processes.
2. Describe the characteristics of normal cognition.
3. Identify the cognitive factors that are a part of each of the stages of the lifespan.
4. Recognize factors that affect normal cognitive function.
5. Identify manifestations of altered cognitive processes.
6. Use the nursing process in the care of the client experiencing altered cognitive processes.
7. Appreciate the types of resources available to families of individuals with altered cognitive processes.

■ Mastering the Information

MATCHING

Match the terms in Column I with a definition, example, or related statement from Column II. Place the letter corresponding to the answer in the space provided. (Use each letter only once; some letters may not be used.)

COLUMN I

1. _______ Attention
2. _______ Comprehension
3. _______ Coma
4. _______ Consciousness
5. _______ Delirium
6. _______ Delusion
7. _______ Dementia

COLUMN II

a. The capacity to understand and reason
b. A state of awareness and full responsiveness to stimuli
c. A clinical syndrome involving progressive impairment of intellectual function and memory
d. The aspect of consciousness that enables one to concentrate on and take in specific sensory stimuli
e. Fixed false belief
f. An acute organic mental disorder characterized by global cognitive impairment, disturbed attention, and disturbed sleep
g. Complete unresponsiveness to incoming stimuli

COLUMN I

1. _______ Intelligence
2. _______ Judgment
3. _______ Memory
4. _______ Perceiving
5. _______ Reality orientation
6. _______ Sundown syndrome

COLUMN II

a. The process by which information and experiences are stored and retrieved
b. The measurable product of intellectual functioning
c. The process of receiving and interpreting the sensory stimuli that function as a basis for understanding, knowing, or learning
d. The ability to process incoming stimuli and determine the complex meanings associated with the many aspects of a situation.
e. An increase in confusion and disorientation at the end of the day
f. Perception of reality; includes the awareness of time, place, situation, and self

FILL IN THE BLANK

Supply the missing term or the information requested.

1. Important factors that play a role in normal cognitive processes include ________________, ________________, ________________, ________________, and ________________.
2. Intact structure and functioning of the ________________ receptors, the ________________ nervous pathways, and the ________________ cortex are required for a person to be able to take in information through the senses and to assimilate and interpret that information.
3. Normal cognitive function consists of ________________, ________________, ________________, ________________, ________________, and ________________.
4. Name five of the nine personal factors that affect normal cognitive function. ________________, ________________, ________________, ________________, and ________________
5. As a person ages, cognitive function remains relatively unchanged in the absence of trauma or specific dysfunction, although the ________________ of information may require more time.
6. Manifestations of altered cognition are often associated with ________________ thinking and ________________ thought processes.

■ Applying Your Knowledge

CASE STUDY

A 12-year-old boy who recently received a diagnosis of leukemia is concerned that he will fall behind his classmates while hospitalized. His mother reports that she often finds him crying. Use your database about pain, sensory perception, and cognition in the following exercises.

1. Describe the factors that may affect the child's cognitive processes.
2. Outline the additional information you will need to develop a nursing care plan.
3. Discuss which professionals should be involved in assisting the boy to cope with his situation and why.

CRITICAL INQUIRY EXERCISE

Prepare a discharge teaching plan for family members of a client exhibiting altered thought processes; include communication techniques and reality orientation techniques.

CRITICAL EXPLORATION EXERCISE

While in the clinical area, select a confused client for whom to provide care. Plan and implement safety measures and measures to facilitate communication and decrease stress.

■ Practicing for NCLEX

MULTIPLE CHOICE QUESTIONS

Circle the letter that corresponds to the best answer for each question.

1. A client with altered cognitive function would benefit from which of the following nursing actions?
   a. Allow the client extended periods of privacy and independent activity to strengthen problem-solving thought processes.
   b. Maintain dim lighting to prevent disturbing environmental glare.
   c. Remove unnecessary obstructions from the room to prevent falls.
   d. Vary routines and activities daily to provide needed diversional distraction.

2. The nurse teaching family members principles of reality orientation would include which of the following instructions?
   a. Change environmental lighting to match the usual day and night cuing.
   b. Ignore all behaviors to minimize the apparent alterations in thought processes.
   c. Reinforce references to delusions if necessary to avoid agitating the client.
   d. Use complex, comprehensive sentences to explain requests to the client.

3. The nurse takes a confused client to the bathroom every night at 9:00 PM prior to helping him to bed for the night. This is an example of
   a. bladder and bowel training.
   b. encouraging client participation.
   c. establishing a consistent routine.
   d. providing orientation cues.

4. The student nurse is planning to teach an 80-year-old client about her medications. The teaching plan should include
   a. additional time to present and explain material and to allow the client to demonstrate understanding.
   b. limited information about side effects because this would be too difficult for the client to comprehend at her age.
   c. instructions to the client to hire a nurse to administer medications because she is too old to learn to do this.
   d. only the names of the medications because, with aging, the older person has decreased ability to learn new things.

5. Which of the following data best supports the nursing diagnosis Impaired Verbal Communication?
   a. Misperception
   b. Altered interpretation/response to stimuli
   c. Absence of eye contact or difficulty attending
   d. Distractibility

6. A client is walking up the hallway in the hospital toward the lounge. The client appears confused and asks for directions to the room he has had for the past 10 days. The client is demonstrating
   a. attention span deficit.
   b. alteration in level of arousal.
   c. delusional thinking pattern.
   d. short-term memory impairment.

7. Which of the following would be an appropriate documentation of a client's cognitive dysfunction?
   a. "Senile and uncooperative"
   b. "Slightly confused"
   c. "Poor attention span"
   d. "Oriented to family only"

8. Stress-management techniques do which of the following?
   a. Accelerate the rate of learning
   b. Decrease concentration
   c. Improve rest and relaxation
   d. Provide needed distraction

9. The nurse caring for a client with an irreversible neurologic deficit should prepare to
   a. administer medical treatment to control the condition.
   b. allow the client to perform all self-care measures to promote the use of remaining mental abilities.
   c. minimize visits from family and friends to minimize irritation to external stimuli.
   d. use clocks and calendars to facilitate reorientation to time.

FILL IN THE BLANK

Supply the missing term or the information requested.

1. The systematic way in which a person thinks, reasons, and uses language is referred to as ____________________.

2. The cognitive developmental work of infancy is carried out through exploration of the environment and through ______________.

MULTIPLE-ANSWER MULTIPLE CHOICE

Circle the letter(s) corresponding to the appropriate answer(s). Circle all that apply.

1. Which of the following interventions are appropriate for the client who is experiencing alterations in cognitive processes?
   a. Assessing a client who is confused about place and person for visual impairment
   b. Deciding that an elderly client who exhibits altered thought processes and confusion is probably just senile
   c. Placing a client identified as being at risk for altered thought processes in restraints every night while hospitalized
   d. Alerting the client and family members that subtle changes in cognition may occur as a result of medications
   e. Assessing alcohol intake when taking a medication history

2. Which of the following interventions are inappropriate for the client who is experiencing alterations in cognitive processes?
   a. Evaluating the client's hemoglobin level when assessing cardiovascular function
   b. Monitoring the sodium, calcium, and glucose levels of a confused client for possible contributing factors
   c. Administering higher levels of medication to clients with poor kidney function to facilitate metabolism of the drug
   d. Promoting regular exercise as a method of improving oxygen perfusion to the brain
   e. Encouraging clients who exhibit sundown syndrome to switch to sleeping in the daytime and being awake at night

3. The characteristics of normal cognition include
   a. intellectual function.
   b. perception of reality.
   c. orientation.
   d. language.
   e. judgment.
   f. recall.
   g. recognition.

4. Which of the following describes the oral expressions that characterize the person with anomic aphasia?
   a. Fluent speech
   b. Disorganized content
   c. Talks around the subject
   d. Meaningless recurrent sounds
   e. Telegraphic

HOT SPOT QUESTIONS

Place an "X" on the area of the brain that is responsible for visual reception.

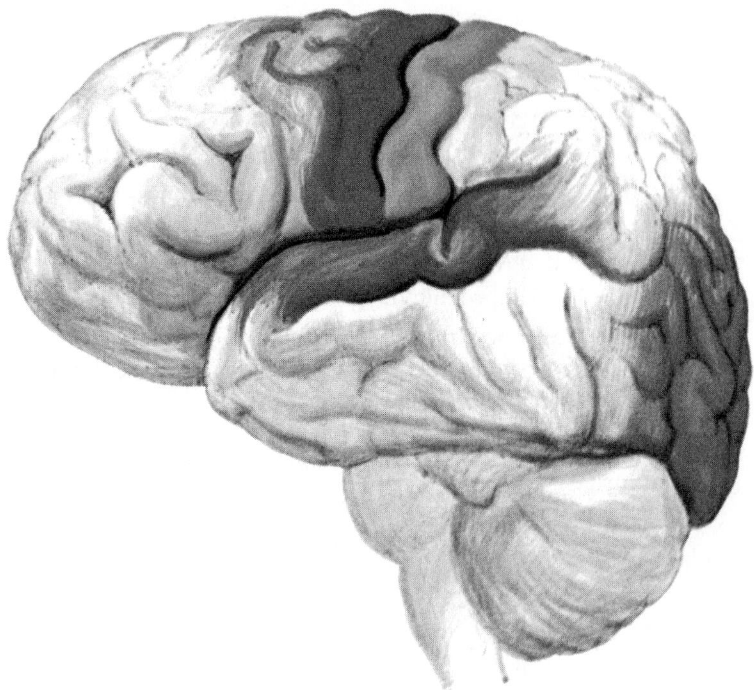

UNIT XIII

SELF-PERCEPTION AND SELF-CONCEPT

CHAPTER 48

Self-Concept

CHAPTER OVERVIEW

Chapter 48 defines self-concept, presents factors affecting self-concept, and discusses planning care for clients with manifestations of altered self-concept.

LEARNING OBJECTIVES

After mastering the content in this chapter, you should be able to do the following:

1. Describe the functions of self and self-concept.
2. Define self-concept, self-perception, self-knowledge, self-expectation, social self, and self-evaluation.
3. Discuss factors that can affect self-concept.
4. Identify the four patterns of self-concept.
5. Identify possible manifestations of altered self-concept.
6. Discuss how self-concept develops throughout the lifespan.
7. Apply the theory to assess for self-concept functioning.
8. Plan care for a person with an altered self-concept.

■ Mastering the Information

MATCHING

Match the terms in Column II with a definition, example, or related statement from Column I. Place the letter corresponding to the answer in the space provided. (Use each letter only once; some letters may not be used.)

COLUMN I

1. ______ A dimension of self-perception that involves setting goals for present and future
2. ______ Conscious self-assessment leading to self-worth or self-respect
3. ______ A mental image one has of oneself
4. ______ Involves basic facts and qualities related to who one is
5. ______ How one pictures and feels about the body
6. ______ How a person explains behavior based on self-observation

COLUMN II

a. Self-evaluation
b. Self-perception
c. Self-knowledge
d. Self-concept
e. Self-expectation
f. Body image

TRUE–FALSE

Indicate if the following statements are true or false.

______ 1. The basis for positive self-concept is established with a newborn when the mother is calm and communicates warmth and acceptance.

______ 2. An example of developmental role transition would be the death of a spouse.

______ 3. A person with high self-esteem accepts others.

______ 4. A person with a cardiac condition may suffer altered body image.

______ 5. Nursing interventions for the school-age child with altered self-concept would include educating the family about identity and body image changes.

FILL IN THE BLANK

Supply the missing term or the information requested.

1. The four dimensions of self-perception are ________________, ________________, ________________, and ________________.
2. The two sources of self-esteem are ________________ and ________________.
3. Two types of role transition are ________________ and ________________.
4. When there is no choice in role performance, this is called an ________________ role, and when a role is selected by choice, it is termed an ________________ role.
5. The mental image of the self is composed of ________________, ________________, ________________, and ________________.
6. List and briefly describe three common problems associated with roles.

   a.

   b.

   c.

■ Applying Your Knowledge

CASE STUDY

A 56-year-old widowed homemaker has recently become involved with the local ladies sewing circle and volunteered to help deliver meals to shut-ins. Her 28-year-old daughter expresses concern to you about her mother's newfound activities and wonders if it is "normal" for a woman her age.

1. Discuss your response based on the client's activities and the outcome to her life changes that she is demonstrating according to Sheehy (1974).
2. Develop a teaching plan that will help the client's daughter understand the impact of her responses to her mother's changes on her mother's self-esteem.
3. In what ways might the client's role transitions affect her family members, and how might they respond?

CRITICAL INQUIRY EXERCISE

1. Write a brief paragraph to address your normal functions and patterns of self-concept.
2. Use the nursing process to plan and provide care for clients with high potential for alteration in body image (e.g., clients with burn injuries, facial scars, or mastectomies).

CRITICAL EXPLORATION EXERCISE

1. Identify three people you know and address their role functions.
2. Give examples of personal role transitions—situational and developmental—experienced during the last 5 years of your life. Identify the coping strategies you used to adapt to these role transitions.

■ Practicing for NCLEX

MULTIPLE CHOICE QUESTIONS

Circle the letter that corresponds to the best answer for each question.

1. A client is being admitted to the hospital for a mastectomy. Which of the following would most directly result from the client's scheduled surgical procedure?
   a. Altered self-esteem
   b. Altered identity
   c. Altered body image
   d. Role ambiguity

2. Select the most appropriate nursing intervention for the client recovering from a mastectomy.
   a. Allow the client to perform all activities.
   b. Remove mirrors from the client's room.
   c. Encourage the client to view the surgical area within the first postoperative hours.
   d. Encourage independence but assist as needed.

3. An adolescent female has begun her menstrual cycle. Which of the following nursing interventions would be most appropriate for the client?
   a. Assist the client with self-control.
   b. Educate the client about sexual health.
   c. Allow privacy and complete independence.
   d. Assist the client with this situational role transition.

4. A 4-year-old preschooler asked the nurse, "What do you call the fat part of your chest?" The most appropriate response by the nurse is to
   a. ignore the preschooler's question.
   b. answer the question by saying, "breasts."
   c. tell the child to ask his or her mother.
   d. tell the preschooler to never ask adults questions like this.

FILL IN THE BLANK

Supply the missing term or the information requested.

1. The awareness that one is a distinct individual separate from others is referred to as

   ____________________.

2. What is the term used to describe the degree of self-confidence a person has about his/her ability to perform specific activities?

   ____

MULTIPLE-ANSWER MULTIPLE CHOICE

Circle the letter(s) corresponding to the appropriate answer(s). Circle all that apply.

1. Which of the following nursing interventions would be appropriate for the client who has just given birth to her first child?
   a. Teach the client about how her socialization needs will change.
   b. Support the family and assist members to maintain self-control.
   c. Limit the number of care choices so that client will not be overwhelmed.
   d. Help the client to adjust to her new role.

2. The nurse is working with a client who is scheduled to be discharged during the next 24 hours. The client had a colon resection and will be discharged home with a colostomy. Which of the following behaviors indicates that the client is accepting responsibility for self-care?
   a. The client lists negative attitudes and their effect on self before discharge.
   b. The client makes eye contact with the nurse during conversation.
   c. The client participates in colostomy care before discharge.
   d. The client verbalizes strategies to support self-care in the home environment.

3. Which of the following questions will assist the nurse to assess the client's self-concept?
   a. How do you get along with your family members?
   b. Are you experiencing changes in your body or the things you can do?
   c. Do you find thins frequently make you feel angry, anxious, frustrated, afraid, sad, or annoyed?
   d. Do you have unrealistic expectations of yourself and others?

ORDERING

Place the Erikson's characteristics of self-concept development in ascending order, beginning with the task that characterizes the infant.

______ Autonomy vs. Shame and Doubt

______ Generativity vs. Self-absorption

______ Identity vs. Role Confusion

______ Industry vs. Inferiority

______ Initiative vs. Guilt

______ Integrity vs. Despair

______ Intimacy vs. Isolation

______ Trust vs. Mistrust

UNIT XIV

Roles and Relationships

CHAPTER 49

Families and Their Relationships

CHAPTER OVERVIEW

Chapter 49 presents characteristics of normal family function, lifespan considerations, factors affecting family function, and manifestations of altered family function. Common nursing diagnoses, goals, and interventions to promote family health are discussed.

LEARNING OBJECTIVES

After mastering the content in this chapter, you should be able to do the following:

1. Describe variations in family structure and function.
2. Identify factors affecting normal family relationships.
3. Discuss common needs that are met in a family unit.
4. Describe manifestations of altered family function.
5. Identify nursing diagnoses and related factors associated with altered family function.
6. Discuss nursing interventions to promote family health and function.
7. Discuss nursing interventions for altered family function.

■ Mastering the Information

MATCHING

Match the terms in Column II with a definition, example, or related statement from Column I. Place the letter corresponding to the answer in the space provided. (Use each letter only once; some letters may not be used.)

COLUMN I

1. ______ Consists of the married adult man and woman with or without children
2. ______ Includes the nuclear family, grandparents, aunts, uncles, and cousins
3. ______ Consists of children living with one birth parent and one nonbirth parent and perhaps an offspring of a nonbirth parent
4. ______ Includes people living together without formal or legal bonds of marriage
5. ______ Includes members who share a common bond, such as religion, ideology, economic, or learning needs

COLUMN II

a. Blended family
b. Communal family
c. Cohabitated family
d. Nuclear family
e. Extended family

COLUMN I

1. ______ Child's perception of his or her own abilities; significant in the development of a sense of industry
2. ______ Encouraging child's independence within established limits fosters the development of autonomy
3. ______ Important to ensure the child that changes, such as illness and death, are not their fault
4. ______ Peer-group identity strongly desired
5. ______ Process of attachment and bonding critical to the developmental task of establishing trust

COLUMN II

a. Infant
b. Toddler
c. Preschooler
d. School-age
e. Adolescent

TRUE–FALSE

Indicate if the following statements are true or false.

_____ 1. Family and social relationships change in response to both acute and chronic illness.

_____ 2. Only objective data are useful in documenting family dysfunction.

_____ 3. Goals for dysfunctional families involve improving communication and coping mechanisms, fulfilling needs of the family, and accomplishing developmental tasks.

_____ 4. Evaluation of nursing care for a family is accomplished by recording statements of individual family members regarding satisfaction with nursing care.

_____ 5. A multidisciplinary approach is most useful when intervening with altered family function.

_____ 6. When a family is in crisis, the nurse is obligated to ensure the safety of individual members through notification and referral to appropriate groups.

_____ 7. Family and marital counseling focuses on members interacting with one another, rather than counseling any one person.

_____ 8. Teaching family members the techniques of care to meet the physical needs of an ill member greatly assists in adaptation to the role of caregiver.

_____ 9. Providing a family with the names and telephone numbers of people to call for answers to various questions can ease adaptation to the home setting.

_____ 10. An understanding of an individual's perspectives of the family is the most important consideration to positively influence family function.

FILL IN THE BLANK

Supply the missing term or the information requested.

1. Families function in their own unique ways but usually have common ________________.
2. Needs that are met in families include ________________ care, ________________ provisions, ________________ intimacy, ________________, ________________, ________________, ________________, and ________________.
3. Identify six of the nine factors that affect family function.
   a.
   b.
   c.
   d.
   e.
   f.
4. Manifestations of altered family function include ________________, ________________, ________________, and ________________ changes.
5. ________________ strain is a manifestation of altered family function in which changes in roles are chosen or forced on family members by changing events or development in the family.

■ Applying Your Knowledge

CASE STUDY

The nurse is interviewing a family that consists of the husband, wife, and three children. The oldest sibling is in college and reportedly doing well. However, the parents tell the nurse that they believe that the two younger adolescent siblings are using drugs. They report that expensive items, such as a watch, the silverware, and other valuables, are missing from the house. Both of the children are in high school.

Recently their grades have been less than average, even though both children were on the honor roll last year. Using your knowledge of family and social relationships, address the following:

1. Describe your feelings when you hear the information and how these feelings might affect your response.
2. Discuss how you will proceed to validate or invalidate the parents' suspicion.
3. Describe the long-term impact the behaviors of each family member could have on the family and on the community.
4. Recommend ways of facilitating family integrity.

CRITICAL INQUIRY EXERCISE

Perform a functional assessment of your own family.

a. Identify family structure.
b. List family strengths.
c. Discuss the family communication pattern.
d. Identify social factors that influence family function.

CRITICAL EXPLORATION EXERCISE

1. Review a family health record at a local health department or home-health agency.
2. Accompany a community health nurse during a home visit.

■ Practicing for NCLEX

MULTIPLE CHOICE QUESTIONS

Circle the letter that corresponds to the best answer for each question.

1. An 8-year-old girl who is extremely playful at the dinner table is constantly distracting her 2-year-old sibling, who is learning to use a spoon and fork. After the girl is admonished several times, she is sent to her room to be alone for a while. This is an example of
   a. informal education.
   b. severe punishment.
   c. child abuse.
   d. severe family dysfunction.

2. Nursing interventions for altered family function focus on
   a. removing barriers to the provision of physical care and a high quality of life, improving economic status, and role development.
   b. improving financial status, physical care, formal education, and spending practices.
   c. reducing spending practices, increasing the perception of health, limiting communication, and providing high-quality physical care.
   d. returning the family to positive outcomes, improving the problem, and supporting family relationships.

3. Immediately after a client is told that her newborn has congenital hip dysplasia, she repeatedly states, "I can't believe it. I just can't believe it." This is likely an expression of which of the following feelings?
   a. Denial, which may be necessary as the family struggles with the initial shock of the child's disability.
   b. Denial, which is always unacceptable in coping with illness or loss and which requires immediate intervention.
   c. Guilt and inadequacy to cope with disappointments in the past.
   d. Anxiety about the future of the family and other children in the extended family.

4. The nurse is interviewing the family of an alcoholic who has recently become unemployed. Very little is required of the unemployed family member by other members of the family. The spouse and siblings now work to pay bills and to support the family. They may now be considered
   a. encouragers, under role strain, who enhance family relationships.
   b. enforcers, under role strain, who support drinking.
   c. rescuers, under role strain, who can impede interactions within the family and between the family and the community.
   d. enablers, under role strain, who can impede interactions within the family and between the family and the community.

5. A 9-year-old child acts out in school by throwing temper tantrums, refusing to do schoolwork, and harassing other students. The school nurse is consulted because such behavior is very likely indicative of
   a. boredom related to a lack of teacher interest.
   b. an emotional problem related to altered family function.
   c. a physical illness that has not been diagnosed.
   d. inadequate nutritional intake to support growth and development.

6. A 39-year-old single parent has just received a diagnosis of breast cancer. In the immediate crisis period following the diagnosis, decisions have to be made regarding
   a. who will pay the rent and take the children to school and to social events.
   b. who will make decisions about discipline, spending money, and organizing the house.
   c. how to share the diagnosis with the children, which family members can provide assistance, and what kind of treatment to choose.
   d. whether to ask the children's father to "keep house," who will cook food, and who will clean the house.

7. The nurse asks a client, "What do you think you may have problems with when you're discharged from the hospital?" The nurse is attempting to identify
   a. strengths of the family for problem solution.
   b. areas of risk for dysfunction.
   c. attitudes about work and rest.
   d. the development stage of the client.

8. Characteristic risk factors for alteration in parenting include
   a. good performance in school and at work, high self-esteem, strong family ties, and a firm support system.
   b. economic and emotional security, good self-concept, adequate role development, and strong group interactions.
   c. a firm support system, good work and school performance, altered self-concept, inadequate role development, and poor group interactions.
   d. unrealistic expectations of self, inappropriate role model, a skill or knowledge deficit, unmet psychological needs, and an inadequate support system.

9. Which one of the following diagnoses would be most directly related to a situation in which the breadwinner for a family has recently become unemployed?
   a. Interrupted family processes related to the inability to meet the usual physical needs of its members
   b. Interrupted family processes related to the inability to meet the emotional needs of family members
   c. Interrupted family processes related to the inability to meet the spiritual needs of family members
   d. Interrupted family processes related to the inability to provide mutual growth and maturation of family members

10. A 15-year-old girl has an 8-month-old son. She lives with her father and two younger siblings. There is no milk or food in the house. She tells the nurse that she does not know what she and her child will eat later in the day but that "everything will be fine." The house is cluttered and filthy. An appropriate nursing diagnosis is
    a. compromised family coping related to inadequate health information.
    b. compromised family coping related to overconcern for herself and her infant.
    c. disabled family coping related to the denial of the existing situation.
    d. disabled family coping related to extreme agitation, depression, and open hostility.

11. A 16-year-old girl who has a 19-year-old sibling and lives with both parents threatens suicide. Which of the following is an appropriate family goal?
    a. Family will demonstrate awareness of other members' needs for physical care, economic security, education, and nurturing.
    b. Family will provide safety and security for the teenage girl and nurturing for all family members.
    c. Family will develop the ability to teach, nurture, educate, and socialize offspring.
    d. Family will be able to adjust to role strain because the daughter cannot adapt if needs are not met.

FILL IN THE BLANK

Supply the missing term or the information requested.

1. What is the phrase used to describe adult children who are faced with meeting their own needs as well as the needs of their children and their parents? ______________________

2. A man tells the nurse that he needs help dressing his wife's foot ulcer because he is not sure which solutions to use or how tight to place the dressing. A likely nursing diagnosis is ______________.

MULTIPLE-ANSWER MULTIPLE CHOICE

Circle the letter(s) corresponding to the appropriate answer(s). Circle all that apply.

1. Behavioral signs of family dysfunction may include
   a. dependence.
   b. labile emotions.
   c. poor eating and sleeping habits.
   d. limited socialization.

2. Nursing interventions that foster problem solving include
   a. identifying the individual family member who is causing the problem.
   b. temporarily taking over the role of decision maker for the family.
   c. recommending a specific problem-solving approach based on the type of problem the family is experiencing.
   d. providing concrete feedback based on nursing observations.

3. The primary goal of a "family-centered" network of care is to
   a. reinforce the current communication pattern.
   b. prevent family member disagreements.
   c. eliminate the negative impact of illness or disability.
   d. provide as "normal" a lifestyle as is possible.

4. When family conflict arises, psychosocial development may be
   a. accelerated at that level.
   b. indifferent from that level.
   c. regressed from that level.
   d. arrested at that level.

5. Family abuse may be physical, sexual, emotional, or economic. It may be aimed at
   a. the spouse.
   b. children.
   c. parents.
   d. grandparents.

CHAPTER 50

Loss and Grieving

CHAPTER OVERVIEW

Chapter 50 addresses loss and the grief experience. Normal grieving and dysfunctional grieving are reviewed. The application of the nursing process to grieving clients is discussed, and the role of hospice programs in facilitating the grief process is outlined.

LEARNING OBJECTIVES

After mastering the content in this chapter, you should be able to do the following:

1. Define selected terms related to loss and grief.
2. Identify the normal function of grief.
3. Compare models of grief related to bereavement and grief related to dying.
4. Evaluate understanding of death and grief reactions across the lifespan.
5. Identify the common manifestations of grief.
6. Discuss the effects of multiple losses on the grief process.
7. Apply the nursing process to grieving clients.
8. Differentiate between normal and dysfunctional grieving.

■ Mastering the Information

MATCHING

Match the terms in Column II with a definition, example, or related statement from Column I. Place the letter corresponding to the answer in the space provided. (Use each letter only once; some letters may not be used.)

COLUMN I

1. ______ Anticipatory grief
2. ______ Bereavement
3. ______ Grief
4. ______ Dysfunctional grief
5. ______ Mourning

COLUMN II

a. The characteristic pattern of psychological responses a person experiences after the loss of a significant person, object, belief, or relationship

b. A state of dissolution that occurs as the result of a loss, particularly the death of a significant other

c. Encompasses the socially prescribed behaviors after the death of a significant other

d. The characteristic pattern of psychological and physiologic responses a person makes to the impending loss (real or imagined) of a significant other, object, belief, or relationship

e. Abnormal response to the loss of a significant other, object, belief, or relationship with little energy left for normal growth and development

TRUE–FALSE

Indicate if the following statements are true or false.

______ 1. Caution must be used to prevent interpreting the grief cycle model too literally because people may vary greatly in their responses to loss and still fall within the normal response range.

______ 2. Factors affecting people's reactions to loss are limited to sociocultural resources and stressors.

______ 3. The impact of a traumatic event and the person's reaction to it depend on the individual's developmental stage.

______ 4. Children tend to grieve more intensely and more continuously but for a relatively shorter period of time than do adults.

______ 5. Behaviors such as the inability to experience joy, inability to form new relationships, and talking and acting as if the deceased is alive that persist beyond 3 years are considered by bereavement experts as abnormal.

_____ 6. Dysfunctional grief by one family member does not affect the family.

_____ 7. Crisis theory states that the outcome of a loss experience is predetermined.

_____ 8. To understand the loss reaction of a client, the nurse needs to know the physical and psychological significance of the lost person or object, whether the loss was expected or unexpected, and if the survivor perceived that he or she contributed to the loss.

_____ 9. Personal stressors and resources that affect grief responses include personality characteristics, coping skills, communication skills, physical health status, spirituality, and previous experiences with loss.

_____ 10. If a person remains in complete denial of a loss or if the person's grief symptoms continue unabated over a long period of time, the person is likely experiencing grief dysfunction.

FILL IN THE BLANK

Supply the missing term or the information requested.

1. List two of the three important functions of grief.

   a.

   b.

2. Loss of a loved one by death, divorce, or termination of a relationship is an example of both a ________________ and ________________ loss.

3. An accidental death is an example of a(n) _______ loss and may result in a higher level of distress.

4. Two popular stage models of grief are those proposed by ______________ and ______________. A third model is the ______________.

5. State and briefly describe the five stages of dying proposed by Kubler-Ross (1969).

   a.

   b.

   c.

   d.

   e.

6. Models of grief are useful in guiding ________________ of clients experiencing loss.

STAGES OF GRIEF

Using the grief cycle model that was derived from Parkes' (1986) theory as a reference, indicate the stage of grief for which the intervention listed is most appropriate. Write "S" for shock, "P" for protest, "D" for disorganization, or "R" for reorganization.

1. ______ Refer the client to self-help groups.
2. ______ Identify new support systems.
3. ______ Help the client to establish coping behaviors used in the past.
4. ______ Provide role models who have successfully coped with similar loss.
5. ______ Refer the client for a complete physical examination.
6. ______ Encourage participation in mourning rituals.
7. ______ Encourage remembering and talking about that which was lost.
8. ______ Refer the client to educational programs.
9. ______ Have someone drive the client home.
10. ______ Refer the client to social activity programs.

■ Applying Your Knowledge

CASE STUDY

A 51-year-old woman who is a former executive secretary now has a malignant brain tumor. She lives with her 25-year-old son and is registered with a home care hospice program. You are the nurse assigned to guide the hospice team. Reflecting on your knowledge base of loss and the grieving process, do the following.

1. Plan additional strategies for obtaining additional information you will need to make a thorough assessment of this client and her family.

2. Consider possible nursing diagnoses for the client and her family.
3. Discuss the role of the hospice program in facilitating the grief process.
4. Identify professional and nonprofessional resources that may be mobilized to assist the family.

CRITICAL INQUIRY EXERCISE

1. Recall the most recent loss you have experienced. What mental and physical symptoms do you remember experiencing during the immediate periods of grief. What symptoms did you notice in the persons around you who were also experiencing grief?
2. What strategies have you used to support an individual (friend/family) during a grief period. Which strategies were effective and which did you notice were not effective?

CRITICAL EXPLORATION EXERCISE

1. Visit a local hospice organization. Interview a nurse regarding strategies used to support families during the death and dying process.
2. Visit a cancer unit for adults and a cancer unit for children. Choose a client with terminal disease from each unit, and observe each client's family and friends. Compare and contrast grief responses noted.

■ Practicing for NCLEX

MULTIPLE CHOICE QUESTIONS

Circle the letter that corresponds to the best answer for each question.

1. A client has recently divorced his wife. Which of the following factors will most likely affect his response to this experience?
   a. Genetic factors related to coping
   b. His ex-wife's attitude toward divorce
   c. His feelings regarding marriage
   d. His job and salary

2. Which of the following descriptions is consistent with the general adult response to loss?
   a. Refraining from dating or beginning a new relationship for the first 3 months after the divorce
   b. Talking about the divorce 4 years later as if it had just happened
   c. Keeping the ex-spouse's clothes and personal items in a special room 2 years after the divorce
   d. Experiencing intermittent periods of grief over a 5-year period after the divorce is final

3. The nurse would find which of the following responses to death inappropriate?
   a. A 16-month-old girl who cries for her mother who died suddenly
   b. A 10-year-old boy who states he will be glad when his dead father comes back to play with him
   c. A 17-year-old girl who cries at night when she thinks about her father who died 8 months ago
   d. A 3-year-old girl who asks when her mother, who died months before, will wake up

4. Cultural and social ties will most likely have which of the following effects on the grieving process?
   a. Family members and friends will always supportively reduce the grieving period.
   b. They will have little or no effect because grieving generally follows the same pattern for all people.
   c. Tradition will dictate the length and type of grieving and mourning.
   d. Sociocultural expectations allow the survivor to proceed in an individual manner and on his or her own time schedule for grieving.

5. To assess personal stressors and resources of the husband of a deceased client, the nurse would need to know
   a. how well the husband coped with previous losses.
   b. medications the client was taking before death.
   c. the history of other family members' coping behaviors.
   d. the medical diagnosis of the person who died.

6. A 70-year-old man has just lost his wife of 50 years through death. He appears calm and shows no signs of grief. The nurse should
   a. assume that the client is handling the loss of his wife well.
   b. determine if the client is demonstrating a dysfunctional grief pattern.
   c. instruct the client that he needs to cry to release his grief.
   d. plan follow-up care for the client, who may have a delayed grief reaction.

7. A client's husband has lung cancer and is terminally ill. She tells the nurse, "The children are so good to me, but I don't know what I'll do when he's gone. I lie awake at night thinking about what's going to happen to me." A likely nursing diagnosis for the client is
   a. dysfunctional grieving evidenced by verbal expressions and lying awake, related to husband's illness.
   b. anticipatory grieving as evidenced by verbal expressions related to her husband's terminal illness.
   c. dysfunctional grieving as evidenced by expressions of care given by children related to selfishness.
   d. all of the above.

FILL IN THE BLANK

Supply the missing term or the information requested.

1. The experience of parting with an object, person, belief, or relationship that one values is defined as ________________.

2. Perception of death as reversible, avoidable, and occurring in degrees is characteristic of the ________________.

MULTIPLE-ANSWER MULTIPLE CHOICE

Circle the letter(s) corresponding to the appropriate answer(s). Circle all that apply.

1. Which of the following models of grief include the stages of disorganization and reorganization?
   a. Engel's model
   b. Grief cycle model
   c. Kubler-Ross' stages of dying
   d. Parkes' model

2. Which of the following behaviors are considered "normal" grief manifestations?
   a. Inability to "have fun" or "a good time" 10 months after the loss
   b. Being unable to remember or talk about a close friend 4 years after his death
   c. Reports of hearing or seeing a deceased friend who died 2 months previously
   d. Demonstrating symptoms of depression 8 months after the death of a favorite pet
   e. Leaving the deceased's belongings intact 3 years after the death

3. Which of the following behaviors are considered "abnormal" grief manifestations?
   a. Failure to form a new relationship 1 year after the death of a spouse
   b. Reporting symptoms similar to those expressed by a spouse who died of cancer 3½ years ago
   c. Crying each time a deceased sibling's name is mentioned 6 months after the death
   d. Preparing a place at the breakfast table for a deceased parent 5 years after the parent's death
   e. Talking about the death, 4 years after it occurred, as if it had just happened

4. Which of the following nursing interventions is appropriate to use to assist a client's move through the shock phase of the grieving process?
   a. Promote appropriate sleep habits.
   b. Protect client from physical harm.
   c. Provide anticipatory guidance regarding the normal grief process.
   d. Provide role models who have successfully coped with similar loss.

UNIT XV

COPING AND STRESS MANAGEMENT

CHAPTER 51

Stress, Coping, and Adaptation

CHAPTER OVERVIEW

Chapter 51 discusses stress and the factors affecting an individual's ability to cope with stress. The psychological and physiologic manifestations and responses of stress are reviewed. Theories relative to stress and coping processes are also reviewed. The use of the nursing process to address the needs of a client faced with stress is discussed.

LEARNING OBJECTIVES

After mastering the content in this chapter, you should be able to do the following:

1. Identify physiologic signs and symptoms of stress.
2. Identify psychological responses to stress.
3. List examples of biophysical and psychosocial stressors.
4. Give examples of variables that affect a person's ability to cope with stress.
5. Describe various types of coping patterns people typically use to handle stress.
6. Identify stress management techniques that nurses can use to help clients adapt to stress.

■ Mastering the Information

MATCHING

Match the terms in Column I with a definition, example, or related statement from Column II. Place the letter corresponding to the answer in the space provided. (Use each letter only once; some letters may not be used.)

COLUMN I

1. ______ Adaptation
2. ______ Allostasis
3. ______ Coping
4. ______ Crisis
5. ______ Homeostasis
6. ______ Stressor

COLUMN II

a. The coordinated physiologic processes that maintain most of the steady states in the organism
b. The attempt to achieve respect or recognition in one activity as a substitute for the inability to achieve in another endeavor
c. A process that a person uses to manage stressors or events encountered
d. A person's capacity to flourish and survive even with adversity
e. The stimulus that evokes a generalized stress response; anything that places a demand on the person
f. Reflects body's capacity to maintain stability in the face of constant change and to adjust to new levels of functioning
g. After a trauma, blood vessels that dilate in the inflamed area
h. Suggests a situation in which the usual coping strategies are ineffective and the person is disorganized or unable to problem solve appropriately

COLUMN I

1. ______ A systematic technique teaching the body and mind to respond to verbal commands, allowing the person to achieve a deep state of relaxation through self-suggestion and self-hypnosis
2. ______ An attempt to affect an unconscious process by using conscious suggestion or a mental picture of the desired change
3. ______ A form of exercise to foster relaxation, mental alacrity, and good health
4. ______ Strong, positive, feeling-rich statements about a desired change to reinforce and increase the effectiveness of visualization; can be silent
5. ______ The person who learns to monitor physiologic processes such as heart rate, translate information about these processes to determine if stress is present, and exert control over automatic functions

COLUMN II

a. Affirmations
b. Autogenic training
c. Biofeedback
d. Massage
e. Medication
f. Visualization and imagery
g. Yoga

TRUE–FALSE

Indicate if the following statements are true or false.

______ 1. Stress has always been part of the human experience.

______ 2. Overeating is an example of a long-term coping mechanism.

______ 3. Making and sticking to a time schedule is an example of problem-oriented coping.

______ 4. To best judge a client's response to stress, the nurse should use his or her own coping expectations as a guide.

______ 5. Health teaching related to the causes of stress can help a client develop strategies for coping and adapting.

______ 6. The preschooler can identify stressors and begin to reason with parents and others about how to cope with them.

______ 7. The infant learns to develop coping strategies for relatively simple stressors, such as a slight delay in getting wants and needs met.

FILL IN THE BLANK

Supply the missing term or the information requested

1. Prior exposure to and past experience with particular stressors influence the person's ________________ and ________________ to current encounters.
2. Two types of coping processes are ________________ and ________________.
3. Stressors may be ________________ and ________________, or ________________ and ________________.
4. People who are most successful in coping need to be ______________ and to use a ______________ of strategies to adapt to new situations and stressors.
5. Families can be a great source of support but can also be the source of ________________ and ________________ coping.

■ Applying Your Knowledge

CASE STUDY

A 16-year-old girl who had diabetes diagnosed approximately 1 year ago is being admitted to your floor for the sixth time. The client tells you, "The diet you told me about makes me look stupid around my friends. I can't eat anything they eat." The client's mother tells you that the client won't eat right and calls her daughter "stupid." The client's mother asks you, "What should I do?"

1. Discuss the stressors you assess the client and her mother are experiencing.

2. Outline the strategies you could teach the family to help them deal with the stress of their situation.
3. Identify community services that might be used in this situation.

CRITICAL INQUIRY EXERCISE

List the changes that have occurred in your life during the last year. Exchange lists with two other classmates, and evaluate your classmates' stressors. Discuss your findings with your classmates for validation.

CRITICAL EXPLORATION EXERCISE

Select a client on one clinical day and assess the coping mechanisms being used by that client relative to hospitalization, medical or surgical treatments, financial demands, and daily life disruptions.

■ Practicing for NCLEX

MULTIPLE CHOICE QUESTIONS

Circle the letter that corresponds to the best answer for each question.

1. Which of the following findings might indicate that the client is experiencing stress?
   a. Bradycardia
   b. Hypotension
   c. Hypoventilation
   d. Tachypnea
2. A common physical response to stress might be
   a. diarrhea.
   b. muscle flaccidity.
   c. sedation.
   d. skin dryness.
3. A client who has been having marital problems is admitted to the hospital with a diagnosis of migraine headaches. Which of the following would the nurse note to be a long-term coping mechanism for the client?
   a. Drinking coffee or cola every 2 to 3 hours
   b. Having a candy bar or cookie to calm her upset nerves
   c. Praying daily in the morning and at night for guidance
   d. Taking a sedative whenever she feels anxious
4. Emotion-focused coping might include which of the following?
   a. Applying for another job because you cannot perform your current job accurately
   b. Blaming the teacher when you fail an exam for which you did not study
   c. Learning about low-sodium diets so you can control your hypertension
   d. Preparing and using a budget to help with money management
5. Which of the following represents lifestyle factors that might affect normal coping?
   a. Adopting a child
   b. Attending school for the first time
   c. Divorce or marital separation
   d. Inadequate or poor dietary intake

FILL IN THE BLANK

Supply the missing term or the information requested.

1. Hospitalization can be a source of stress for any client because it is a form of which type of relocation? ________________
2. Which developmental stage is characterized by dependence on reflex responses for coping with environment and stressors? ________________
3. Release of libido in socially acceptable behavior rather than using it to obtain sexual gratification is known as ________________.
4. Consciously dismissing something from the mind and thoughts is known as ________________.
5. Taking into one's personality the characteristics of another is known as ________________.
6. Concealing the motive for behavior by giving some socially acceptable reason for the action is known as ________________.
7. Immersing something in the subconscious or unconscious level of thought is known as ________________.

MULTIPLE-ANSWER MULTIPLE CHOICE

Circle the letter(s) corresponding to the appropriate answer(s). Circle all that apply.

1. The benefits of exercise include
   a. decreasing the absorption of food.
   b. decreasing general anxiety and depression.
   c. improving appearance and self-image.
   d. increasing the resting heart rate.

2. The use of previous exposure to stressful situations to cope with similar situations more constructively is characteristic of which developmental stage?
   a. Adolescent
   b. Adult
   c. Child
   d. Older adult

3. Which of the following nursing interventions would be appropriate to use with a patient experiencing stress and to facilitate effective coping?
   a. Using the North American Nursing Diagnosis Association (NANDA) diagnosis of Ineffective Coping to address a client who uses forms of coping that impede adaptive behavior
   b. Helping a person with high self-expectations to plan methods for becoming the perfect person that person seeks to be
   c. Encouraging a person who is experiencing stress to avoid activity and exercise for at least 1 month to allow the body to unwind
   d. Instructing clients to avoid conflict by not being assertive
   e. Teaching deep-breathing exercises to clients for use before, during, or after encountering a stressful situation
   f. Referring a client discharged with a debilitating illness and the family to a community support group

ORDERING

Place the "uplifts," from Lazarus' Everyday Hassles Scale, in ascending order (greatest contributor to stress management to least contributor).

1. ______ Completing a task
2. ______ Eating out
3. ______ Feeling healthy
4. ______ Getting enough sleep
5. ______ Meeting responsibilities
6. ______ Relating well to spouse or lover
7. ______ Relating well with friends
8. ______ Spending time with family
9. ______ Taking pleasure in one's home
10. ______ Visiting, telephoning, or writing someone

UNIT XVI

SEXUALITY AND REPRODUCTION

CHAPTER 52

Human Sexuality

CHAPTER OVERVIEW

Chapter 52 discusses concepts of human sexuality, the nursing process as it relates to the client with altered sexual functioning, and self-examination of the breast and testicles.

LEARNING OBJECTIVES

After mastering the content in this chapter, you should be able to do the following:

1. Describe the structures of the male and female reproductive systems.
2. Discuss sexual expression, menstruation, and reproduction as functions of human sexuality.
3. Compare the male and female sexual response cycles.
4. Relate sexuality to all stages of the life cycle.
5. Identify factors that affect sexual functioning.
6. Describe common risks and alterations in sexuality.
7. Understand the nursing process as it relates to sexual functioning.
8. Perform breast self-examination or testicular self-examination.

■ Mastering the Information

MATCHING

Match the terms in Column II with a definition, example, or related statement from Column I. Place the letter corresponding to the answer in the space provided. (Use each letter only once; some letters may not be used.)

COLUMN I

1. ______ The actual biologic gender not coinciding with gender identity
2. ______ Painful intercourse
3. ______ The function as well as one's perceptions of sexual organ, sexual expression, and sexual preference
4. ______ Self-stimulation with or without a partner
5. ______ The permanent cessation of menstrual activity
6. ______ An involuntary contraction of the muscles surrounding the vaginal orifice
7. ______ The period between middle age and old age during which significant changes occur in sexuality

COLUMN II

a. Menopause
b. Vaginismus
c. Climacteric
d. Transsexual
e. Human sexual response
f. Sexuality
g. Dyspareunia
h. Masturbation

TRUE–FALSE

Indicate if the following statements are true or false.

_____ 1. An XX chromosome combination becomes a male.

_____ 2. Masturbation usually begins during toddlerhood.

_____ 3. Infants often explore their genitalia, and it is important for parents to recognize this as a normal developmental process.

_____ 4. Impotency is the inability to obtain or maintain an erection long enough to have satisfactory sexual intercourse.

_____ 5. Sexual difficulties may lend themselves to interpersonal difficulties.

_____ 6. Nurses working in institutional settings should exclude sexual concerns from the nursing care plan.

FILL IN THE BLANK

Supply the missing term or the information requested.

1. The predominant pattern of sexual response as described by Masters and Johnson (1966) includes the _______________ phase, the _______________, _______________, and _______________.
2. Three elements of sexual well-being are:
   a.
   b.
   c.
3. List five factors that affect sexuality.
   a.
   b.
   c.
   d.
   e.
4. Factors that may predispose a person to disruption of normal patterns of sexuality include _______________, _______________, and _______________; alteration in _______________, identification; _______________; _______________; and _______________.
5. Alterations in normal patterns of sexuality can be seen in the following manifestations _______________, _______________, _______________, _______________, _______________, _______________, and _______________.
6. An assessment of risk factors for sexual dysfunction or present sexual dysfunction can be made by asking direct questions, observing _______________, and evaluating information obtained through diagnostic and _______________ tests.

■ Applying Your Knowledge

CASE STUDY

Michelle Yui is 40 years old and has been married for a year to her 46-year-old husband. She and her husband would like to have a child. Mrs. Yui and her husband Paul arrive at the family planning clinic to discuss their concerns that after 6 months of trying, she has been unable to conceive. They relate that sometimes Mr. Yui has problems with erections and ask if they will need to use artificial means of fertilization.

1. What history would be important to obtain to better explore the concerns of Michelle and her husband?
2. What physical assessments and laboratory data would provide beneficial information?
3. What information might the nurse anticipate would need to be provided in teaching when addressing the couple's concerns?
4. What referrals might be appropriate?

CRITICAL INQUIRY EXERCISE

You are invited to speak to a group of high school students in a biology class on the topic of "safe sex."

1. Determine how your personal attitudes regarding sexuality and your personal expertise and limitations with regard to counseling in sexual matters might affect your speech.
2. Discuss physiologic and psychological components of sexual experiences that are affected by the stage of development for most high school students.
3. Develop an outline for teaching the class.

CRITICAL EXPLORATION EXERCISE

In a clinical setting, include sexuality as part of your assessment. Compare the age groups of clients interviewed to the sexual alteration (if any) experienced.

■ Practicing for NCLEX

MULTIPLE CHOICE QUESTIONS

Circle the letter that corresponds to the best answer for each question.

An 18-year-old girl visits the clinic to obtain a contraceptive. She elected to use the intrauterine device (IUD) as a method of birth control.

1. The major concern with the use of the IUD is
   a. thrombophlebitis.
   b. pain on intercourse.
   c. infection.
   d. abnormal bleeding and hemorrhage.

2. The client begins to question the nurse about sexuality and becoming sexually active. During sexual counseling, the nurse should place a major point of emphasis on
   a. douching after sexual intercourse.
   b. sex during menstruation.
   c. performing Kegel exercises.
   d. safe and responsible sex.

3. The appropriate position in which to place the client for examination of genitalia is
   a. lithotomy.
   b. side-lying.
   c. prone.
   d. supine.

4. The nurse assisting the client informs her that a bimanual examination will be performed. Which of the following statements would enhance the client's understanding of this procedure?
   a. "A speculum will be placed into your vagina by the doctor."
   b. "The doctor will expose your abdomen and feel for uterus tenderness."
   c. "Two fingers of one of the doctor's hands will be placed into your vagina, and the doctor's other hand will be placed on your lower abdomen."
   d. "The rectum will be examined by the doctor through the vaginal wall."

5. A nursing intervention to promote sexual health and function is
   a. encouraging myths.
   b. discouraging homosexuality.
   c. encouraging women to examine themselves with a mirror.
   d. teaching the use of abdominal muscles during pregnancy.

6. A natural-planning contraceptive method in which a woman is taught to differentiate the dryness and wetness of the vagina is the
   a. calendar rhythm method.
   b. hormonal method.
   c. symptothermal method.
   d. cervical-mucus method.

7. Both males and females experience an increase in heart rate and blood pressure during which one of the following phases of the human sexual response?
   a. Excitement
   b. Plateau
   c. Orgasm
   d. Resolution

8. One specific technique that nurses can use when working with clients with altered sexual function is the
   a. PLISSIT model.
   b. P-IXIS model.
   c. PUBEER model.
   d. All of the above

FILL IN THE BLANK

Supply the missing term or the information requested.

1. The external organs of the male reproductive system include the penis and scrotum. The penis is covered with loose skin called the ________________.
2. In the female, the small erectile body lying just above the urinary meatus corresponding to the male penis in its physiologic function of orgasm is called the ________________.
3. The woman who has a regular menstrual cycle should perform the breast self-examination ________________________.

MULTIPLE-ANSWER MULTIPLE CHOICE

Circle the letter(s) corresponding to the appropriate answer(s). Circle all that apply.

1. Which of the following suggestions would be appropriate when giving the older adult guidance on maintaining an active sexual life?
   a. Assist patient to explore alternate forms of sexual expression.
   b. Suggest that patient decrease the amount of foreplay.
   c. Suggest that the patient use a lubricant.
   d. Suggest that the patient decrease the frequency of having sexual intercourse.
2. Which of the following categories of drugs may adversely affect sexual function?
   a. Antibiotics
   b. Antihypertensives
   c. Hormones
   d. Nonsteroidal anti-inflammatory drugs
3. Which of the following guidelines should be discussed when teaching a patient about testicular self-examination?
   a. Both testicles should be examined simultaneously.
   b. Discovery of a hard lump or nodule should be reported to the doctor promptly.
   c. Most lumps and nodules found on the testicle are benign.
   d. The best time to perform the exam is after a warm bath or shower.
   e. An x-ray study may be ordered to assist with making an accurate diagnosis.

HOT SPOT QUESTIONS

Place an "X" on the two glands that produce and store most of the seminal fluid.

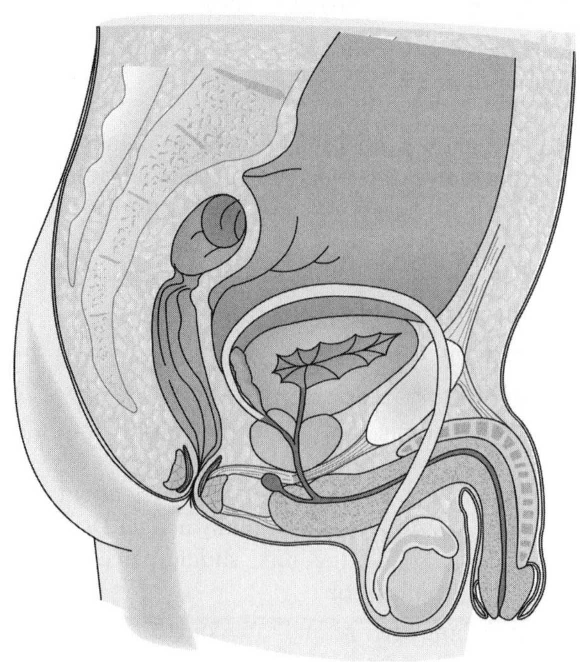

UNIT XVII

Values and Beliefs

CHAPTER 53

Spiritual Health

CHAPTER OVERVIEW

Chapter 53 discusses spiritual needs, major religious faiths, and religious traditions. The nursing process is applied to assess spiritual needs and to provide appropriate interventions.

LEARNING OBJECTIVES

After mastering the content in this chapter, you should be able to do the following:

1. Explore philosophic questions about life.
2. Discuss your personal spiritual journey.
3. Identify spiritual needs in yourself and others.
4. Identify major local religious faiths and their traditions.
5. Incorporate age-appropriate spiritual-assessment questions into the nursing assessment.
6. Use appropriate nursing diagnoses in writing plans of care for clients with spiritual problems.
7. Plan how to use yourself in spiritual support.
8. Develop a resource library of "spiritual" literature.

■ Mastering the Information

MATCHING

Match the terms in Column II with a definition, example, or related statement from Column I. Place the letter corresponding to the answer in the space provided. (Use each letter only once; some letters may not be used.)

COLUMN I

1. ______ A quality or essence that pervades, integrates, and transcends one's biopsychosocial nature
2. ______ A condition in which a person experiences peace, harmony, and a sense of interconnectedness with God, self, community, and environment
3. ______ A quality that goes beyond religious affiliation that strives for inspiration, reverence, awe, meaning, and purpose
4. ______ Represents a normal expression of a person's inner being that seeks meaning in all experience and a dynamic relationship with self, others, and to the supreme others as defined by the person
5. ______ The position of viewing the universe as a system of harmonious interconnectedness, which integrates mind, body, and spirit
6. ______ Acting out beliefs to make meaning in one's life

COLUMN II

a. Spiritual well-being
b. Holism
c. Spiritual dimension
d. Faith
e. Spirituality
f. Spiritual needs
g. Spiritual distress

TRUE–FALSE

Indicate if the following statements are true or false.

______ 1. The three main branches of Judaism are Reformed, Conservative, and Orthodox.

______ 2. Christians, Jews, and Muslims are usually atheists or agnostics.

______ 3. Inappropriate nursing care may be provided by a nurse who hesitates to encourage clients to speak of spirituality.

______ 4. Beliefs, faith, and values are interconnected because what one believes in, or lives out, is also what one values.

______ 5. A nurse should encourage clients not to allow their practice of spirituality to interfere with medical treatment.

FILL IN THE BLANK

Supply the missing term or the information requested.

1. The major religious faiths of the world are ____________, ____________, ____________, ____________, and ____________.

2. The seven areas of spiritual needs are ____________, ____________, ____________, ____________, ____________, ____________, and ____________.

3. Identify the two manifestations of altered spiritual function, and give examples of objective and subjective client data that would include these manifestations.

   a. ____________________________

   ____

   b. ____________________________

   ____

■ Applying Your Knowledge

CASE STUDY

A 24-year-old client is admitted to the hospital with a diagnosis of bowel obstruction. Surgery is required. The client may also need to have a blood transfusion. The client expresses concern about consenting to the surgery and a blood transfusion. The client shares with the nurse that she has had past affiliations with the Christian Science Church and is currently a Jehovah's Witness.

1. Explain how you would encourage the client to discuss her spiritual concerns.
2. Discuss the connections that might exist between the client's concerns about the planned therapies and prior religious affiliations.
3. Discuss how you would respond if the client indicates a desire not to have surgery or a blood transfusion.

CRITICAL INQUIRY EXERCISE

Write a paper on your own spiritual needs and personal spiritual journey.

CRITICAL EXPLORATION EXERCISE

During clinical experiences, use spiritual assessment to obtain information regarding the client's spiritual needs. Apply the nursing process to any spiritual distress noted.

■ Practicing for NCLEX

MULTIPLE CHOICE QUESTIONS

Circle the letter that corresponds to the best answer for each question.

1. Seeking answers to life's philosophic questions and seeking a higher level of consciousness or a deeper awareness of spiritual life is
   a. spiritual well-being.
   b. spiritual quest.
   c. spiritual distress.
   d. spiritual dimension.

2. The nurse caring for clients in this age group during illness knows that their priorities are the development of a personal style and interaction with peers. This age group is
   a. older adult.
   b. adult.
   c. toddler and preschooler.
   d. adolescent.

3. A 47-year-old client is experiencing altered spiritual functioning. Which of the following manifestations should alert the nurse that the client is experiencing spiritual concerns?
   a. Statements of feeling "no good anymore"
   b. Quiet and calm appearance
   c. Well-organized and clear conversation
   d. Sleeping well through the night

4. Which of the following nursing interventions would the nurse caring for this client select to promote spiritual health?
   a. Building a relationship of pity and sympathy
   b. Encouraging the treatment regimen, even if variation in spiritual practice is required
   c. Active listening and using good communication skills
   d. Relying only on the nurse's own spiritual tradition

FILL IN THE BLANK

Supply the missing term or the information requested.

1. Wholeness and harmony within oneself, with others, and with God or one's higher power is a major characteristic of ________________.
2. An impaired ability to experience and integrate meaning and purpose in life through the individual's connectedness to self, others, art, music, literature, nature, or a power greater than oneself is referred to as ____________________.

MULTIPLE-ANSWER MULTIPLE CHOICE

Circle the letter(s) corresponding to the appropriate answer(s). Circle all that apply.

1. Which of the following is/are subjective components of the spiritual assessment?
   a. Importance of faith to the client
   b. Presence of religious reading materials
   c. Significance of God to the client
   d. Visits from church members

2. The spiritual dimension is a quality that is relevant to the
   a. Atheists
   b. Buddhists
   c. Christians
   d. Hindus
   e. Jews
   f. Muslims

3. Expression of spirituality is influenced by
   a. background.
   b. culture.
   c. stereotypes.
   d. religion.
   e. society.

4. Spiritual beliefs and practices fulfill which of the following needs?
   a. Drive acceptance or rejection of others
   b. Give meaning to life
   c. Guide daily living habits
   d. Provide total satisfaction with life

ORDERING

Place the stages of faith development in ascending order.

1. ______ Conjunctive
2. ______ Individuative—Reflective
3. ______ Intuitive—Projective
4. ______ Mythic—Literal
5. ______ Synthetic—Conventional
6. ______ Undifferentiated—Primal
7. ______ Universalizing

Answers

Chapter 1

MASTERING THE INFORMATION

MATCHING

1. c, 2. e, 3. d, 4. a, 5. f, 6. b

TRUE–FALSE

1. False. The story indicated nurses focus on many aspects of care delivery and many client populations.
2. True
3. True
4. False. The story indicated the nursing home as an enjoyable practice area.
5. True
6. False. The story discussed executive positions requiring nursing skills.
7. True

FILL IN THE BLANK

1. Economic; social
2. Scope
3. Assess; consult; design; implement
4. Promotion/maintenance; prevention; supportive care
5. Right

PRACTICING FOR NCLEX

MULTIPLE CHOICE

1. c, 2. d, 3. b, 4. b

ALTERNATIVE FORMAT: FILL IN THE BLANK

1. Put dollar value; client outcomes
2. Broadening scope
3. Informed; analyzed judgments
4. Complex matrix
5. Cultural diversity

ALTERNATIVE FORMAT: MULTIPLE-ANSWER MULTIPLE CHOICE

1. d
2. b
3. a, c, d
4. b, d, e
5. a, b, c, d, e

Chapter 2

MASTERING THE INFORMATION

MATCHING

1. a, 2. d, 3. b, 4. e, 5. c

1. b, 2. a, 3. c, 4. b, 5. a, 6. c, 7. b, 8. c

TRUE–FALSE

1. False. The desire for each was almost equal.
2. True
3. True
4. True
5. False. The focus of nursing care is the same.
6. True

FILL IN THE BLANK

1. Actively
2. Specific
3. Physical; mental
4. Chronic; acute
5. Comprehensive; person

PRACTICING FOR NCLEX

MULTIPLE CHOICE

1. b, 2. c, 3. d

FILL IN THE BLANK

1. The late 1800s
2. Family conference
3. Discharge planner; skilled nursing facility or long-term care facility
4. Nursing care
5. Specific population

MULTIPLE-ANSWER MULTIPLE CHOICE

1. a, b, c, e
2. b
3. b
4. c

Chapter 3

MASTERING THE INFORMATION

MATCHING

1. f, 2. c, 3. h 4. g, 5. e, 6. i, 7. d

1. b, 2. d, 3. a, 4. c

FILL IN THE BLANK

1. a. Diploma, b. Associate, c. Baccalaureate
2. a. Healthcare cost containment, b. Scientific and technical advances, c. Women's movement
3. Any four of the following would be correct: a. Caregiver and communicator; b. Decision maker; c. Client advocate; d. Manager and coordinator; e. Educator
4. Client advocate
5. Collaboratively; independently

TRUE–FALSE

1. False. It is regulated by the Nurse Practice Act
2. True
3. False. The diploma degree nursing programs were the first.
4. True

PRACTICING FOR NCLEX

MULTIPLE CHOICE

1. a, 2. d, 3. c, 4. a, 5. d

FILL IN THE BLANK

1. Independent
2. Independent
3. Collaborative
4. Independent
5. Collaborative

MULTIPLE-ANSWER MULTIPLE CHOICE

1. a, b, c, d
2. b
3. c, d
4. c
5. a, b, c

Chapter 4

MASTERING THE INFORMATION

MATCHING

1. c, 2. a, 3. d, 4. b

1. c, 2. a, 3. b

TRUE–FALSE

1. False. Concepts and propositions are abstract and general.
2. True
3. False. Theory should guide nursing research.
4. True
5. True

FILL IN THE BLANK

1. Theory provides the foundation for nursing knowledge, gives direction to practice, and guides the future direction of nursing research.
2. Family; community
3. Gordon's health perception–health management pattern focuses on health values and beliefs and the resources in the community available to meet health needs.
4. Conceptual framework
5. Person—human beings; environment—internal and external client factors; health—the person's state of being; and nursing—what nursing is, what nurses do, and the nurse's role in client care.

PRACTICING FOR NCLEX

MULTIPLE CHOICE

1. a, 2. d, 3. a, 4. c, 5. d

ALTERNATIVE FORMAT: FILL IN THE BLANK

1. Unfreezing
2. Hypothalamus
3. Health
4. Nursing theory
5. Movement

ALTERNATIVE FORMAT: MULTIPLE-ANSWER MULTIPLE CHOICE

1. a, d
2. a
3. d

Chapter 5

MASTERING THE INFORMATION

MATCHING

1. d, 2. e, 3. c, 4. b, 5. f, 6. a

1. c, 2. a, 3. b, 4. d, 5. b, 6. c, 7. a, 8. d, 9. a, 10. c

FILL IN THE BLANK

1. Attitudes; beliefs; behaviors
2. Respect for people and human dignity
3. Any three of the following would be appropriate: a. Reward and punishment by parents, family, and caregivers; b. Language; c. Modeling by significant others; d. Media influence; e. Unspoken expectations
4. Socialization; classroom study; clinical study
5. Value clarification is a method of self-discovery of personal values, and value inquiry is a method of examining social issues and values that motivate human choices.
6. a. General human needs: All human beings have in common certain functional health patterns. Assessment of health patterns helps the nurse to identify functional and dysfunctional patterns.
   b. Culture/social group: The culture/social group influences or contributes to a person's perception of health.
   c. Individual/personal needs: Each person is unique and thus has individual values and needs that the nurse should include as part of the basic assessment to have a complete database of the client's value system as it relates to health.

TRUE–FALSE

1. True
2. False. Behavior is the most significant indicator of a value.
3. True
4. False. Attitudes and beliefs about nutrition are influenced by cultural background.
5. True

PRACTICING FOR NCLEX

MULTIPLE CHOICE

1. a, 2. d, 3. b, 4. b, 5. d

FILL IN THE BLANK

1. Modeling
2. Behavior
3. Conformity
4. Intimacy; generativity
5. Perception; language

MULTIPLE-ANSWER MULTIPLE CHOICE

1. a, c, e
2. a, b, c, d, e, all human beings
3. c, e
4. d, e
5. b

Chapter 6

MASTERING THE INFORMATION

MATCHING

1. g, 2. a, 3. c, 4. e, 5. h, 6. b, 7. d, 8. f
1. a, 2. d, 3. b, 4. c

TRUE–FALSE

1. False. Torts must be intentional acts to qualify for damages.
2. True
3. True
4. False. The *Code of Ethics* delineates nurse's conduct and responsibilities.
5. True
6. False. The major type of administrative law that governs nursing is licensing law.
7. False. State nurse practice acts provide one set of guidelines for the standard of care; however, standards of care are also defined on the national level by the American Nurses Association and other specialty organizations.
8. False. State and national regulations provide the standards of care to be followed.
9. True
10. True

FILL IN THE BLANK

1. Think; act
2. Beneficence; nonmaleficence; autonomy; justice
3. Veracity; fidelity; confidentiality; privacy
4. a. Duty; b. Failure to meet the standard of care/breach of duty; c. Causation; d. Damages
5. Personal morals; personal values
6. a. A client's current medical status and the general course of the illness; b. The proposed treatment and its rationale; c. Risks and benefits of the proposed treatment; d. Risk of not consenting to the treatment; e. Alternatives to the proposed treatment and their associated risks and benefits, including nontreatment and associated risks and benefits

PRACTICING FOR NCLEX

MULTIPLE CHOICE

1. b, 2. b, 3. b, 4. d, 5. d

FILL IN THE BLANK

1. Neurologic
2. Informed consent
3. Civil
4. Liability
5. Good Samaritan Law

MULTIPLE-ANSWER MULTIPLE CHOICE

1. a, c, d
2. a, b, c, d, e, f, g, all of them
3. b, c, e
4. b
5. a, c, e

Chapter 7

MASTERING THE INFORMATION

MATCHING

1. b, 2. h, 3. i, 4. g, 5. c, 6. a, 7. j, 8. e

TRUE–FALSE

1. False. Staff members usually dislike and resist change.
2. False. The clinical nurse specialist usually practices in the hospital or hospital-clinic setting.
3. True
4. False. In managed care, the nurse and physician plan care jointly.

FILL IN THE BLANK

1. Human; financial; information
2. Leadership focuses on people and on inspiring them to perform or change, whereas management focuses on getting the job done by planning, organizing, directing, and controlling people's activities.
3. Directive leadership is most appropriate in an emergency because there is no time for group discussion and decision making.
4. In team nursing, team members are assigned to provide specific care functions for all clients in their group under the coordination of a team leader for one shift. In primary nursing, one professional nurse assumes total responsibility for the quality of client care for one or more clients by developing a 24-hour nursing care plan and coordinating the implementation of that plan. Advantages of team nursing include cost-effectiveness, naturally facilitated group discussions and group decision making, and experienced nurses being able to teach less-experienced nurses. Advantages of primary nursing include increased continuity of care, improved interdisciplinary communication, and enhanced coordination of the total therapy plan. Disadvantages of team nursing include fragmentation of care, decreased accountability and delivery of care, and decreased nurse–client/family rapport. Disadvantages of primary

nursing include the need for a large number of professional nurses, decreased nurse-to-nurse consultation, and the possible economic inefficiency.
5. Any three of the following: problem solving; communication; managing change; planning; delegation.
6. The team leader assumes responsibility for the care given to an assigned group of clients in the nursing unit, whereas the charge nurse assumes responsibility for the functioning of the entire nursing unit for a particular work shift.
7. Managed care

PRACTICING FOR NCLEX

MULTIPLE CHOICE

1. c, 2. d, 3. b, 4. c, 5. d, 6. d, 7. b

FILL IN THE BLANK

1. Three
2. Determine
3. Five
4. Identify; analyze
5. Fourth

MULTIPLE-ANSWER MULTIPLE CHOICE

1. b
2. b
3. a, b
4. c, f
5. a, b, c, d, e

Chapter 8

MASTERING THE INFORMATION

MATCHING

1. d, 2. e, 3. c, 4. g, 5. a, 6. f, 7. h, 8. b

TRUE–FALSE

1. False. Florence Nightingale performed many research steps.
2. True
3. False. Research has aided in improving client health.
4. False. The National Institutes of Health is the parent organization from which the National Center for Nursing Research was established.
5. True

FILL IN THE BLANK

1. Nursing research generates fundamental knowledge to guide nursing practice.
2. Identical
3. Any three of the following would be correct: a. An explanation of the study; b. Procedures to be followed and their purposes; c. Clear description of physical and mental discomforts, any invasion of privacy, and any threat of dignity; d. Methods used to protect anonymity and ensure confidentiality
4. Any three of the following would be correct:
   a. The focus of nursing research must be on a variance that makes a difference in improving client care.
   b. Nursing research has the potential for contributing to theory development and the body of scientific nursing knowledge.
   c. A research problem is a nursing research problem when nurses have access to control over phenomena being studied.
   d. A nurse interested in research must have an inquisitive, curious, and questioning mind.

PRACTICING FOR NCLEX

MULTIPLE CHOICE

1. b, 2. d, 3. c, 4. d, 5. d, 6. b, 7. b, 8. c, 9. d, 10. b

FILL IN THE BLANK

1. Master's
2. Conduct
3. Translational
4. Variables
5. Variance

MULTIPLE-ANSWER MULTIPLE CHOICE

1. a, c
2. c
3. a, c, d
4. b

Chapter 9

MASTERING THE INFORMATION

MATCHING

1. d, 2. a, 3. b, 4. f, 5. e

1. c, 2. a, 3. b

TRUE–FALSE

1. True
2. False. This is the definition of deduction.
3. True
4. False. These phases are part of the systems theory.
5. True
6. False. Yura and Walsh first identified these four steps of the nursing process.
7. False. Active listening involves verbal and nonverbal cues.

FILL IN THE BLANK

1. Assessment; diagnosis; outcome identification; planning; implementation; evaluation
2. Nursing process
3. Systems theory; problem-solving process; decision-making process; information-processing theory; diagnostic
4. Functional health patterns
5. Attainment; outcome

PRACTICING FOR NCLEX

MULTIPLE CHOICE

1. b, 2. c, 3. d, 4. c, 5. b

FILL IN THE BLANK

1. Summarize
2. Implementation
3. Nursing process
4. Collecting
5. Secondary

MULTIPLE-ANSWER MULTIPLE CHOICE

1. c
2. b
3. a
4. a
5. c

Chapter 10

MASTERING THE INFORMATION

MATCHING

1. b, 2. c, 3. d, 4. a

1. a, 2. c, 3. b, 4. d

TRUE–FALSE

1. True
2. True
3. False. Intuitive decisions are based on insight, instinct, and experience.
4. True
5. False. This is a barrier to communication.
6. False. Assessment involves collecting, validating, and organizing data.
7. False. This defines auscultation.
8. True
9. True
10. False. This is a secondary source of data.

FILL IN THE BLANK

1. a. Initial assessment; b. Time-lapse assessment; c. Focus assessment; d. Emergency assessment
2. a. Observation; b. Interviewing; c. Physical examination; d. Intuition
3. Physical examination
4. Subjective; objective
5. Intuition
6. Primary sources; secondary sources
7. Health team members; family members or significant others; laboratory/diagnostic procedures; the health record; review of pertinent literature
8. Body systems model; functional health model; head to toe model

SUBJECTIVE VS. OBJECTIVE DATA

1. S
2. S
3. O
4. O
5. S
6. O
7. S
8. O
9. O
10. S

PRACTICING FOR NCLEX

MULTIPLE CHOICE

1. c, 2. b, 3. d, 4. a, 5. c, 6. b

FILL IN THE BLANK

1. Touch
2. Subjective
3. Assessment
4. Third
5. Palpation
6. Intuition
7. Environmental

MULTIPLE-ANSWER MULTIPLE CHOICE

1. c
2. c
3. a, b, c
4. d, e
5. b, g

ORDERING

a. 3, b. 2, c. 1, d. 4

Chapter 11

MASTERING THE INFORMATION

MATCHING

1. c, 2. a, 3. b, 4. e, 5. d

TRUE–FALSE

1. False. Data clustering refers to the bringing together of several objective or subjective cues that are then interpreted and validated.
2. True
3. True
4. True
5. True
6. False. The purpose of the NDEC is to evaluate and revise existing NANDA diagnoses, develop new diagnostic terms, and organize NANDA diagnoses.

FILL IN THE BLANK

1. Diagnostic; two
2. Any five of the following would be appropriate:
   a. Diagnostic concept; b. Time; c. Unit of care; d. Age; e. Health status; f. Descriptor; g. Topology

3. Coding; computerized; direct
4. Diagnostic label; defining characteristics; related factors
5. Any five of the following would be appropriate:
   a. Provide a means of communicating nursing requirements for client care to other nurses, the healthcare team, and the public
   b. Serve as shorthand for specific client problems
   c. Help to ensure that clients receive quality nursing care
   d. Increase the specificity of nursing interventions for each client
   e. Allow for direct reimbursement of nurses
   f. Help to articulate the scope of nursing practice
   g. Assist in bridging the gap between knowledge and practice

PRACTICING FOR NCLEX

MULTIPLE CHOICE

1. c, 2. a, 3. b, 4. a, 5. d

ALTERNATIVE FORMAT: FILL IN THE BLANK

1. 173
2. Medical diagnosis
3. Validation
4. Shorthand

ALTERNATIVE FORMAT: MULTIPLE-ANSWER MULTIPLE CHOICE

1. d
2. d, e
3. b
4. d
5. b

Chapter 12

MASTERING THE INFORMATION

MATCHING

1. c, 2. a, 3. b, 4. e, 5. f, 6. d

TRUE–FALSE

1. False. Plans of care must be developed by a registered nurse.
2. True
3. False. At least one goal must be stated for each nursing diagnosis.
4. True
5. False. Instructional client plans include nursing diagnoses, goals or outcome criteria, interventions, scientific rationale, and evaluations.

FILL IN THE BLANK

1. a. Provide individualized care; b. Promote client participation; c. Plan care that is realistic and measurable; d. Allow for involvement of support people
2. Life threatening; immediate action
3. Days; less than a week; weeks; months
4. Who; what actions; what circumstances; how well; when
5. Any three of the following would be accurate: a. Direct client activities; b. Promote continuity of care; c. Focus charting requirements; d. Allow for delegation of specific activities
6. a. Planning nursing interventions; b. Writing the client plan of care
7. a. Monitor health status; b. Prevent, resolve, or control a problem; c. Assist with activities of daily living; d. Promote optimum health and independence
8. Any five of the following would be correct:
   a. Psychomotor (positioning, inserting, applying)
   b. Psychosocial (supporting, exploring, encouraging)
   c. Educational (demonstrating, teaching, observing, return demonstrations)
   d. Maintenance (skin care, hygiene)
   e. Surveillance (detecting changes)
   f. Supervisory (other healthcare providers)
   g. Sociocultural (spending time, incorporating cultural differences into care regimen)

PRACTICING FOR NCLEX

MULTIPLE CHOICE

1. b, 2. a, 3. b, 4. b, 5. b

FILL IN THE BLANK

1. Physicians
2. Grid; intermediate
3. Specific; realistic
4. Variances
5. Always

MULTIPLE-ANSWER MULTIPLE CHOICE

1. b, d, e
2. a, e
3. b
4. a, b, d
5. a

Chapter 13

MASTERING THE INFORMATION

MATCHING

1. d, 2. a, 3. e, 4. b, 5. c

TRUE–FALSE

1. False. Technical competence means being able to use equipment, machines, and supplies in a particular specialty.
2. True
3. True
4. False. Some clients and families respond to stress by joking, teasing, and laughing about it. The nurse can use humor as a way to relieve stress and give the client examples of difficult situations and ways to resolve them.
5. False. The goal of maintenance nursing interventions is to help the client retain a certain state of health.
6. True
7. True

FILL IN THE BLANK

1. Reassessing; setting priorities; performing nursing interventions; recording actions
2. Problem solving; decision making; teaching
3. Any four of the following would be correct:
   a. The client's condition
   b. New information from reassessment
   c. Time and resources available for nursing interventions
   d. Feedback from the client, family, and healthcare staff
   e. The nurse's experience in assessing situations and setting priorities.
4. Nursing Interventions Classification (NIC)
5. Cognitive; interpersonal; technical
6. Supervisory
7. Coordination; supportive; psychosocial
8. Evaluation

PRACTICING FOR NCLEX

MULTIPLE CHOICE

1. b, 2. c, 3. d, 4. d, 5. a, 6. b

FILL IN THE BLANK

1. Nursing Interventions Classification (NIC)
2. Reassessment
3. Technical
4. Implementation
5. Objective
6. a. Collect, analyze, and synthesize
   b. Outcome criteria
   c. Completely met
   d. Delete
   e. A potential
   f. Reassess

MULTIPLE-ANSWER MULTIPLE CHOICE

1. b
2. a, b, c, d, e
3. a, b, c, e, f
4. b
5. d

Chapter 14

MASTERING THE INFORMATION

MATCHING

1. b, 2. d, 3. e, 4. a, 5. c

TRUE–FALSE

1. False. Students should build on existing thinking skills.
2. False. Memorization-style thinking cannot keep up with these nursing tasks.
3. True
4. False. Curiosity is important to critical thinking.
5. True

FILL IN THE BLANK

1. Conscious; deliberate
2. Clinical
3. Information; evidence
4. All reasoning
   a. Has purpose
   b. Is an attempt to figure something out
   c. Is based on assumption
   d. Is done from one point of view
   e. Is based on data/information/evidence
   f. Is expressed through and shaped by concepts and ideas
   g. Contains inferences or interpretations
   h. Leads somewhere or has implications and consequences
5. Reflection is the intellectual and effective actions in which individuals engage to explain their experiences.

PRACTICING FOR NCLEX

MULTIPLE CHOICE

1. b, 2. d, 3. e, 4. a, 5. b

FILL IN THE BLANK

1. Clinical
2. Paralleled
3. Kinesthetic
4. Essential
5. Interactions

MULTIPLE-ANSWER MULTIPLE CHOICE

1. e
2. c
3. d
4. a, b, c, d, e
5. a, d, e

Chapter 15

MASTERING THE INFORMATION

MATCHING

1. g, 2. k, 3. b, 4. a, 5. e, 6. j, 7. f, 8. c, 9. i, 10. d

TRUE–FALSE

1. False. Nursing discharge plans are started at the initiation of care.
2. True
3. True
4. True
5. False. Nurses may initiate consults based on their assessments.

FILL IN THE BLANK

1. Communicates; continuity
2. Randomly; documented
3. Incident
4. Erasing
5. Computer-based personal

PRACTICING FOR NCLEX

MULTIPLE CHOICE

1. c, 2. b, 3. c, 4. d, 5. c

ALTERNATIVE FORMAT: FILL IN THE BLANK

1. Admitted
2. Dose
5. Standardization

ALTERNATIVE FORMAT: MULTIPLE-ANSWER MULTIPLE CHOICE

1. a, c
2. b
3. c
4. c, d
5. a, c, d, e, f

Chapter 16

MASTERING THE INFORMATION

MATCHING

1. b, 2. d, 3. a, 4. c, 5. e

1. c, 2. a, 3. b, 4. e, 5. d

TRUE–FALSE

1. True
2. True
3. False. It is useful for people at various developmental levels.
4. False. Health is interpreted as the absence of signs and symptoms of disease in the clinical model.
5. True
6. True
7. True
8. False. Nurses in all settings can use wellness nursing diagnoses to focus on promoting health.

FILL IN THE BLANK

1. Expectations; values
2. Any four of the following: clinical; agent–host environment; health belief; high-level wellness; holistic

NURSING ACTIONS

1. H
2. R
3. H
4. H

PRACTICING FOR NCLEX

MULTIPLE CHOICE

1. b, 2. a, 3. d, 4. a, 5. a, 6. d

FILL IN THE BLANK

1. Rescuer
   Holism
   Self-knowing
   Responsibility
   Control
   Disease
   Response
   Illness

MULTIPLE-ANSWER MULTIPLE CHOICE

1. a, c, d
2. b
3. d
4. a, c
5. c

Chapter 17

MASTERING THE INFORMATION

MATCHING

1. c, 2. f, 3. a, 4. e, 5. b, 6. d

TRUE–FALSE

1. False. Meditation is considered the cornerstone.
2. False. All are true of Yang, except that neither force is considered superior to the other.
3. False. This study revealed that most clients do not share this information with their physicians.
4. True
5. False. Centering is first. Assessment is second.
6. True
7. False. Studies have shown that acupuncture is safe and effective.
8. False. Nursing has had a tradition of holistic care since its founding by Florence Nightingale.
9. True
10. True

FILL IN THE BLANK

1. a. Promote relaxation; b. Alter pain perception; c. Decrease anxiety; d. Accelerate healing; e. Promote comfort in dying
2. Naturopaths; herbal
3. Food and Drug Administration (FDA)
4. Atomistic
5. a. Concentrative; b. Receptive; c. Reflective; d. Expressive

PRACTICING FOR NCLEX

MULTIPLE CHOICE

1. c, 2. e, 3. b, 4. d, 5. c

FILL IN THE BLANK

1. Integrative
2. Taoist
3. Therapeutic; prevention
4. Energy field
5. Cloning; infertility; legal

MULTIPLE-ANSWER MULTIPLE CHOICE

1. b, c, f
2. e
3. a, b, c, d, f, g, h
4. all
5. a, b, d, e

CHAPTER 18

MASTERING THE INFORMATION

MATCHING

1. b, 2. d, 3. e, 4. c, 5. f, 6. a

1. g, 2. e, 3. i, 4. b, 5. h, 6. a, 7. j, 8. d, 9. f, 10. c

FILL IN THE BLANK

1. Genetics; environment
2. Moment; conception
3. Last
4. Malnutrition; oxygen
5. Organized
6. a. Toddler/Preschooler
   b. Adult/Older Adult
   c. Newborn/Infant
   d. School Age/Adolescent

PRACTICING FOR NCLEX

MULTIPLE CHOICE

1. d, 2. b, 3. d, 4. b, 5. d, 6. a, 7. a , 8. c, 9. d, 10. c

FILL IN THE BLANK

1. Development
2. Instability

MULTIPLE-ANSWER MULTIPLE CHOICE

1. a, b, c
2. a, b, c, d, e
3. a, c, d

ORDERING

a. 2
b. 8
c. 7
d. 5
e. 4
f. 3
g. 6
h. 1

Chapter 19

MASTERING THE INFORMATION

MATCHING

1. e, 2. c, 3. a, 4. b

TRUE–FALSE

1. True
2. False. Less than 20% of people 65 years and older were minorities.
3. False. Living arrangements vary widely based on gender.
4. True
5. True
6. False. Depression often goes unrecognized or is misdiagnosed.
7. False. Numerous community agencies are available to provide assistance.
8. False. Normal changes result in increased awakenings and less restful sleep.
9. True

FILL IN THE BLANK

1. Cognitive, sensory, language

PRACTICING FOR NCLEX

MULTIPLE CHOICE

1. c, 2. b, 3. c, 4. a, 5. d, 6. b, 7. c, 8. d

FILL IN THE BLANK

1. Interplay/interaction
2. Decreases
3. Higher
4. Falls

MULTIPLE-ANSWER MULTIPLE CHOICE

1. a, e

ORDERING

1. H
2. L
3. L
4. H
5. H

Chapter 20

MASTERING THE INFORMATION

MATCHING

1. d, 2. b, 3. d, 4. c, 5. a

TRUE–FALSE

1. True
2. False. Higgs and Gustafson believe that communities are social units and have a hierarchy of needs.
3. True
4. False. Systems theory suggests that the community has responsibilities toward the family, but the family also is responsible for taking an active part in community activities and promoting good services.
5. True
6. True
7. True
8. False. In a closed system, no exchange occurs.
9. True
10. True

FILL IN THE BLANK

1. Craven and others define family as "a social group whose members share common values, occupy specific positions, and interact with each other over time. Adults bear and rear children, engage in economic and political cooperation, and care for the elders."

2. Tucker views a community "as a spatial unit, as an ethnic group with a common culture, and as an aggregate of people with shared values, interests, and goals." Craven and others define community as "a social group whose members may or may not share common geographic boundaries, yet who interact because of common interests or shared values to meet their needs within a larger society."
3. Family; community
4. Conceptual
5. Tasks; role
6. Family systems
7. Observation; comparison; interview
8. A method the client finds acceptable; a method to use community resources for the maximum benefit
9. Developmental stage; wholeness; communication; support
10. Emotional; structural; functional
11. Wholeness; circular interaction; lack of an identified client; holistic perspective; family themes; family roles
12. Space; institution; interaction; people; distribution; social system

PRACTICING FOR NCLEX

MULTIPLE CHOICE

1. c, 2. b, 3. d, 4. a, 5. b, 6. c, 7. c, 8. b, 9. a

FILL IN THE BLANK

1. Eight
2. Greater
3. Community
4. Resources
5. Well-being

MULTIPLE-ANSWER MULTIPLE CHOICE

1. a, b, c, e, f
2. a, b, c, d, e, f, g, h, j

Chapter 21

MASTERING THE INFORMATION

MATCHING

1. d, 2. c, 3. b, 4. a

1. b, 2. f, 3. e, 4. c, 5. d, 6. a

TRUE–FALSE

1. True
2. True
3. True
4. False. Nurses should minimize ethnocentric tendencies and maximize cultural sensitivity.
5. True
6. False. Sometimes understanding a person's culture and beliefs requires long-term contact. Although the approach of anthropologists, it usually takes too long for most nurses.
7. True
8. False. If the nurse and the client speak the same language but do not share the same culture, about two thirds of the messages or information shared may be misconstrued.
9. True
10. True

FILL IN THE BLANK

1. Any 10 of the following would be accurate: a. learned from other people; b. learned over time; c. shared by people; d. shared unequally by its members; e. always changing; f. learned; g. diversified; h. reasonable; i. not easily described by its members; j. habituated assumptions; k. ethnocentric; l. relative; m. pervasive and holistic; n. ritualistic; o. stabilizing; p. recognizable at many levels
2. Blueprint
3. Culture shock
4. Key informant technique
5. Cultural habituation
6. Advantageous; expert
7. Social power; size of the population
8. Open-ended questions; clarification of responses; documentation
9. Client
10. Observation over time; use of client's language

PRACTICING FOR NCLEX

MULTIPLE CHOICE

1. c, 2. b, 3. d, 4. d, 5. c, 6. a, 7. b, 8. a, 9. c, 10. d, 11. b, 12. a, 13. b, 14. d, 15. c

FILL IN THE BLANK

1. Anthropologists
2. Adulterating/contaminating
3. White
4. Self-conscious
5. Disparate behaviors

MULTIPLE-ANSWER MULTIPLE CHOICE

1. a, b, c
2. b
3. b, c
4. a, c, d, e

Chapter 22

MASTERING THE INFORMATION

MATCHING

1. c, 2. d, 3. a, 4. b, 5. e, 6. f, 7. g, 8. i, 9. h, 10. j

TRUE–FALSE

1. True
2. True
3. False. Effective communication in the nurse–client relationship is a learned skill.
4. True
5. False. The main subject in the nurse–client relationship should be the client and his or her experiences and problems.
6. True
7. True
8. True
9. False. The main goal of communication between the nurse and the client is improvement in the client's health status and well-being.
10. True
11. True
12. True
13. False. The nurse should listen for content and feelings that are expressed.
14. True
15. True

FILL IN THE BLANK

1. Sending; receiving
2. The client; client experiences; problems
3. A sender; a message; a receiver; encoding; decoding; feedback
4. Client; goal-directed; parameters
5. Orientation; working; termination
6. Words; gestures; facial expressions; posture; body movement; voice tone
7. Empathy; positive regard; comfortable sense of self
8. Nurse–client; therapeutic

PRACTICING FOR NCLEX

MULTIPLE CHOICE

1. c, 2. d, 3. b, 4. b, 5. a, 6. d, 7. d, 8. b, 9. c, 10. b, 11. a, 12. b, 13. a, 14. a, 15. b

FILL IN THE BLANK

1. Nontherapeutic
2. Empathy

MULTIPLE-ANSWER MULTIPLE CHOICE

1. a, d
2. a
3. b, d, e
4. a, c
5. a, c

Chapter 23

MASTERING THE INFORMATION

MATCHING

1. c, 2. a, 3. e, 4. b, 5. d

TRUE–FALSE

1. True
2. True
3. False. The client with a plan to commit suicide is more likely to commit suicide.
4. True
5. False. The behavior should be addressed by explaining which behavior is inappropriate and specifically why.

FILL IN THE BLANK

1. Malfeasance
2. Hours
3. a. H — Hear the person out
   b. E — Empathize with the person's feelings
   c. A — Accept some responsibility
   d. T — Take action to ameliorate the situation
4. Any five of the following would be correct: a. Respect personal space; b. Do not provoke the client; c. Be concise and repeat yourself; d. Recognize the client's wants and feelings; e. Listen; f. Agree with the client; g. Set limits; h. Offer choices; i. Debrief the client and staff

PRACTICING FOR NCLEX

MULTIPLE CHOICE

1. d, 2. b, 3. a, 4. d, 5. c

FILL IN THE BLANK

1. Suicidal ideation
2. De-escalation
3. Delirium

MULTIPLE-ANSWER MULTIPLE CHOICE

1. a, b, c, e, f
2. b, d

Chapter 24

MASTERING THE INFORMATION

MATCHING

1. c, 2. b, 3. b, 4. a, 5. c

TRUE–FALSE

1. False. Friends are sometimes more willing and supportive than family members.
2. False. It may be necessary to delay teaching until the client desires to actively participate.
3. False. A person's spoken language does not indicate literacy level.
4. True
5. True

FILL IN THE BLANK

1. a. Pedagogy—instruction of children; teacher in control; learner participates passively
   b. Andragogy—instruction of adults; client teaching around client's needs and goals
2. Learning
3. Environment
4. a. Client focus; b. Holism; c. Negotiation; d. Interaction
5. Motivation

PRACTICING FOR NCLEX

MULTIPLE CHOICE

1. d, 2. b, 3. c, 4. c, 5. a, 6. d

FILL IN THE BLANK

1. Role playing
2. Repetition

MULTIPLE-ANSWER MULTIPLE CHOICE

1. a, b, c
2. a, e

Chapter 25

MASTERING THE INFORMATION

MATCHING

1. b, 2. c, 3. a, 4. e, 5. d

1. b, 2. e, 3. d, 4. a, 5. c

TRUE–FALSE

1. False. Harris encourages home health nurses to welcome the increasing use of technology.
2. True
3. True
4. False. Telenursing is a highly effective strategy to supplement home visits.
5. True
6. False. When home management is not feasible, placement in a community facility may be necessary to provide a safe environment where adequate support can be given.

FILL IN THE BLANK

1. Activities; daily living
2. Reimbursable; acute; chronic
3. Initiation; previsit; in-home; termination; postvisit
4. Mind; body; spirit
5. Supports; resources

PRACTICING FOR NCLEX

MULTIPLE CHOICE

1. b, 2. d, 3. a, 4. d, 5. c, 6. b, 7. c, 8. a, 9. d, 10. c

FILL IN THE BLANK

1. OASIS
2. Home health nurse
3. Rice

MULTIPLE-ANSWER MULTIPLE CHOICE

1. a, b, c, d, e, g, h, j

Chapter 26

MASTERING THE INFORMATION

MATCHING

1. c, 2. e, 3. j, 4. b, 5. f, 6. a, 7. i, 8. d, 9. g, 10. h

TRUE–FALSE

1. True
2. True
3. False. Does not provide direct data about the cardiovascular system.
4. True
5. False. Does not assess the cardiovascular area.

FILL IN THE BLANK

1. Database; abilities; risk factors; alteration
2. Inspection; palpation; percussion; auscultation
3. Preventing disease; living healthy lifestyles
4. Posture; gait; movement
5. Any three of the following would be acceptable: memory; language; awareness; thought process; judgment; attention span
6. Family; work; social
7. Comprehensive health assessment
8. After birth; 24
9. Any six of the following would be acceptable: penlight; tuning fork; Snellen chart; tongue blade; reflex hammer; cotton applicator; vials of hot and cold water; vials of salt, sugar, and lemon; vials with coffee, vanilla, or clove extract; sterile toothpick

PRACTICING FOR NCLEX

MULTIPLE CHOICE

1. a, 2. d, 3. c, 4. c, 5. d, 6. c, 7. c, 8. c

FILL IN THE BLANK

1. Least
2. Values

MULTIPLE-ANSWER MULTIPLE CHOICE

1. b, d, e, f, i,
2. c
3. a

HOT SPOT

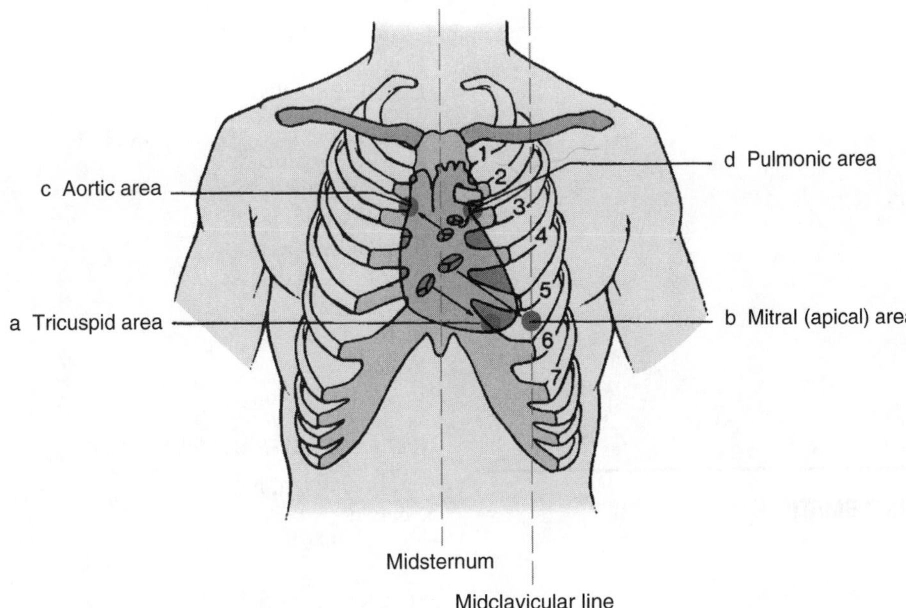

Chapter 27

MASTERING THE INFORMATION

MATCHING

1. e, 2. f, 3. d, 4. h, 5. b, 6. g, 7. a, 8. j, 9. i, 10. c

TRUE–FALSE

1. True
2. False. Pulse pressure is the mathematical difference between systolic pressure and diastolic pressure.
3. True
4. False. Immediately return the client to the supine position.
5. True
6. True
7. True
8. False. Hypercapnia is the normal stimulus for breathing.
9. False. Respiratory rate and depth increase because O_2 concentration decreases at high elevation.
10. False. Respiratory rate increases in infants because of decreased lung capacity.

FILL IN THE BLANK

1. Smoking; oxygen administration; drinking hot or cold liquids
2. 3 AM; 5 PM; 7 PM
3. Any four of the following would be accurate:
   a. Temporal: Most easily palpated just in front of the upper part of the ear
   b. Carotid: Most easily palpated along the medial border of the sternocleidomastoid muscle in the lower half of the neck
   c. Apical: Palpated or auscultated over the left ventricle at the level of the fifth intercostal space in the midclavicular line
   d. Brachial: Located on the inner aspect of the upper arm and most easily palpated with a client's arm flexed at the elbow and supported by the examiner
   e. Radial: Palpated on the thumb side of the inner aspect of the wrist
   f. Femoral: Palpated in the anterior medial aspect of the thigh just below the inguinal ligament; deep palpation may be required
   g. Popliteal: Palpated behind the knee on the lateral aspect of the popliteal fossa and best assessed with the knee flexed, leg relaxed, and client in the supine or prone position
   h. Pedal: Palpated on the top surface of the foot, lateral to the tendon that runs from the great toe toward the ankle
   i. Posterior tibial: Palpated by hooking the fingertips behind the malleolus bone
4. Any four of the following would be accurate: a. age; b. stress; c. altitude; d. fever; e. medication; f. exercise; g. gender; h. body position

PRACTICING FOR NCLEX

MULTIPLE CHOICE

1. c, 2. b, 3. a, 4. c, 5. c, 6. a, 7. b, 8. c, 9. d, 10. d

FILL IN THE BLANK

1. 15 minutes
2. 2 minutes
3. 1
4. 37.2°C
5. 12 to 20/minute

MULTIPLE-ANSWER MULTIPLE CHOICE

1. a., b, c

ORDERING

a. 1
b. 2
c. 10
d. 8
e. 3
f. 4
g. 9
h. 5
i. 7
j. 6

Chapter 28

MASTERING THE INFORMATION

MATCHING

1. e, 2. d, 3. a, 4. c, 5. b

1. f, 2. b, 3. a, 4. d, 5. e, 6. c

1. d, 2. a, 3. b, 4. e, 5. c

TRUE–FALSE

1. False. Infectious exposure and risks of contracting infectious disease change during a person's lifespan. Infants, toddlers, and the elderly are at higher risk for infection.
2. True
3. True
4. True
5. True
6. True
7. True
8. True
9. True
10. True

FILL IN THE BLANK

1. Local/state, regional, provincial, and national
2. Written; procedures; infection
3. Monitor; counsel
4. Healthcare personnel; client; care provider
5. Methods; agents
6. Dirty; untouchable
7. Agent; source; exit; mode; transmission; entry; susceptible host
8. Environment; therapeutic regimen; resistance
9. Any six of the following would be correct: blood and blood products; pathology laboratory specimens; laboratory cultures; body parts from surgery; contaminated equipment; food; infant and adult unrinsed diapers
10. Chlorine; formaldehyde (formalin); glutaraldehyde

PRACTICING FOR NCLEX

MULTIPLE CHOICE

1. d, 2. a, 3. b, 4. b, 5. c, 6. c, 7. d, 8. b, 9. c, 10. b

FILL IN THE BLANK

1. Sterile
2. Microorganisms
3. Fingernails
4. Antiseptic
5. Handwashing
6. Infectious disease
7. Parasites
8. Needle-sticks
9. Spores
10. Cleaned

MULTIPLE-ANSWER MULTIPLE CHOICE

1. a, b, c, d, f, g, h
2. b, c, d

Chapter 29

MASTERING THE INFORMATION

MATCHING

1. d, 2. c, 3. a, 4. f, 5. e, 6. b, 7. g

TRUE–FALSE

1. False. A medication is a drug administered for its therapeutic effect.
2. False. It can be given as ordered after the verbal or telephone order is received, and it is usually signed by the doctor within 48 hours of receiving the order.
3. True
4. True
5. False. Place ophthalmic medications in conjunctival sacs.
6. False. Liquid medications are instilled rectally using an enema.
7. True
8. True
9. False. Intermittent infusion is used for intermittent time periods over 20 minutes to 1 hour.
10. True
11. False. This is the definition for tolerance.
12. True

FILL IN THE BLANK

1. a. Clinical composition; b. Clinical actions; c. Therapeutic affect on body systems
2. a. Four times a day; b. As needed, according to necessity; c. Subcutaneously; d. Right eye; e. Before meals

3. Healthcare facility personnel perform a count of controlled medications at specified times (e.g., at each change of shift or when removed from an automated dispensing machine). Before a controlled medication is administered, the count in the drawer must be verified, and the control sheet must be signed (handwritten or electronic) to indicate that the medication has been removed. If all or part of a dose is discarded, a second nurse must witness the discarding and countersign the control record.
4. Metric; apothecary; household
5. a. Accurately interpret the prescriber's instructions.
   b. Incorporate five rights when administering medications.
   c. Accurately calculate the dosage.
   d. Document medication administration according to agency policy.
6. a. Client's name; b. Date and hour given; c. Physician's name; d. Amount given; e. nurse's name
7. a. Right dose; b. Right client; c. Right time; d. Right route; e. Right medication
8. a. Greater trochanter; b. Posterior superior iliac spine
9. Client record; cover of record; any other location mandated by agency policy
10. Bar-code system; unit dose; automated medication dispensing system; self-administered supply

PRACTICING FOR NCLEX

MULTIPLE CHOICE

1. c, 2. c, 3. b, 4. d, 5. d, 6. c, 7. b, 8. d, 9. c, 10. b, 11. c, 12. b, 13. c, 14. a

FILL IN THE BLANK

1. 0.75 mL
2. Pharmacodynamics
3. Therapeutic effect
4. Pharmacokinetics
5. Allergic reactions
6. Generic

MULTIPLE-ANSWER MULTIPLE CHOICE

1. a

ORDERING

a. 2
b. 3
c. 1
d. 5
e. 4

Chapter 30

MASTERING THE INFORMATION

MATCHING

1. e, 2. a, 3. f, 4. b, 5. d, 6. g, 7. c

TRUE–FALSE

1. False. This definition describes a hemolytic reaction.
2. False. Povidone-iodine is a better bactericide.
3. False. Implanted vascular accesses do not protrude from the skin.
4. True
5. True
6. False. Hypotonic solutions are administered when a client requires cellular hydration.
7. False. Alarms should never be turned off.
8. False. Absence of backflow could be attributed to the type of catheter or location of the needle level.

FILL IN THE BLANK

1. a. Isotonic—Lactated Ringers (LR); 0.9% NaCl (normal saline-NS)
   b. Hypotonic—0.45% NaCl (1/2 NS); 5% dextrose and water (D5W)
   c. Hypertonic—3% NS and 5% NS
2. Any three of the following would be accurate:
   a. Peripheral insertion devices
   b. Intermittent infusion devices
   c. Central venous catheters
   d. Tunneled central venous catheters
   e. Peripherally inserted central catheters
   f. Implanted vascular access devices
3. Any three of the following would be accurate:
   a. Maintain adequate fluid intake
   b. Maintain normal electrolyte balance
   c. Provide the client with glucose to use for energy
   d. Provide an access route to administer medication
   e. Provide an access route to administer blood components
   f. Provide an access route to administer treatment if an emergency situation should occur
4. Any four of the following would be accurate:
   a. Height of the IV bottle
   b. Patency of the catheter
   c. Clogged air vent
   d. Position of the extremity
   e. Position of the needle or catheter in the vein
   f. Constriction or kink in the tubing

PRACTICING FOR NCLEX

MULTIPLE CHOICE

1. a, 2. b, 3. d, 4. c, 5. a

FILL IN THE BLANK

1. Parenteral nutrition
2. Central

MULTIPLE-ANSWER MULTIPLE CHOICE

1. c, d
2. b, c
3. a, c

ORDERING

a.	3	g.	5
b.	7	h.	2
c.	1	i.	8
d.	4	j.	10
e.	6	k.	12
f.	11	l.	9

Chapter 31

MASTERING THE INFORMATION

MATCHING

1. f, 2. d, 3. i, 4. c, 5. b, 6. j, 7. a, 8. e, 9. g, 10. h

FILL IN THE BLANK

1. Preoperative; intraoperative; postoperative
2. Sponges; instruments
3. Any five of the following would be accurate:
   Decreased ambient temperature in the OR
   Vasodilation secondary to certain anesthetic agents
   Intravenous fluid administration
   Exposure of body surface area
   Skin preparation solutions that are cool
   Decreased consciousness that may lead to a decreased ability to maintain body temperature
   Blood loss
   Prematurity
   Advanced age
4. 30; 60
5. IV; NPO; preoperative; skin
6. Muscle relaxants
7. Any five of the following would be accurate:
   a. Surgical procedure—type and extent
   b. Anesthesia—type and status (e.g., intubated/extubated or level of spinal)
   c. Medications administered—time and dosage
   d. Blood loss—amount and replacement
   e. Complications—surgical or anesthetic
   f. Inpatient or outpatient
8. a. Void
   b. Be able to ambulate
   c. Be alert and oriented
   d. Have minimal nausea and vomiting
   e. Require no pain medication within the last hour
   f. Exhibit no excess bleeding or drainage
9. 3
10. Any two of the following would be correct: positioning; distraction; emotional support; back massage

PRACTICING FOR NCLEX

MULTIPLE CHOICE

1. d, 2. b, 3. c, 4. d, 5. a, 6 c, 7. a, 8. c, 9. b, 10. c

FILL IN THE BLANK

1. 1
3. 15
4. 8

MULTIPLE-ANSWER MULTIPLE CHOICE

1. a, b, d
2. b, e
3. a, b

Chapter 32

MASTERING THE INFORMATION

MATCHING

1. b, 2. c, 3. d, 4. e, 5. a

1. c, 2.d, 3. b, 4. a, 5. e

TRUE–FALSE

1. True
2. True
3. False. Nursing interventions to promote safety fall into two broad categories: providing a safe environment in the healthcare facility and safety education.
4. True
5. True
6. True
7. True
8. True
9. False. The Occupational Safety and Health Administration (OSHA) is required to investigate worker reports of unsafe working conditions.
10. False. Safety concerns in the community include crime, noise levels, poor lighting, presence of landfills, busy intersections, dilapidated houses, cliffs, clean air, clean water supply, and extremes in temperature.
11. True
12. False. Filing of an incident report should not be documented in the client's medical record.

FILL IN THE BLANK

1. Injuries
2. Prevention
3. Anxiety; depression
4. Altered safety
5. Bathroom
6. Education
7. Safety precautions
8. Fire evacuations

PRACTICING FOR NCLEX

MULTIPLE CHOICE

1. b, 2. a, 3. d, 4. c, 5. c, 6. a, 7. d, 8. b, 9. a, 10. a, 11. b, 12. c

FILL IN THE BLANK

1. Falls
2. Dysfunctional
3. "What if"
4. Nursing interventions

MULTIPLE-ANSWER MULTIPLE CHOICE

1. a, c, d
2. b, c, d, e, f, h
3. a, d

ORDERING

1. a. 3
   b. 4
   c. 2
   d. 1

2. a. 3
   b. 2
   c. 1
   d. 4
   e. 5
   f. 6

Chapter 33

MASTERING THE INFORMATION

MATCHING

1. b, 2. a, 3. c

TRUE–FALSE

1. True
2. False. Individuals in this group are more likely to pursue healthy behaviors.
3. True.
4. False. Health promotion is characterized by approach behaviors only.
5. True
6. True

FILL IN THE BLANK

1. a. Perception of health: A person's beliefs related to their health status. Perception influences how a person rates personal health. The person's perception, therefore, will determine his or her behavior and actions in relation to health.
   b. Motivation: When a person is strongly motivated toward achieving an optimal level of wellness, the person will actively seek information and activities for health promotion and is more likely to achieve the goal of optimal health, whereas the opposite is true of the person with a low level of motivation.
   c. Adherence to management goals: Identifying and adhering to a realistic plan to change lifestyle and break old habits. It is very important for the individual to set realistic and achievable goals.
   d. Available social and economic resources to change direction and adhere to goals.
2. Any two of the following would be accurate:
   a. High risk of infection
   b. High risk of injury
   c. Knowledge deficit
   d. Noncompliance
3. Any of the items listed in each of the following categories would be accurate:
   Infancy: prenatal care, immunizations, proper nutrition, health checkups
   Toddlerhood: safety, immunizations, proper sleep and nutrition, avoiding second-hand tobacco smoke
   Adolescence: safe driving, prevention of pregnancy and sexually transmitted diseases, avoiding drugs and alcohol, maintaining mental health, primary health maintenance, and avoiding gang-related violence

PRACTICING FOR NCLEX

MULTIPLE CHOICE

1. c, 2. b, 3. a, 4. d, 5. a, 6. b, 7. a, 8. c

FILL IN THE BLANK

1. Tobacco use/smoking
2. Family history/genetics

MULTIPLE-ANSWER MULTIPLE CHOICE

1. a, b, d

Chapter 34

MASTERING THE INFORMATION

MATCHING

1. a, 2. c, 3. b, 4. d
1. b, 2. a, 3. a, 4. b, 5. a, 6. b

TRUE–FALSE

1. False. Regression is a normal coping mechanism that should be permitted because it allows the child to withdraw, conserve energy, and regain control.
2. True
3. True
4. False. Filing is usually safe; however, cutting the toenails should be avoided.
5. False. A different washcloth should be used if an infection is suspected.
6. True
7. False. Dentures should be removed at night so that tissues are exposed to air.
8. True
9. False. Asepsis is important and is not the same as sterile technique.

FILL IN THE BLANK

1. Any five of the following would be correct:
   a. Culture, values, and beliefs
   b. Environment
   c. Motivation
   d. Emotional disturbance and depression
   e. Cognitive abilities
   f. Energy
   g. Acute illness and surgery
   h. Pain
   i. Neuromuscular function
   j. Sensorimotor deficits

2. a. Sitz
   b. Hot water
   c. Warm water
   d. Cool water
   e. Soaks
3. Any three of the following would be correct:
   a. Turn on the bathroom tap water.
   b. Have the client visualize his or her bathroom at home.
   c. Warm the bedpan.
   d. Have the client assume a comfortable position.
   e. Provide analgesics.
   f. Pour warm water over the perineum.
   g. Always provide the call light within easy reach.
4. Any four of the following would be correct:
   a. Impaired skin integrity
   b. Altered nutrition: less than body requirements
   c. Fluid volume deficit
   d. Impaired oral mucous membrane
   e. Ineffective individual coping
   f. Anxiety
   g. Powerlessness
   h. Interrupted family process
   i. Caregiver role strain

PRACTICING FOR NCLEX

MULTIPLE CHOICE

1. b, 2. c, 3. a, 4. d, 5. b, 6. c, 7. a, 8. a, 9. c, 10. b

FILL IN THE BLANK

1. 110°F to 115°F
2. Meals on Wheels
3. Lindane (Kwell)

MULTIPLE-ANSWER MULTIPLE CHOICE

1. b, e, f

ORDERING

a. 1	k. 5
b. 20	l. 6
c. 8	m. 12
d. 15	n. 9
e. 7	o. 10
f. 17	p. 18
g. 13	q. 3
h. 11	r. 14
i. 2	s. 19
j. 4	t. 16

Chapter 35

MASTERING THE INFORMATION

MATCHING

1. d, 2. h, 3. j, 4. i, 5. c, 6. b, 7. f, 8. g, 9. e, 10. a

TRUE–FALSE

1. True
2. False. Impairment of the nervous system often hinders functional mobility.
3. False. Chronic health problems limit the oxygen and nutrients delivered to the muscles.
4. False. Paraplegia is decreased motor and sensory function to the legs; quadriplegia is paralysis of the arms and legs.
5. False. Severe affective disorders hinder mobility because the person lacks the desire to move.
6. True
7. True
8. False. Movement promotes the formation of new connective tissue.
9. False. Flexion contractures are most common.
10. True

FILL IN THE BLANK

1. Body alignment; posture; balance; coordinated movement
2. Safe; efficient; mechanics
3. Stance; swing
4. Any five of the following would be accurate:
   a. An intact musculoskeletal system
   b. Nervous system control
   c. Adequate circulation and oxygenation
   d. Adequate energy
   e. Appropriate lifestyle values
   f. Suitable emotional state
5. Any four of the following would be accurate: decreased muscle strength or tone; lack of coordination; altered gait; decreased joint flexibility; pain on movement; decreased activity tolerance
6. Any two of the following three most common diagnoses would be accurate: activity intolerance; impaired physical mobility; high risk for disuse syndrome.
7. Optimum; endurance; tolerance; immobility; adapting
8. Immobility
9. Gangly; awkward
10. Random; reflexive activity
11. a. To prevent injury to the nurse's musculoskeletal system or to the client during transfer
    b. Using body mechanics to save musculoskeletal function and help the nurse maintain balance without muscle strain
12. Mechanical lifts/aids; assistance/personnel
13. Any three of the following would be accurate:
    a. Assess the situation carefully before acting.
    b. Use the large muscle groups of the legs whenever possible.
    c. Perform work at the appropriate height for body position.
    d. Use mechanical lifts or assistance whenever needed to facilitate the movement of a client.
14. Transfer; ambulation; equipment

PRACTICING FOR NCLEX

MULTIPLE CHOICE

1. d, 2. b, 3.d, 4. a, 5.c, 6. c, 7. d, 8. c, 9. d, 10. d, 11. a, 12. c, 13. d, 14. b

FILL IN THE BLANK

1. Plan
2. a. Flexion; b. Adduction; c. Rotation, external; d. Supination; e. Eversion; f. Circumduction; g. Extension

MULTIPLE-ANSWER MULTIPLE CHOICE

1. c, d, e
2. a, b, f, g, h
3. a, c, i

Chapter 36

MASTERING THE INFORMATION

MATCHING

1. b, 2. d, 3. e, 4. c, 5. a

TRUE–FALSE

1. True
2. False. This is abnormal; apneic period should not exceed 20 seconds.
3. True
4. False. The rate would increase due to the increased oxygen demand and increased carbon dioxide production.
5. False. Chest pain can be associated with a wide variety of conditions, including some respiratory conditions.
6. True
7. True
8. True

FILL IN THE BLANK

1. a. Makes oxygen available to the blood
   b. Allows carbon dioxide to be removed from the blood
   c. Helps to maintain acid–base balance
2. Rate; pattern
3. a. Clear or white without odor and of medium consistency
   b. Stringy like thickened egg white
   c. Yellow or greenish with putrid or musky odor
4. Any four of the following would be correct:
   a. Chest x-rays
   b. Pulmonary function test
   c. Arterial blood gases
   d. Bronchoscopy
   e. Pulse oximetry
   f. Skin test
   g. Sputum culture
5. a. Ineffective breathing pattern
   Definition: The state in which an individual's inhalation or exhalation pattern does not enable adequate ventilation.
   Defining characteristics: Decreased inspiratory/expiratory pressure, decreased minute ventilation, dyspnea, shortness of breath, tachypnea, fremitus, abnormal arterial blood gas values, cyanosis, cough, nasal flaring, respiratory depth changes, assumption of three-point position, pursed-lip breathing or prolonged expiratory phase, increased anteroposterior diameter, use of accessory muscles, altered chest excursion, and decreased vital capacity
   Related factors: Hyperventilation, hypoventilation, obesity, spinal cord injury, neuromuscular dysfunction, pain, musculoskeletal impairment, perceptual or cognitive impairment, anxiety, decreased energy/fatigue, respiratory muscle fatigue, and neurological immaturity
   b. Impaired gas exchange
   Definition: The state in which a person experiences an excess or deficit in oxygenation and/or carbon dioxide elimination at an alveolar-capillary level
   Defining characteristics: Confusion, somnolence, restlessness, irritability, hypercapnia/hypercarbia, dyspnea, abnormal rate rhythm, depth of breathing, and/or hypoxia/hypoxemia, abnormal skin color, cyanosis in the neonate, nasal flaring, abnormal arterial pH, visual disturbance or headache upon awakening
   Related factors: Imbalance of ventilation and perfusion and alveolar-capillary membrane changes contribute to impaired gas exchange
6. Color; breathing effort; heart rate; alertness
7. a. Individual can walk 1 mile at own pace before experiencing shortness of breath.
   b. Individual becomes short of breath after walking 100 yards on level ground or after climbing a flight of stairs.
   c. Individual becomes short of breath while talking or performing activities of daily living.
   d. Individual becomes short of breath during periods of no activity.
   e. Individual experiences shortness of breath while lying down.
8. Fingernail polish; acrylic nails

PRACTICING FOR NCLEX

MULTIPLE CHOICE

1. a, 2. c, 3. a, 4. c, 5. c, 6. b, 7. c, 8. c, 9. a, 10. b, 11. b, 12. b

FILL IN THE BLANK

1. Carbon dioxide
2. Smoking
3. Allergens
4. Pursed lip breathing

MULTIPLE-ANSWER MULTIPLE CHOICE

1. a, d, e
2. a, b, c, d
3. c, d, e, f
4. a, b, c

ORDERING

a. 8	e. 5	i. 4	m. 12
b. 9	f. 7	j. 3	n. 2
c. 6	g. 13	k. 11	
d. 14	h. 1	l. 10	

HOT SPOT

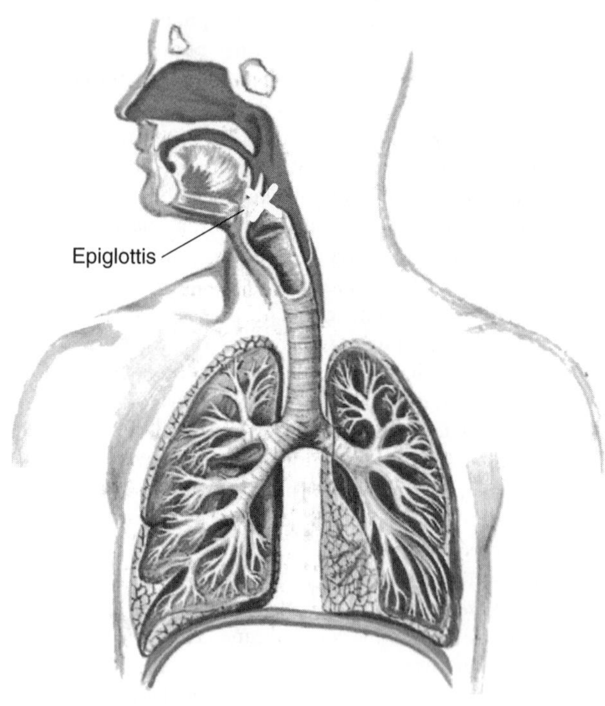

6. a. Changes in vital signs
   b. Decreased tissue perfusion
   c. Changes in the color or temperature of the skin or color of mucous membranes
   d. Decreased cardiac output
   e. Altered blood flow to vital organs
7. Examples include the following:
   a. Dysrhythmias; muscle damage; valve dysfunction
   b. Atherosclerosis; vein problems; clots; emboli
   c. Anemia; low blood volume
8. Cardiac arrest; morbidity; mortality

PRACTICING FOR NCLEX

MULTIPLE CHOICE

1. b, 2. a, 3. d, 4. a, 5. c, 6. c, 7. d, 8. a, 9. a, 10. b

FILL IN THE BLANK

1. Waste
2. Cardiac arrest

MULTIPLE-ANSWER MULTIPLE CHOICE

1. a
2. a, b, c, d, e
3. b, c, d
4. c, e, f, g
5. c, d, e

ORDERING

a.	5	e.	8
b.	2	f.	6
c.	3	g.	7
d.	1	h.	4

CHAPTER 37

MASTERING THE INFORMATION

MATCHING

1. g, 2. l, 3. h, 4. i, 5. e, 6. j, 7. k, 8. a, 9. d, 10. c

TRUE–FALSE

1. True
2. True
3. False. Plaque formation narrows the lumen of vessels and results in high blood pressure
4. True
5. False. Venous pooling increases myocardial work and decreases stroke volume.

FILL IN THE BLANK

1. Healthy heart; blood volume, blood vessels
2. Major arteries
3. Any two of the following would be correct: ineffective tissue perfusion; decreased cardiac output; activity intolerance
4. Teaching risk modification for the general public
5. Cardiovascular dysfunction can decrease a person's ability to perform activities of daily living and may necessitate lifestyle changes.

Chapter 38

MASTERING THE INFORMATION

MATCHING

1. e, 2. b, 3. a, 4. c, 5. d

TRUE–FALSE

1. False. Mental-status changes are early indicators of fluid and electrolyte imbalances, and stress increases the risk for imbalances.
2. False. Weight gain is the early sign. A significant excess body fluid must be present before edema is apparent.
3. False. It is handled by the lungs, not the kidneys.
4. True
5. True
6. True
7. False. The pulse would be bounding.
8. False. Water loss is proportionately greater in the young child.

FILL IN THE BLANK

1. Any three of the following would be accurate:
   a. Kidneys
   b. Lungs
   c. Skin
   d. Gastrointestinal tract
2. Age; gender; body fat
3. Any three of the following would be accurate:
   a. Self-care deficit
   b. High risk for injury
   c. Knowledge deficit
   d. Activity intolerance
   e. Impaired skin integrity
   f. Noncompliance
   g. Alteration in bowel function
4. a. Prevent or treat fluid imbalances; b. Prevent or treat electrolyte imbalance

PRACTICING FOR NCLEX

MULTIPLE CHOICE

1. b, 2. a, 3. d, 4. d, 5. c, 6. c, 7. b, 8. c, 9. b, 10. b

FILL IN THE BLANK

1. 10%
2. 480

MULTIPLE-ANSWER MULTIPLE CHOICE

1. a, c, e
2. a, b, c
3. a, b, c, d, e, f, g
4. a, e

Chapter 39

MASTERING THE INFORMATION

MATCHING

1. f, 2. j, 3. i, 4. g, 5. a, 6. k, 7. h, 8. e, 9. b, 10. d, 11. c

TRUE–FALSE

1. True
2. False. Clients with impaired nutritional status may require therapies, such as nasogastric tube feedings, percutaneous endoscopic gastrostomy tube feedings, peripheral parenteral nutrition, or total parenteral nutrition, to maintain optimal nutritional status.
3. True
4. True
5. True
6. False. Therapeutic diets are often used to promote health, manage disease, or to “encourage” healing.
7. True
8. True
9. True
10. True

FILL IN THE BLANK

1. Fats; carbohydrates; proteins; vitamins; minerals; water
2. Liver; lean meats; dried beans; fortified cereals
3. Any four of the following would be accurate: Physiologic factors; lifestyle and habits; culture and beliefs; economic resources; drug and nutrient interactions; gender; surgery; cancer and cancer treatment; alcohol and drug abuse; psychological state
4. Milk and diary; green leafy vegetables; whole grains; nuts; legumes; seafood
5. Milk; meat; poultry; fish; eggs; salt; salt compounds
6. Protein-rich foods; bread; cereal; fruits; vegetables
7. Digestion; absorption; metabolism; excretion
8. a. Body mass index
   b. Ideal body weight
   c. Physical status: alertness, skin tone and turgor, moist pink membranes, and so forth
   d. Normal laboratory values
9. a. Ability to acquire or prepare food
   b. Knowledge
   c. Swallowing impairment
   d. Discomfort during or after eating
   e. Anorexia
   f. Nausea and vomiting
   g. Excessive intake of calories and fat
10. a. Overweight
   b. Obesity
   c. Decreased energy level
   d. Underweight
   e. Recent significant weight increase or decrease
   f. Altered bowel pattern
   g. Altered appearance: hair, teeth, mucous membranes

PRACTICING FOR NCLEX

MULTIPLE CHOICE

1. b, 2. a, 3. d, 4. c, 5. c, 6. c, 7. d, 8. d, 9. a, 10. c

FILL IN THE BLANK

1. 80 mg/dL
2. 1300 mg/dL
3. Food diary

MULTIPLE-ANSWER MULTIPLE CHOICE

1. a, c, d
2. c, d
3. a, b, c, d
4. b, d
5. a, b, c, d, e

Chapter 40

MASTERING THE INFORMATION

MATCHING

1. b, 2. e, 3. d, 4. g, 5. a, 6. h, 7. f, 8. c

1. e, 2. d, 3. b, 4. a, 5. c

TRUE–FALSE

1. True
2. False. A characteristic odor is normal with perspiration, especially in the axilla and groin areas.
3. False. Healing by first intention occurs when there is minimal tissue loss and the wound edges are approximated, such as in clean surgical incisions or shallow, sutured wounds. Healing by third intention is described.
4. True
5. False. Planned nursing interventions are very important to prevent pressure sore development or trauma to skin for all bedridden clients, whether hospitalized or homebound.
6. True
7. True
8. True
9. True

FILL IN THE BLANK

1. Blood flow, nutrition, epidermis, hygiene
2. a. Protection
   b. Thermoregulation
   c. Sensation
   d. Metabolism
   e. Communication
3. Pruritus; rashes; lesions; inadequate wound healing; pain
4. Assessment; management
5. Any five of the following would be correct: Circulation, nutrition, condition of epidermis, allergy, infections, abnormal growth rate, systemic disease, trauma, excessive exposure, mechanical forces, abnormal growth rates
6. Any five of the following would be accurate: Intact skin is the body's first line of defense against tissue trauma and infection; breakdown of skin must be prevented; skin must be adequately nourished; adequate circulation is needed to maintain cells; skin hygiene is necessary; skin sensitivity varies among people and according to one's health and developmental status
7. a. Normal skin status
   b. Risk of skin impairment
   c. History of existing skin alterations or development of prior wound problems and their prior management
8. Vasodilation; waste

PRACTICING FOR NCLEX

MULTIPLE CHOICE

1. c, 2. a, 3. b, 4. c, 5. b, 6. a, 7. c, 8. a

FILL IN THE BLANK

1. Normal saline
2. 7 to 10 days
3. Hemovac
4. School-age children and adolescents

MULTIPLE-ANSWER MULTIPLE CHOICE

1. a, d
2. b, c, e
3. a
4. a, b, c, e, f

ORDERING

a.	9	f.	5
b.	6	g.	3
c.	7	h.	2
d.	8	i.	4
e.	1		

HOT SPOT

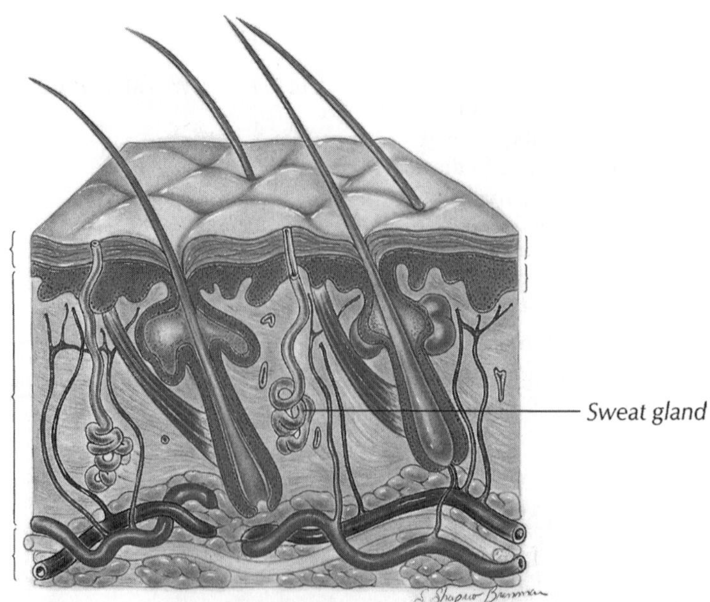

Chapter 41

MASTERING THE INFORMATION

MATCHING

1. e, 2. f, 3. a, 4. g, 5. c, 6. h, 7. b, 8. d

1. b, 2. d, 3. a, 4. c

TRUE–FALSE

1. False. Intact skin and mucous membranes are the most important barriers to infection.
2. True
3. True
4. False. Antibiotics are given to kill or slow the growth of infecting organisms.
5. True
6. True

FILL IN THE BLANK

1. Urinary tract infections; surgical or traumatic wound infections; respiratory tract infections; bacteremias (associated with IV lines)
2. Anatomic, chemical, and mechanical barriers; WBCs, inflammatory response; fever; culture
3. Breaks in skin and mucous membrane; invasive devices; stasis of bodily fluids; inadequate nutrition; stress; immune system dysfunction; coexisting medical problems; drug therapy
4. Redness; warmth; swelling; pain
5. Incubation period; prodromal period; acute phase of illness; convalescent period

PRACTICING FOR NCLEX

MULTIPLE CHOICE

1. a, 2. c, 3. b, 4. b, 5. a, 6. c, 7. b, 8. b, 9. a, 10. d

FILL IN THE BLANK

1. Aspirin
2. 30
3. Early morning

MULTIPLE-ANSWER MULTIPLE CHOICE

1. a, b
2. a, b, d, e, g
3. a, b, c, d, e
4. a, d
5. a, b, c, e

Chapter 42

MASTERING THE INFORMATION

MATCHING

1. c, 2. e, 3. b, 4. a

1. h, 2. j, 3. f, 4. b, 5. a, 6. g, 7. d, 8. e, 9. i, 10. c

TRUE–FALSE

1. False. Clients find it more difficult to describe their normal elimination patterns.
2. True.
3. False. Often these words are better understood by clients.
4. False. These conditions could result in alterations in urinary elimination.
5. True
6. True
7. False. The time of voiding may indicate certain pathology (e.g., nocturia as an indication of heart failure).
8. False. Urinary retention should be suspected and the lower abdomen palpated and percussed for bladder distention.
9. False. Ultrasound is the most precise method for determining the degree of bladder distention, followed by percussion.
10. True

FILL IN THE BLANK

1. Volume; extracellular fluid
2. Nephron; filtration; reabsorption; secretion
3. Assessment of client allergy to iodine
4. Hematuria as a sign of hemorrhage; signs of infection; bladder spasms; urinary retention or other dysuria
5. Any of the following three goals would be accurate: client will strengthen or maintain adequate perineal muscle control; client will reestablish control over voiding; client will verbalize understanding of procedures necessary to promote optimal urinary function.

PRACTICING FOR NCLEX

MULTIPLE CHOICE

1. b, 2.c, 3. b, 4. c, 5. d, 6. a, 7. d, 8. d, 9. a, 10. b, 11. d, 12. b

FILL IN THE BLANK

1. Detrusor muscle
2. Bladder ultrasonic scan

MULTIPLE-ANSWER MULTIPLE CHOICE

1. b, d
2. c
3. c, d, e, f
4. a, b, c
5. a, c
6. a, b, c, d, e

Chapter 43

MASTERING THE INFORMATION

MATCHING

1. d, 2. a, 3. c, 4. b

1. e, 2. f, 3. b, 4. d, 5. a, 6. c

TRUE–FALSE

1. True
2. False. It is seen in newborns.
3. True
4. False. These are typical infectious organisms.
5. True
6. False. This surgery is called colostomy.
7. True
8. True
9. True
10. False. Special attempts are made to separate stool and urine.

FILL IN THE BLANK

1. Any five of the following would be accurate: nutrition; fluid intake; activity and exercise; body position; ignoring urge to defecate; lifestyle; pregnancy; medications; diagnostic procedures; surgery; fecal diversion.
2. Motility; absorption; defecation
3. Constipation; fecal impaction; diarrhea; fecal incontinence; flatulence; distention
4. Any of the following would be correct: a normal pattern of bowel elimination; an absence of preventable complications form altered bowel elimination; participation in a program to maintain and promote an acceptable pattern of bowel elimination.

PRACTICING FOR NCLEX

MULTIPLE CHOICE

1. d, 2. b, 3. c, 4. d, 5. c, 6. b

FILL IN THE BLANK

1. Blue
2. Administer laxative
3. Pink

MULTIPLE-ANSWER MULTIPLE CHOICE

1. a, b, d
2. b, c
3. a, b, c, d

ORDERING

a. 4
b. 7
c. 2
d. 6
e. 1
f. 5
g. 3

Chapter 44

MASTERING THE INFORMATION

MATCHING

1. d, 2. c, 3. b, 4. e, 5. a

TRUE–FALSE

1. True
2. False. Getting the toddler or preschooler to fall asleep is the most frequently reported problem.
3. True
4. False. Healthcare providers are among the most frequent disturbers of sleep in institutional settings.
5. True
6. True
7. True
8. True

FILL IN THE BLANK

1. Electrophysiologic; neurotransmitter
2. a. Stage 1 is the transition between drowsiness and sleep. Muscles relax, respirations are even, and pulse decreases. This stage lasts only a few minutes.
   b. Stage 2 is relatively light sleep from which a person is easily awakened.
   c. Stage 3 is when muscles are very relaxed. In this stage, stronger stimuli are required to awaken the person.
   d. Stage 4 is deep sleep. Blood pressure and temperature are decreased.
   e. REM sleep closely resembles wakefulness except for very low muscle tone.
3. Sleep latency
4. Taking longer to fall asleep, awakening more frequently, feeling sleepy during the daytime, and needing longer to adjust to changes in schedule

PRACTICING FOR NCLEX

MULTIPLE CHOICE

1. c, 2. a, 3. d, 4. b, 5. b, 6. c

FILL IN THE BLANK

1. Circadian rhythms
2. Fatigue

MULTIPLE-ANSWER MULTIPLE CHOICE

1. a, b, d
2. a, b, d

Chapter 45

MASTERING THE INFORMATION

MATCHING

1. d, 2. c, 3. a, 4. e, 5. b

1. b, 2. a, 3. d, 4. c, 5. f, 6. e

TRUE–FALSE

1. True
2. False. Endogenous opioids are produced by the body, and exogenous opioids are administered to the person.
3. True
4. True
5. True
6. True
7. False. As with physiologic signs, behavioral responses often adapt with time.
8. False. Clients of all ages experience pain, but the way they express it differs.
9. True
10. True

FILL IN THE BLANK

1. Protective
2. Ascending; descending
3. Peripheral; spinal cord; brain
4. Sensory; emotional; behavioral; cognitive
5. Location; intensity; quality; temporal (onset and duration)

PRACTICING FOR NCLEX

MULTIPLE CHOICE

1. d, 2. c, 3. c, 4. b, 5. b, 6. a, 7. d, 8. c, 9. d, 10. c

FILL IN THE BLANK

1. 4000 mg
2. 72 hours
3. 15 mg

MULTIPLE-ANSWER MULTIPLE CHOICE

1. b, c, e, f
2. a, b, c, d, e
3. a, b, c

HOT SPOT

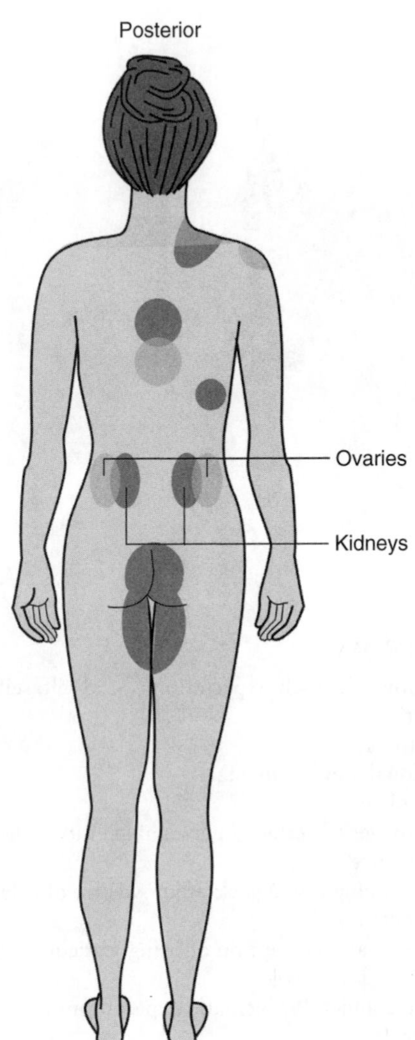

Chapter 46

MASTERING THE INFORMATION

MATCHING

1. f, 2. g, 3. a, 4. c, 5. d

TRUE–FALSE

1. True
2. False. Sudden loss of sensory perception may cause total disorientation.
3. True
4. True
5. True
6. False. Assessment for sensory perception focuses on the client, the environment, and interactions between the client and others.
7. True
8. True
9. False. Depression and withdrawal result from sensory deficits or sensory deprivation
10. False. Sensory aids may be situational, and when one sense is lost, the client can be taught to enhance other senses.

FILL IN THE BLANK

1. Pathways
2. Sight; hearing; smell; taste; touch
3. 20/20; field; tricolor (red, green, blue)
4. Lead time; afterburn
5. Experience; environment; lifestyle and habits; illness; age; medications; variation in stimulation
6. Touch; feel
7. Developmental

PRACTICING FOR NCLEX

MULTIPLE CHOICE

1. a, 2. b, 3. a, 4. b, 5. b

FILL IN THE BLANK

1. Sensory perception
2. Sensoristasis
3. Antibiotics

MULTIPLE-ANSWER MULTIPLE CHOICE

1. a, b, c, d
2. b, d
3. a, c
4. d

Chapter 47

MASTERING THE INFORMATION

MATCHING

1. d, 2. a, 3. g, 4. b, 5. f, 6. e, 7. c

1. b, 2. d, 3. a, 4. c, 5. f, 6. e

FILL IN THE BLANK

1. Consciousness; thinking; memory; learning; remembering; communicating
2. Sensory; afferent; cerebral
3. Attending; perceiving; thinking; learning; remembering; communicating
4. Any five of the following would be correct: blood flow; nutrition and metabolism; fluid and electrolyte balance; sleep and rest; self-concept; infectious processes; degenerative processes; pharmacologic agents; head trauma.
5. Processing
6. Disorganized; impaired

PRACTICING FOR NCLEX

MULTIPLE CHOICE

1. c, 2. a, 3. c, 4. a, 5. c, 6. d, 7. d, 8. c, 9. d

FILL IN THE BLANK

1. Cognition
2. Play

MULTIPLE-ANSWER MULTIPLE CHOICE

1. a, d, e
2. c, e
3. a, b, c, d, e, f, g
4. a, c,

HOT SPOT

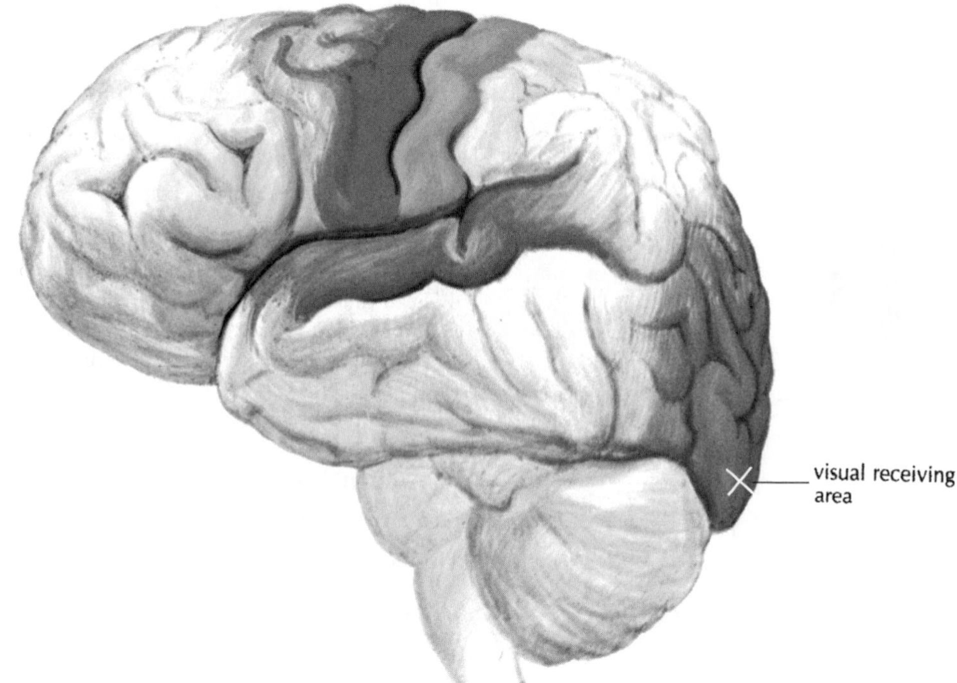

Chapter 48

MASTERING THE INFORMATION

MATCHING

1. e, 2. a, 3. d, 4. c, 5. f, 6. b

TRUE–FALSE

1. True
2. False. This is an example of situational role transition.
3. True
4. True
5. False. The adolescent requires intervention for identity and body image changes.

FILL IN THE BLANK

1. Self-knowledge; self-expectation; social self; self-evaluation
2. Self; others
3. Situational; developmental
4. Ascribed; assumed
5. Body image; self-esteem; personal identity; role performance
6. a. Role ambiguity: A lack of knowledge of role expectation
   b. Role strain: Perception of being inadequate or unsuited for a role
   c. Role conflict: Problematic expectations concerning the role

PRACTICING FOR NCLEX

MULTIPLE CHOICE

1. c, 2. d, 3. b, 4. b

FILL IN THE BLANK

1. Identity
2. Self-efficacy
3. School-age child and adolescent

MULTIPLE-ANSWER MULTIPLE CHOICE

1. d
2. a, b, c, d
3. b, c

ORDERING

2, Autonomy vs. Shame and Doubt
7, Generativity vs. Self-absorption
5, Identity vs Role Confusion
4, Industry vs. Inferiority
3, Initiative vs. Guilt
8, Integrity vs. Despair
6, Intimacy vs. Isolation
1, Trust vs. Mistrust

Chapter 49

MASTERING THE INFORMATION

MATCHING

1. d, 2. e, 3. a, 4. c, 5. b

1. d, 2. b, 3. c, 4. e, 5. a

TRUE–FALSE

1. True
2. False. Both objective and subjective data are useful in identifying and documenting family dysfunction.
3. True
4. False. Evaluation of nursing care for a family is accomplished by comparing the outcome criteria with the actual outcome.
5. True
6. True
7. True
8. True
9. True
10. False. Nurses must understand the importance of family functioning for positive influence on the health of the individual and the family. This involves each family member's ideas and actions.

FILL IN THE BLANK

1. Goals
2. Physical; economic; sexual; reproduction; education; socialization; nurturing; support
3. Any six of the following would be correct:
   a. Culture, values, beliefs
   b. Lifestyle
   c. Economic resources
   d. Previous life experiences
   e. Coping and stress tolerance
   f. Acute illness
   g. Chronic illness
   h. Traumatic experiences
   i. Substance abuse
4. Structural; functional; developmental; systems
5. Role

PRACTICING FOR NCLEX

MULTIPLE CHOICE

1. a, 2. d, 3. a, 4. d, 5. b, 6. c, 7. b, 8. d, 9. a, 10. c, 11. a

FILL IN THE BLANK

1. Sandwich generation
2. Compromised family coping related to knowledge deficit

MULTIPLE-ANSWER MULTIPLE CHOICE

1. a, b, c
2. d
3. d
4. d
5. a, b, c, d

Chapter 50

MASTERING THE INFORMATION

MATCHING

1. d, 2. b, 3. a, 4. e, 5. c

TRUE–FALSE

1. True
2. False. Factors affecting people's reactions to loss include meaning of the loss itself, personal resources, personal stressors, and circumstances of the loss.
3. True
4. False. Adults tend to grieve more intensely and more continuously for a shorter period of time.
5. True
6. False. Dysfunctional grief by one family member can greatly affect family functions, especially if the grieving one is the parent.
7. False. The outcome is determined by the balance of stressors and resources present during the grief period.
8. True
9. True
10. True

FILL IN THE BLANK

1. Any two of the following would be accurate:
   a. To make the outer reality of the loss into an internally accepted reality
   b. To sever the emotional attachment to the lost person or object
   c. To make it possible for the bereaved person to become attached to another person or object
2. Material; psychological
3. Unexpected
4. Engle; Parkes; grief cycle
5. a. Denial–ranges from denial of illness to denial of effects of dying on self and others
   b. Anger–directed toward God, family members, healthcare providers, or others
   c. Bargaining–seeking to delay the dreaded event
   d. Depression–acknowledgment of the reality and inevitability of impending death
   e. Acceptance–coming to terms with the loss; beginning to detach from supportive people and to lose interest in worldly activities.
6. Nursing care

STAGES OF GRIEF

1. D	6. S
2. P	7. P
3. S	8. R
4. P	9. S
5. P	10. R

PRACTICING FOR NCLEX

MULTIPLE CHOICE

1. c, 2. a, 3. b, 4. c, 5. a, 6. d, 7. b

FILL IN THE BLANK

1. Loss
2. Preschoolers

MULTIPLE-ANSWER MULTIPLE CHOICE

1. b, d
2. a, c, d
3. b, d, e
4. b

Chapter 51

MASTERING THE INFORMATION

MATCHING

1. d, 2. f, 3. c, 4. h, 5. a, 6. e

1. b, 2. f, 3. g, 4. a, 5. c

TRUE–FALSE

1. True
2. False. Overeating is a short-term coping mechanism.
3. True
4. False. The nurse should not let personal coping expectations affect assessment of a client.
5. True
6. False. The child and adolescent can identify stressors and begin to reason with parents and others about how to cope with them.
7. False. The toddler and preschooler learn to develop coping strategies for relatively simple stressors such as a slight delay in getting wants and needs met.

FILL IN THE BLANK

1. Response; adaptation
2. Problem-oriented; emotion-focused
3. Negative; bad; good; useful
4. Flexible; variety
5. Distress; altered

PRACTICING FOR NCLEX

MULTIPLE CHOICE

1. d, 2. a, 3. c, 4. b, 5. d

FILL IN THE BLANK

1. Involuntary
2. Newborn and infant
3. Sublimation
4. Suppression
5. Introjection
6. Rationalization
7. Repression

MULTIPLE-ANSWER MULTIPLE CHOICE

1. b, c
2. b, d
3. a, e, f

ORDERING

1. 3
2. 6
3. 4
4. 5
5. 7
6. 1
7. 2
8. 9
9. 10
10. 8

Chapter 52

MASTERING THE INFORMATION

MATCHING

1. d, 2. g, 3. f, 4. h, 5. a, 6. b, 7. c

TRUE–FALSE

1. False. XX is female and XY is male.
2. True
3. True
4. True
5. False. Sexual functioning is crucial for all human.
6.

FILL IN THE BLANK

1. Excitement; plateau; orgasm; resolution
2. a. A capacity to enjoy and control sexual behavior in accordance with a social and personal ethic
   b. Freedom from fear, shame, guilt, false beliefs, and other psychological factors inhibiting sexual response and impairing sexual relationships.
   c. Freedom from organic disorder, disease, and deficiencies that interfere with sexual and reproductive functions.
3. Any five of the following would be accurate:
   a. Self-concept
   b. Relationships
   c. Cognition and perception
   d. Culture, values, and beliefs
   e. Pregnancy
   f. Environment
   g. Gender identification
   h. Illness and disability
   i. Previous experience
   j. Medication
   k. Surgery
4. Pregnancy; infertility; abortion; gender; environment; illness; surgery
5. Sexual abuse; inhibited sexual desire; impotence; ejaculatory dysfunction; organic dysfunction; dyspareunia; vaginismus
6. Nonverbal behaviors; laboratory

PRACTICING FOR NCLEX

MULTIPLE CHOICE

1. c, 2. d, 3. a, 4. c, 5. c, 6. d, 7. b, 8. a

FILL IN THE BLANK

1. Foreskin
2. Clitoris
3. 1 week after her period

MULTIPLE-ANSWER MULTIPLE CHOICE

1. a, c
2. b, c
3. b, d, e

HOT SPOT

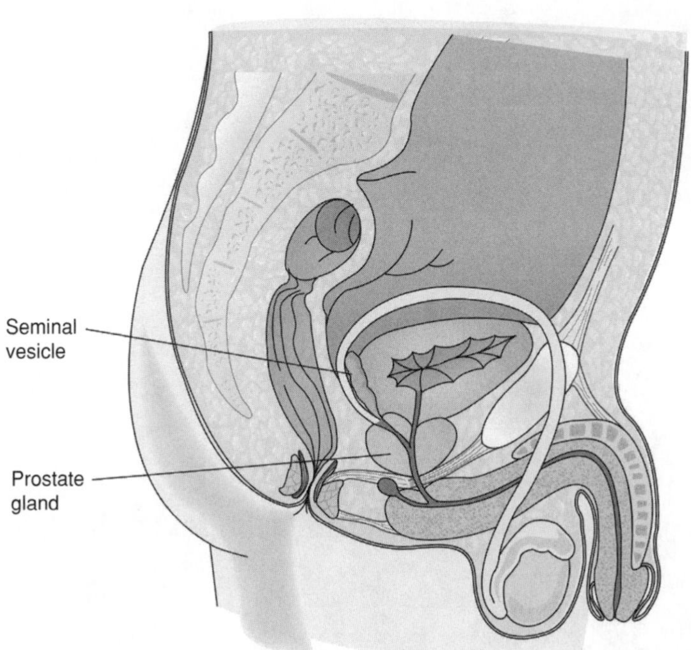

Chapter 53

MASTERING THE INFORMATION

MATCHING

1. e, 2. a, 3. c, 4. f, 5. b, 6. d

TRUE–FALSE

1. True
2. False. Christians, Jews, and Muslims are theists.
3. True
4. True
5. False. Every client has a right to practice spirituality.

FILL IN THE BLANK

1. Christianity; Judaism; Hinduism; Islam; Buddhism
2. Trust; creativity and hope; meaning and purpose; grace; forgiveness; love and relatedness; faith
3. a. Verbalization of distress: Rambling speech about life, death, and worth; person may state that he or she misses Sunday church services and the beautiful music of the choir, or say "I've never missed a service in 20 years"
   b. Altered behavior: Guilt, fear, and depression, nervousness, anger, introspective, emotional; others show no outward signs

PRACTICING FOR NCLEX

MULTIPLE CHOICE

1. b, 2. d, 3. a, 4. c

FILL IN THE BLANK

1. Spirituality
2. Spiritual distress

MULTIPLE-ANSWER MULTIPLE CHOICE

1. a, c
2. a, b, c, d, e, f
3. a, b, d, e
4. b, c

ORDERING

1. 6
2. 5
3. 2
4. 3
5. 4
6. 1
7. 7